APPLIED CLINICAL INFORMATICS
FOR NURSES

Edited by

Susan Alexander, DNP, ANP-BC, ADM-BC
Associate Professor
College of Nursing
University of Alabama in Huntsville

Karen H. Frith, PhD, RN, NEA-BC
Associate Dean for Undergraduate Programs
Professor
College of Nursing
University of Alabama in Huntsville

Haley Hoy, PhD, ACNP
Associate Dean for Graduate Programs
Associate Professor
College of Nursing
University of Alabama in Huntsville

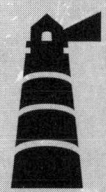

JONES & BARTLETT
LEARNING

World Headquarters
Jones & Bartlett Learning
5 Wall Street
Burlington, MA 01803
978-443-5000
info@jblearning.com
www.jblearning.com

Jones & Bartlett Learning books and products are available through most bookstores and online booksellers. To contact Jones & Bartlett Learning directly, call 800-832-0034, fax 978-443-8000, or visit our website, www.jblearning.com.

13844-3

Production Credits

VP, Product Management: David D. Cella
Director, Product Management: Amanda Martin
Product Manager: Rebecca Stephenson
Editorial Assistant: Kirsten Haley
Product Assistant: Anna-Maria Forger
Production Manager: Carolyn Rogers Pershouse
Director of Vendor Management: Amy Rose
Vendor Manager: Juna Abrams
Senior Marketing Manager: Jennifer Scherzay
Product Fulfillment Manager: Wendy Kilborn

Composition: S4Carlisle Publishing Services
Project Management: S4Carlisle Publishing Services
Cover Design: Scott Moden
Director of Rights & Media: Joanna Gallant
Rights & Media Specialist: Wes DeShano
Media Development Editor: Troy Liston
Cover Image (Title Page, Part Opener, Chapter Opener, Design Element):
   © nednapa/Shutterstock
Printing and Binding: Edwards Brothers Malloy
Cover Printing: Edwards Brothers Malloy

Library of Congress Cataloging-in-Publication Data
Names: Alexander, Susan, 1969- editor. | Frith, Karen H., editor. | Hoy,
   Haley M., editor.
Title: Applied clinical informatics for nurses/edited by Susan Alexander,
   Karen H. Frith, Haley Hoy.
Description: Second edition. | Burlington, Massachusetts : Jones & Bartlett
   Learning, [2019] | Includes bibliographical references and index.
Identifiers: LCCN 2017034523 | ISBN 9781284129175 (pbk. : alk. paper)
Subjects: | MESH: Nursing Informatics
Classification: LCC RT50.5 | NLM WY 26.5 | DDC 610.730285--dc23 LC record available at https://lccn.loc.gov/2017034523

6048

Printed in the United States of America
21 20 19 18 17   10 9 8 7 6 5 4 3 2 1

Contents

SECTION I Concepts and Issues in Clinical Informatics   1

Chapter 1 Overview of Informatics in Health Care 3

Chapter 2 Information Needs for the Healthcare Professional of the 21st Century 15

Chapter 3 Informatics and Evidence-Based Practice 25

SECTION II Use of Clinical Informatics in Care Support Roles   43

Chapter 4 Human Factors in Computing 45

SECTION III Use of Clinical Informatics Tools in Care Delivery Systems   161

Chapter 11 The Electronic Health Record. 163

Chapter 12 Clinical Decision-Support Systems 183

Chapter 13 Telehealth Nursing 191

Chapter 14 Mobile Health Applications. 207

Chapter 15 Informatics and Public Health. 223

Chapter 16 Digital Patient Engagement and Empowerment 243

Preface

▶ For Whom Is This Text Written?

The text is designed for nurses entering the healthcare field who must be prepared to apply clinical informatics knowledge and skills to:

- increase quality and satisfaction in patients' perception of care,
- enhance the health of populations,
- reduce the cost of health care, and
- improve the work life of healthcare providers.

The chapters are written by a diverse group of contributors with experience in both designing and using health informatics applications. The content is broad in scope, beginning with an overview of basic concepts in informatics and proceeding to a discussion of application of the concepts in selected healthcare delivery settings. Though advanced concepts are included in the text, they are discussed in a manner that is highly readable for nursing students. The text includes multiple examples and case studies that will aid students in immediately linking the content to the clinical environment.

The text begins by introducing concepts and issues relevant to the field of clinical informatics. A review of the culture of health care and the use of health information technology in the United States, with a summary of information science principles, sets the stage for a discussion of the nurse's role in healthcare informatics in the 21st century. The reader is presented with strategies to obtain, evaluate, and apply evidence for nursing practice with the use of informatics tools.

Other chapters contain more isolated concepts, which could be used "as needed" in multiple areas of the nursing curricula. A brief description of more advanced concepts will stimulate the interest of the reader, serving as a way to initiate discussion and interaction between students and teachers on the enormous possibilities for the use of healthcare technologies, now and in the future.

▶ Why Is This Text Important for the Student Nurse?

The text stems from the need for improvements in nurses' skill sets in using health information technology. Nursing is an increasingly high-tech field, requiring a wide variety of competencies that range from basic computer abilities to advanced skills with medical devices and lifesaving equipment. Nurses are the largest group of healthcare providers in the United States, with statistics from the U.S. Department of Labor, Bureau of Labor Statistics, indicating that there are more than 2.8 million nurses employed in the United States (in 2016). The potential impact of nurses who are prepared to use health information technologies safely and efficiently to improve patient care cannot be ignored. Minimum levels of competency in utilizing health information technologies are needed by nurses regardless of practice setting.

Perhaps the most appropriate place to begin the integration of technology and informatics in patient care is for the prelicensure nurse. If this group of nurses enters the workforce with the skill sets, clinical experience, and an expectation to integrate health information technologies into practice, many of the issues that confound healthcare organizations now may cease to exist. This is not an unusual phenomenon. Consider the example of universal precautions for blood and body fluids. The use of universal precautions began in response to the HIV and hepatitis B outbreaks in the 1980s, causing great upheaval in healthcare practice. Millions of dollars were spent in reeducating healthcare providers, redesigning hospital rooms and units, and revising nursing curricula to teach the foundational practice of universal precautions. The hurdles of adopting universal precautions in health care have largely been surmounted. Today's nursing graduates enter the workforce with the needed training and practice patterns that prevent transmission of communicable diseases. Likewise, as informatics knowledge and skills become more embedded in nursing education and in practice settings, the more informatics will be accepted as an indispensable component of nursing practice and patient care.

▶ What Makes This Text Unique?

Designed with the need for flexibility across curricula, the text is written primarily for the prelicensure or RN-BSN student who has experience in the use of diverse hardware and software applications and who is now ready to apply those skills in the healthcare setting. While the text could be used in a focused informatics course, it would also be pertinent for a nursing program that elects to teach designated informatics concepts at different points throughout the program. Course instructors will also find the text useful due to its inclusion of the competencies described in the American Association of Colleges of Nursing's *Essentials of Baccalaureate Education for Professional Nursing Practice* (2008).

▶ Acknowledgments

In this second edition, the editors remain grateful to those who have played a role in making the text become a reality. The study of nursing in the 21st century requires more than learning basic skills of bedside care. Our students, whose rich blend of backgrounds and talents make life endlessly interesting, helped us to understand the need for creating a textbook that could build on existing computer skills and enhance informatics competencies to improve patient care. Technology is interwoven into many of the nurses' tasks, and we applaud those nurses who realize the importance of competence with technology and informatics early in their careers. This is not an easy undertaking, but effective use of health information technologies will lead to important advancements in patient care. We are also thankful for instructors who have adopted the text for use in their educational programs, providing valuable feedback and informing us of surprising and unanticipated methods of using the book's content for their students. Meeting the needs of nursing students, who demonstrate great diversity in technological competence and comfort, is not an easy task. As editors, we hope that our text can continue to assist instructors in encouraging students' interest in the growing field of clinical informatics.

We would like to thank the staff at Jones & Bartlett Learning for their encouragement and guidance, which has been consistently displayed in our work to create a new edition. The production team is a pleasant and talented group. Special thanks also go to Amanda Martin, our optimistic and supportive Director of Product Management, who continues to share our vision of crafting a book that would integrate informatics content into nursing curricula in a manner both clinically relevant and exciting for nursing students. Amanda has been unfailingly gracious over the development of the first and second editions, while managing to keep the book on course! We also acknowledge the numerous other staff members of Jones & Bartlett Learning who assisted with copyediting, permissions, and artwork. Bringing a book to print is truly a team endeavor.

Once again, we are appreciative of the chance to work with the diverse group of authors who contributed their expertise to the writing of this text. Though their positions range from computer scientists to physicians and, of course, nurses, each of our contributors understands the role that informatics will continue to play in achieving high-quality patient care. They also understand the need to challenge our nursing students to apply more advanced informatics concepts in varied healthcare settings.

Finally, we must acknowledge the unceasing support from our families. They remain a positive and calming force in our lives. Alan, Kendal, Ashley, and Trey—we love you all.

Susan Alexander

Karen H. Frith

Haley Hoy

About the Editors

Susan Alexander, DNP, ANP-BC, ADM-BC, is an Associate Professor of Nursing at The University of Alabama in Huntsville. With more than 20 years of experience in nursing, she has extensive clinical experience in a variety of both inpatient and outpatient settings, having earned her doctor of nursing practice degree in 2009. In addition to her faculty responsibilities, she is certified by the American Nurses Credentialing Center as an Adult Health Nurse Practitioner and in Advanced Diabetes Management. She is a member of a research team that is studying how large datasets can be used to demonstrate the impact of environmental changes upon public health and chronic diseases in selected geographical areas. Dr. Alexander serves as a peer reviewer for multiple nursing and nonnursing journals, and is a member of the editorial board for *CIN: Computers, Informatics, Nursing,* where she is also the editor of *CIN Plus.* She is the column editor for the "Nurse Entrepreneur" section of *CNS: The Journal for Advanced Nursing Practice.* Her publications include articles on topics including implementation of software applications for health professionals, the use of online teaching strategies and mobile applications for healthcare providers in transplant, and the challenges of using big data in health care. In addition, she is a contributor to *Distance Education in Nursing, Third Edition* (2013, Springer). Dr. Alexander was the recipient of a 2013 American Association of Nurse Practitioners State Award for Excellence. In 2015, she was awarded the Suzanne B. Smith Mentoring Award by the International Association of Nurse Editors.

Karen H. Frith, PhD, RN, NEA-BC, is a Professor of Nursing and Associate Dean for Undergraduate Programs at The University of Alabama in Huntsville. She has been a nurse educator since 1992 and has an active program of research in clinical informatics and health services. She has received nearly $2 million in grants for research and programs. She is a member of Healthcare Information and Management Systems Society (HIMSS), Sigma Theta Tau International, Honor Society of Nursing, and the Southern Nursing Research Society. She serves as a reviewer (of grants and articles) for Sigma Theta Tau, Health Resources and Services Administration, *Journal of Nursing Administration, Online Journal of Issues in Nursing, Computers, Informatics, Nursing,* and *Nurse Educator,* among others. She has authored more than 40 articles in peer-reviewed journals, authored the book *Distance Education in Nursing, Third Edition,* contributed chapters to four other books, and presents nationally. Her previous clinical experience is in cardiovascular surgical intensive care, coronary intensive care, and orthopedics. She is board certified by the American Nurses Credentialing Center as Nurse Executive, Advanced (NEA-BC).

Haley Hoy, PhD, ACNP, is an acute care nurse practitioner and Associate Dean of Graduate Programs at The University of Alabama in Huntsville. She has been a nurse practitioner for nearly 20 years and has been a leader in technology and transplant nursing. Her current research interests include the role of technology and web- and mobile-based applications for the transplant community, in addition to nurse and community attitudes toward organ donation. She has held research grants from the North American Transplant Coordinators Organization (NATCO) and from The University of Alabama in Huntsville (Faculty Distinguished Research grant recipient). She is an active member of the American Association of Nurse Practitioners, a board member of the North American Transplant Coordinators Organization, and was inducted as a fellow in the American Association of Nurse Practitioners. She was the recipient of the 2011 American Association of Nurse Practitioners State Award for Excellence and the Advanced Transplant Provider Award from the American Society of Transplant Surgeons. She is board certified by the American Nurses Credentialing Center and continues to practice as a nurse practitioner at Vanderbilt Medical Center in the Department of Lung Transplantation.

Contributors

Ellise D. Adams, PhD, RN, CNM
Associate Professor
University of Alabama in
  Huntsville
Huntsville, Alabama

Marsha Howell Adams, PhD, RN, CNE, ANEF, FAAN
Professor and Dean
College of Nursing
University of Alabama in Huntsville
Huntsville, Alabama

Susan Alexander, DNP, ANP-BC, ADM-BC
Associate Professor
University of Alabama in
  Huntsville
Huntsville, Alabama

Dorothy Alford, MSN, RN, CEN, CHI
Director of Education
Clear Lake Regional Medical Center
Mainland Medical Center
Houston, Texas

Faye E. Anderson, DNS, RN, NEA-BC
Associate Professor Emeritus
University of Alabama in
  Huntsville
Huntsville, Alabama

Gennifer Baker, DNP, RN, CCNS
Assistant Professor
Martin Methodist College
Pulaski, Tennessee

Janie T. Best, DNP, RN, ACNS-BC, CNL
Associate Professor
Blair College of Health
Presbyterian School of Nursing
Queens University of Charlotte
Charlotte, North Carolina

Jane M. Carrington, PhD, RN
Assistant Professor
Community & Systems Health Science Division
College of Nursing
University of Arizona
Tucson, Arizona

Heather Carter-Templeton, PhD, RN-BC
Assistant Professor
Capstone College of Nursing
University of Alabama in Huntsville
Huntsville, Alabama

Yeow Chye Ng, PhD, RN
Assistant Professor
College of Nursing
University of Alabama in Huntsville
Huntsville, Alabama

Crayton Fargason, Jr., MD, MBA
Professor
University of Alabama at Birmingham
Medical Director
Children's of Alabama
Birmingham, Alabama

Karen H. Frith, PhD, RN, NEA-BC
Professor
University of Alabama in Huntsville
Huntsville, Alabama

Donna Guerra, EdD, MSN, RN
Assistant Professor
College of Nursing
University of Alabama in Huntsville
Huntsville, Alabama

Joni Hall, MSN, RN
Nurse Informaticist
Children's of Alabama
Birmingham, Alabama

Diana Hankey-Underwood, MS, WHNP-BC
Nurse Practitioner
Huntsville, Alabama

Haley Hoy, PhD, ACNP
Associate Professor
University of Alabama in Huntsville
Nurse Practitioner
Vanderbilt Medical Center
Nashville, Tennessee

Emil Jovanov, PhD
Associate Professor
Department of Electrical and Computer
　Engineering
University of Alabama in Huntsville
Huntsville, Alabama

Steffi Kreuzfeld, Dr. med.
Research Associate
Deputy Director
Institute for Preventive Medicine
University of Rostock
Rostock, Germany

Manil Maskey, MS
Research Scientist
Marshall Space Flight Center
National Aeronauts and Space Administration
Huntsville, Alabama

Aleksandar Milenkovic, PhD
Professor
Department of Electrical and Computer
　Engineering
University of Alabama in Huntsville
Huntsville, Alabama

Mladen Milosevic, PhD
Senior Scientist
Acute Care Solutions Department
Philips Research North America
Cambridge, Massachusetts

Stephanie Norman-Lenz, MSN, RN
Director of Nursing Informatics
Children's of Alabama
Birmingham, Alabama

Louise C. O'Keefe, PhD, CRNP, RN
Assistant Professor
College of Nursing
University of Alabama in Huntsville
Huntsville, Alabama

Pamela V. O'Neal, PhD, RN
Associate Professor
College of Nursing
University of Alabama in Huntsville
Huntsville, Alabama

Rahul Ramachandran, PhD
Research Scientist
Informatics and Data Management
National Aeronautics and Space
　Administration
George C. Marshall Space Flight Center
Huntsville, Alabama

Ron Schwertfeger, MLIS
Instruction, Outreach & Assessment Librarian/
　Lecturer
M. Louis Salmon Library
University of Alabama in Huntsville
Huntsville, Alabama

Kimberly D. Shea, PhD, RN
Associate Clinical Professor of Nursing
Community & Systems Health Science
　Division
College of Nursing
University of Arizona
Tucson, Arizona

Darlene Showalter, DNP, RN, CNS
Clinical Associate Professor
College of Nursing
University of Alabama in Huntsville
Huntsville, Alabama

Regina Stoll, Dr. med. habil.
Director
Institute of Preventive Medicine
University of Rostock
Rostock, Germany

Brenda Talley, PhD, RN, NEA-BC
Associate Professor
College of Nursing
University of Alabama in Huntsville
Huntsville, Alabama

Xiaohua Sarah Wu, MSN, RN, FNP-BC
University of Rochester Medical Center
Strong Memorial Hospital
Rochester, New York

Reviewers

Kim Siarkowski Amer, PhD, RN
Associate Professor
School of Nursing
DePaul University
Chicago, Illinois

Judith Bailey, MS, RN
Cedar Crest College
Allentown, Pennsylvania
Lehigh Valley Health Network
Allentown, Pennsylvania

Margaret Benham-Hutchins, PhD, RN
Texas Woman's University
College of Nursing
Denton, Texas

Ann M. Bowling, PhD, RN, CPNP-PC, CNE
Wright State University
Miami Valley College of Nursing and Health
Dayton, Ohio

Deborah Cheater, MS, RN, CNE
Nursing Instructor
Carl Albert State College
Poteau, Oklahoma

Mary Anne Blum Condon, PhD
Chair and Professor
Averett University
Danville, Virginia

David J. Crowther, PhD, RN, CNS
Associate Professor
Angelo State University
San Angelo, Texas

Kathleen Dunemn, PhD, APRN, CNM
Associate Professor
University of Northern Colorado
Greeley, Colorado

Tresa Kaur Dusaj, PhD, RN-BC, CNE, CHSE, CTN-A
Monmouth University
Long Branch, New Jersey

Beth Elias, PhD, MS
Assistant Professor
University of Alabama
School of Nursing
Birmingham, Alabama

Sally K. Fauchald, PhD, RN
The College of St. Scholastica
Department of Graduate Nursing
Duluth, Minnesota

Rebecca Hill, DNP, MSN, FNP-C
Assistant Professor
Massachusetts College of Pharmacy and
  Health Sciences
Boston, Massachusetts

Janice M. Jones, PhD, RN, CNS
Clinical Professor
University at Buffalo School of Nursing
Buffalo, New York

Lynn M. Klima, MSN, RN
Faculty
School of Nursing
Siena Heights University
Adrian, Michigan

Barbara A. Miller, PhD, RN, ACNS-BC
Assistant Professor
Darton State College
Albany, Georgia

Catherine S. Moe, MS, RN, CNE
Assistant Professor
Lakeview College of Nursing
Danville, Illinois

Angela Mountain, RN, MS, CMSRN
Assistant Professor
Texas A&M Health Sciences Center

Colleen Neal, MS, RN
Assistant Professor
Texas A&M Health Science College of Nursing

Anita K. Reed, MSN, RN
Department Chair Adult and Community
    Health Practice
Saint Joseph's College
St. Elizabeth School of Nursing
Lafayette, Indiana

Tina Reinckens, RN, MA
Coppin State University
Baltimore, Maryland

Annette M. Weiss, PhD, RN, CNE
Assistant Professor and RN to BSN
    Program Director
Misericordia University
Dallas, Pennsylvania

Marisa L. Wilson, DNSc, MHSc, RN-BC
University of Maryland School of Nursing
Baltimore, Maryland

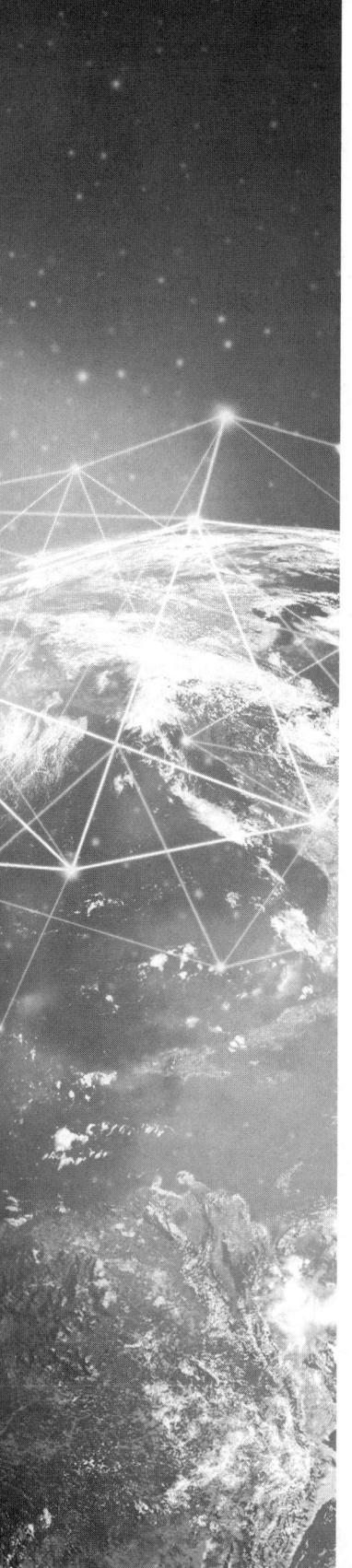

SECTION I

Concepts and Issues in Clinical Informatics

CHAPTER 1

Overview of Informatics in Health Care

Haley Hoy, PhD, ACNP

Susan Alexander, DNP, ANP-BC, ADM-BC

LEARNING OBJECTIVES

1. Review the history of the development of clinical informatics in the United States.
2. Define and discuss key concepts relating to clinical informatics and information science.
3. Describe the present culture of health care in the United States.
4. Describe the role of clinical informatics in contemporary health care in the United States.

KEY TERMS

Clinical informatics	Healthcare providers (HCPs)	Nursing informatics (NI)
Communication technologies	Information	Wisdom
Data (datum)	Information systems	
Fragmentation	Knowledge	

▶ Chapter Overview

The purposes of this chapter are to provide an overview of health information technology (IT) used in contemporary nursing practice and briefly describe the history of clinical informatics using the culture of health care in the United States as a framework. Clinical informatics can provide possible solutions to existing problems in the U.S. healthcare system including fragmentation, access to care, and care of special populations. Nurses who understand clinical informatics will likely improve healthcare delivery and patient safety.

▶ # Informatics in Nursing Practice

The role of the 21st century nurse is complex, requiring interaction with multiple medical devices and health IT. Nurses at all levels of educational preparation and in all healthcare settings use technology every day in practice. In addition to becoming expert users, it is increasingly likely that nurses, because of their rich experience in patient care, will be called on to participate in the design of new clinical systems for delivering high-quality and efficient care. The case study that follows illustrates how technology is integral to all parts of healthcare delivery for **healthcare providers (HCPs)**, patients, and healthcare settings (see **BOX 1-1**).

BOX 1-1 Case Study

Cody arrives for her scheduled 12-hour hospital shift as a circulating surgical registered nurse (RN). After she swipes her name badge at the double doors, the doors slowly swing open for her to proceed to the same-day surgery unit. Another swipe of her badge through the time clock yields a "beep," and Cody knows her day has officially begun. At the desk, Cody greets her coworkers and glances at the large monitor hanging on the wall in the nurses' station where the day's schedule of patients, procedures, their providers, and other notes are posted.

The day's first case is a tonsillectomy for a 3-year-old boy. Proceeding to the child's room, she introduces herself to the little boy and his parents and begins preparations needed for the surgical procedure. After scanning the child's barcoded wrist band and barcodes on the admission paperwork, Cody transmits the codes to the patient's gurney, so that the staff can track the patient's movement throughout the surgical suite and recovery area. She offers additional wristbands to the parents. These wristbands are coded to allow movement in and out of the same-day surgical unit and have a unique six-digit identification number that will allow the parents to watch their son's progress through pre-op, the operating room (OR), and recovery, without breaching privacy rules.

She begins to interview the parents about the child's health and family history and to reconcile the child's medications with the computerized list. Once completed, she uses the computer's touch screen to notify anesthesia services that the patient is ready for the anesthesiologist's exam.

After the anesthesiologist enters the room and introduces herself, she scans the child's wristband, comparing it with the barcoded anesthesia assessments and surgical consent she has collected. Once she has completed her interview and examination, she taps a button on the computer screen in the patient's room, notifying the OR staff that the patient is ready for the surgical procedure. Thirty minutes later, the patient's name begins to blink on the screen, letting the staff and the parents know that the patient will soon be moved to the OR suite.

At the patient's bedside, the transport staff and anesthetist once again compare the code on the child's wristband with their coded documents, confirming the child's name and date of birth verbally with the parents. Releasing the brakes on the patient's gurney, they slowly move the patient to the OR, followed by the child's parents. Along the way, the transport staff points out the location of large monitor screens on which the parents can track their child's progress as they wait for the procedure to conclude. As the child's gurney moves into the OR, a transponder that is embedded in the gurney is detected by a scanner immediately inside the OR door. This information on the patient's location is imported directly into the electronic health record (EHR) and used to update the monitor in the nurses' station. In the OR, the patient is transferred to the OR table, which is again synchronized with barcodes on the wristband and documents, as the OR staff comfort the patient. The anesthesiologist begins her work, and as the child sleeps, he is intubated, intravenous access is obtained, and the surgery begins.

Less than 40 minutes later, the surgery is complete, and the patient is returned to the gurney, which registers movement to the recovery room. Prior to transport, a blanket made of smart fabric, able to monitor vital signs and communicate wirelessly with recovery room monitors, is placed over the child. The child's vital signs, oxygen saturation, and heart rhythm will be monitored until he is awake and able to be discharged later in the day.

Three hours later, the patient is awake and ready for discharge. As orders are again reconciled with the patient's wristband, and the discharge status is updated on the patient's gurney. The child leaves the same-day surgery unit in the arms of his father, along with further instructions and a follow-up appointment already scheduled with the surgeon.

Check Your Understanding

1. How can the use of informatics make the daily work of a nurse easier or harder?
2. Does the addition of informatics and technological tools have an impact on patient care and satisfaction? How? What other tools and devices commonly used by nurses could be integrated into a seamless system to improve the quality of patient care or the efficiency of processes?

▶ History of Clinical Informatics Development

In the 21st century, it is difficult to imagine providing patient care in any setting without the use of computer technology. It is surprising that the word "computer" can be traced to 1646, meaning "one who computes" (Merriam-Webster, 2013). In the 19th century, the word "computer" was used to describe the activities of humans who labored to create tables of numerical values used in science, mathematics, and engineering. Despite painstaking work, the tables contained a high rate of errors, a phenomenon recognized by Charles Babbage, an English mathematician and scholar. In 1821, Babbage began construction of the first mechanical computer, known as the "Analytical Engine" (The Great Idea Finder, 1997–2007), designed to compute the values of polynomial functions, which eventually earned him the title of "Father of Computing" (Hyman, 1982). Babbage's colleague, Augusta Ada Lovelace (Countess Lovelace), a mathematician, is attributed with the first efforts at programming a computer when she authored the first algorithm intended to be processed by a computer (San Diego Computer Science Center, 1997). Though the Analytical Engine did not have the capability for practical daily use, it possessed many features found in modern computers such as the ability to read data from punch cards, store data, and perform arithmetic operations (The Great Idea Finder, 1997–2007). The Analytical Engine helped users begin to understand the potential value of more sophisticated means of collecting and using data.

Over time, the value of computers and technology in the collection and manipulation of data became readily apparent. Through its work in establishing and maintaining ongoing population records, the United States (U.S.) Census Bureau recognized the ability of digital computers to process large amounts of information. The Universal Automatic Computer (UNIVAC) was designed especially for the Census Bureau's needs (see **FIGURE 1-1**). The first version of UNIVAC (UNIVAC I) was used to conduct a portion of the population census in 1950 and then the entire economic census in 1954 (U.S. Census Bureau, n.d.). UNIVAC is widely viewed as the first successful civilian computer, ushering in the dawn of the computer age in information processing.

Although a full history of the development of computers into the handheld models we use today is not within the scope of this text, a brief review of significant changes in the use of computers and technology in health care is

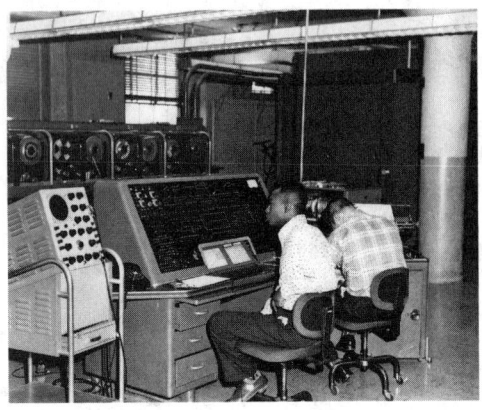

FIGURE 1-1 A UNIVAC 1105 used in the 1960 census, at the Census Bureau.

Courtesy of U.S. Census Bureau. Retrieved from http://www.census.gov/history/www/innovations/technology/univac_i.html

warranted. Radiology is one of the first healthcare fields in which informatics concepts were adopted. Robert Ledley, a dentist who also studied physics, is credited with inventing the first full-body computed tomography (CT) scanner. Dr. Ledley had a deep interest in how the fields of pattern recognition and image analysis could be applied to patient care through the use of computers and founded the National Biomedical Research Foundation in 1960, a nonprofit organization dedicated to the promotion of computing methods among biomedical scientists. He was also a founding fellow of the American College of Medical Informatics. Dr. Ledley foresaw the role of technology in issues of patient care such as record keeping, imaging, and diagnosis in settings ranging from private office practices to acute care facilities. Today, the use of technologically driven devices such as electrocardiogram machines, ventilators, and intravenous pumps necessitates a degree of technical skill in every clinician.

The increasing incorporation of technology into health care quickly resulted in an accumulation of data as HCPs realized that not only could computers be used at the point of patient care, but could collect and store data useful for determining the impact of many factors on patient care. The field of clinical informatics is an example of a specialty field developed by those with interests in manipulation and application of data to patient care. Data storage and maintenance are also of interest to the federal government because huge databases containing billions of data points on patients are available for researchers to answer clinical questions.

A review of the history of clinical informatics would not be complete without a discussion of nursing's contribution to the field and to the development of nursing informatics (NI) as a science in the public and private sectors. In the late 1950s, Harriet Werley became the first nurse researcher at the Walter Reed Army Research Institute and was asked to join a small group of people who were consulting about the possibilities of using computers in health care. Werley was instrumental in promoting research on what would later emerge as the field of NI (Ozbolt & Saba, 2008). The American Medical Informatics Association (AMIA) recognizes many important nurse leaders as NI pioneers. While this text cannot highlight all, it is important to understand the contributions that have shaped the discipline of NI.

Dr. Patricia Abbott, who might be best known for her work in helping to develop NI as a specialty field, was a member of the team of authors who crafted the initial American Nurses Association Scope and Standards of Practice for Nursing Informatics (AMIA, n.d.). Dr. Abbott also worked with the American Nurses Credentialing Center to develop the first certification exam in NI. Dr. Virginia Saba, another pioneer of NI, actively participated in initiating academic technology programs and healthcare IT systems (AMIA, n.d.). Dr. Saba has coordinated distance learning projects for nurses and served on national healthcare standards committees. Dr. Kathleen McCormick has been a clinical trial researcher and NI scientist within the National Institutes of Health Clinical Center and the National Institute on Aging, and she is an elected member of the National Academy of Sciences, Institute of Medicine (IOM) now called the National Academy of Medicine (AMIA, n.d.).

Activities of NI pioneers are not limited to the field of nursing. Dr. Marion Ball has provided service to the public sector as a member of the National Academy of Medicine and on the Board of Regents of the National Library of Medicine (AMIA, n.d.). She has worked with multiple national and international committees, including serving as president of the International Medical Informatics Association and as a board member of the AMIA. Dr. Ball was also invited to serve as an international advisor to the Board of the China Hospital Information Management Association. Roy L. Simpson, vice president, NI, Cerner Corporation, worked with colleagues to develop the Nursing Minimum Data Set and to develop online nursing administration and NI master's programs (AMIA, n.d.).

NI pioneers are also active in the areas of educating and fostering the NI workforce of tomorrow. Dr. Linda Thede is professor emeritus at the College of Nursing at Kent State University, where she has developed and taught NI programs (AMIA, n.d.). Dr. Susan K. Newbold, a healthcare informatics consultant based in Franklin, Tennessee, worked to found CARING, an NI group that was established in 1982. She also participates in teaching NI to nursing students at multiple curricular levels (AMIA, n.d.). Dr. Susan J. Grobe developed the Nursing Education Module Authoring System, which consists of a set of software programs that faculty can use to create modules on the nursing process. Dr. Grobe was one of the first of two nurse fellows elected to the American College of Medical Informatics (AMIA, n.d.).

▸ Clinical Informatics and Nursing Informatics Defined

Clinical informatics is a broad term that encompasses all medical and health specialties, including nursing, and addresses the ways **information systems** (e.g., EHRs, barcode medication administration systems, radiology imaging system, and patient-care devices) are used in the day-to-day operations of patient-care. The domains of clinical informatics include health systems, clinical care, and information and **communication technologies** (see **FIGURE 1-2**). The purpose of clinical informatics is to improve patient care by using methods and technologies from established disciplines such as computer science and information science.

Nursing informatics is a specialty in the discipline of nursing, and it is classified as a special interest group in professional organizations whose focus is clinical informatics. NI is defined by the International Medical Informatics Association's Nursing Informatics Special Interest Group (2009) as the "science and practice [that] integrates nursing, its information and knowledge, with management of information and communication technologies to promote the health of people, families, and communities worldwide." Because of the emphasis on promoting health, the study of NI is a natural fit for nurses who are dedicated to quality care for patients. As described in this book, the understanding of NI concepts is not a "nice to know" set of knowledge, skills, and values; rather, it is a requirement for effective nursing practice (Thede, 2012).

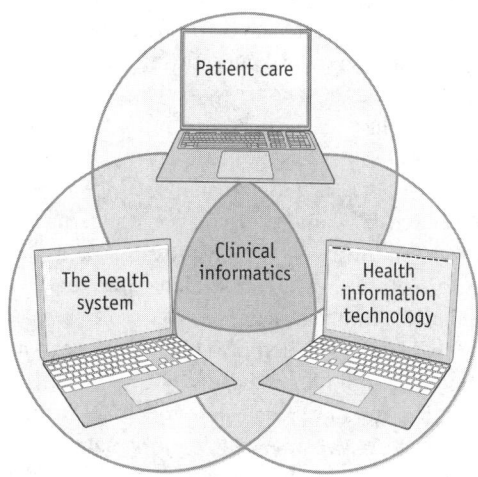

FIGURE 1-2 Domains of clinical informatics.

Data from Gardner, R. M., Overhage, J. M., Steen, E. B., Munger, B. S., Holmes, J. H., Williamson, J. J., & Detmer, D. E., for the AMIA Board of Directors. (2009). Core content for the subspecialty of clinical informatics. *Journal of the American Medical Informatics Association, 16*(2), 153–157.

The role of clinical informatics is becoming increasingly important and can be seen in almost every aspect of patient care, from the bedside to the patient's bill. The use of powerful clinical informatics tools can support processes of care, such as promoting the flow of information between those who are involved in the delivery of care across HCPs in large delivery systems. At the macro-system level, clinical informatics tools can be used to assess specific outcomes of care for groups, such as the efficacy of annual influenza vaccinations or fall prevention programs.

▶ Clinical Informatics Concepts

Informatics is a multidisciplinary science, with its beginnings in how **data** are processed and communicated between systems. What are data? Data are values or measurements, bits of information that can be collected and transformed, allowing a person to answer a question or to create an end product, such as an image. In health care, data may be created with every patient encounter. Nurses and other HCPs use their education and experience to assemble data in a clinical context to create **information,** which gives insight about patient care. Information can then be used to plan care for patient aggregates, increase the efficiency of organizations, improve quality of care, prevent medical errors, increase efficiency of care, and potentially reduce unnecessary costs. Knowledge creation concerns the ways that nurses and HCPs use the data and information they create to better understand and manage their practice. Graves and Corcoran provided a classic definition of **knowledge** as "information that has been synthesized so that relationships are identified and formalized" (1989, p. 230). For example, information is a trend of a patient's vital signs and lab results after surgery, and knowledge is recognition that elevation in a patient's temperature and white blood cell count could mean a post–operative

infection is developing. The proper use of knowledge to solve real-world problems and aid continuous improvement is what is known as **wisdom** (McGonigle & Mastrian, 2012).

Many different systems support the movement from data to information, information to knowledge, or knowledge to wisdom. Systems that support the transfer from data to information are known as information systems. Systems that support the transition from information to knowledge are decision-support systems, and those that apply knowledge through wisdom are known as expert systems (McGonigle & Mastrian, 2012). At each level, these systems contain computer, communications, and human elements.

Principles of informatics can apply to many different fields, from economics to health care. However, in clinical informatics, people with a background in health care use informatics tools, such as health information databases, medical imaging software, or point-of-care technologies to capture information and present it to other members of healthcare teams. The implementation of clinical informatics tools has the potential to create vast improvements in patient care by improving efficiency and reducing errors, which is a top priority for the United States.

▶ The Culture of Health Care in the United States

The United States spends more per capita on health care than any other country in the world. Health expenditures in the United States neared $3.2 trillion in 2015—accounting for 17.8% of the overall share of the economy (Centers for Medicaid and Medicare Services [CMS], Office of the Actuary, National Health Statistics Group, 2015). While the intent of the Affordable Care Act (ACA), enacted in 2010, was to reduce healthcare spending, the ACA is typically associated with the expansion of health care to underserved individuals. Though cost containment has been demonstrated in areas of health care, costs continue to rise at a rate of 5.4% annually through 2024 (Altarum Institute, 2017).

Despite continued increases in healthcare spending, a public opinion poll on the quality of health care in the United States would yield a variety of responses. A report from the IOM (2011) draws attention to the poor health of U.S. citizens. Though the United States has the highest rate of per capita spending on health care, comparing our population of citizens under the age of 75 to those of peer countries finds that ours have higher rates of chronic diseases and disabilities (IOM, 2011). According to the Commonwealth Fund, the United States ranks poorly, and frequently last, when compared with 11 other industrialized countries on factors of health care including healthy lives, access to care, healthcare quality, efficiency, and equity (The Commonwealth Fund, 2014). On measures of quality, the United States ranks near the top in two of four aspects of quality, effective care, and patient-centered care, but ranks much lower in providing safe and coordinated care (2014). **Fragmentation**, occurring when healthcare professionals focus on momentary issues with patients and failing to look at the "big picture" is a serious issue in today's healthcare environment.

The Impact of Fragmentation

Missing medical information can be a detriment to care in many settings, but perhaps more so in areas of high acuity, in which HCPs may be forced to make rapid decisions that may be challenging to patient safety. A retrospective review of 3.6 million patient visits to acute care sites in Massachusetts from 2002 to 2007 revealed that 56.5% of the patients were multisite users or had used more than one acute care site within the 5-year period (Bourgeois, Olson, & Mandl, 2010). Fragmentation of care ultimately places patients at greater risk for poor outcomes, particularly if those patients have multiple or chronic conditions. Patients with chronic diseases such as type 2 diabetes mellitus (T2DM) are at risk for multiple complications that often

necessitate management by subspecialists such as ophthalmologists, nephrologists, podiatrists, and cardiologists. Initiating such referrals and follow ups for patients with T2DM, while consistent with evidence-based guidelines, can be an arduous task for an HCP. Patients who do not receive needed referrals for treatment of complications may be forced to seek care in settings that are more expensive and less appropriate for chronic management, such as an emergency department (ED). Liu, Einstadter, and Cebul (2010) studied the effects of care fragmentation on a group of 683 adult patients with diabetes and chronic kidney disease. The primary outcome variable was the number of ED visits made during a 2-year period. Findings from the study revealed that patients who had fewer visits to primary HCPs had higher numbers of ED visits.

For optimal protection against transmissible diseases such as measles, mumps, and pertussis, childhood immunizations must be given at specified intervals and ages. Tracking the administration of childhood immunizations for each child, which may total 24 timed vaccinations during the first 18 months of life, is another area at risk for fragmentation and subsequent elevation in risk of acquiring childhood diseases (Centers for Disease Control and Prevention [CDC], 2013). The effects of fragmented health care have also been studied in immunization rates of children aged 19–35 months residing in four geographical areas (northern Manhattan, San Diego, Detroit, and rural Colorado), which have received federal designation as health professional shortage areas (Yusuf et al., 2002). HCPs must have reliable information in order to offer necessary immunizations; otherwise children may miss opportunities for vaccinations if providers decide to delay based on inaccurate or incomplete records from parents or other HCPs. Incomplete information from recent HCPs was associated with both overimmunization and underimmunization in this study (Yusuf et al., 2002). The utilization of community-wide immunization registries, containing information from all immunization providers in a community, was suggested as a solution to the dilemma of clinical questions regarding vaccinations (Yusuf et al., 2002).

Inaccurate or incomplete transfer of information, another example of the fragmentation that permeates health care today, can put vulnerable patients at risk of adverse events, hospital readmission, and even death in the transition from inpatient to home care (Davis, Depoe, Kansagara, Nicolaidis, & Englander, 2012). HCPs have identified the need for improved communication between healthcare systems, particularly for those patients who have conditions that have been identified as high risk for hospital readmission. In a qualitative study of 75 healthcare professionals, representing physicians, nurses, pharmacists, and other allied health professionals, poor cross-site communication was noted as a major gap in helping patients to transition from hospital to home (Davis et al., 2012). These gaps were amplified by the lack of interoperability between EHR systems of the facility and outpatient practice, and this was especially troubling to primary care providers who cited:

> A patient's there in front of me [after discharge], they've had a life changing event, and I'm sitting there without the information. You feel like an idiot. . . . I would think, "What kind of system do you guys have here? I almost died, and you don't even have the information." . . . That's embarrassing and I don't think it engenders a lot of confidence for your patients. (Davis et al., 2012, p. 1653)

▶ Introducing Information Science

The Promises of Clinical Informatics Systems

The adoption of clinical informatics systems has the potential to address issues of fragmentation by integrating healthcare delivery across groups of HCPs, health systems, and insurers. The full potential of clinical informatics tools remains to be realized. Improving efficiency of care for specific disease states, care settings, and populations is an area in which clinical informatics tools can make a positive impact. For example, a survey of 40 hospital infection preventionists suggests that expansion of the hospital EHR's capabilities, in order to provide clinical decision prompts on patients who need closer inspection, would be of benefit in detecting and providing timely care for patients with hospital-associated infections. Improved awareness of regional health initiatives and public health reporting capabilities would increase communication and earlier detection (McKinney, 2013).

Improved Efficiency

Defragmentation, a strategy long used in fields such as engineering, computer science, and manufacturing, is a means of managing limited resources while improving the performance of a system. A myriad of applications for health IT and informatics systems incorporating defragmentation can be used to improve efficiency, even in the office environment, where millions of patients schedule appointments with HCPs every day. Conventional appointment scheduling, in which a block of time is scheduled to accommodate a patient's needs, is a trade-off between the need to maximize the productivity of an HCP while minimizing the wait time for a patient. A ranked list of most preferred to least preferred appointment time slots for providers was created for schedulers, designed to offer guidance on how to best schedule patient appointments to prevent provider schedule fragmentation (Lian, Distefano, Shields, Heinichen, Giampietri, & Wang, 2010). A computer model was developed to measure efficiency using two metrics: "acceptance rate (the number between the number of accepted appointments and the total number of appointment requests), and the utilization rate (the health care provider's actual service time divided by the total work time)" (Lian et al., 2010, p. 128). The advanced appointment scheduling process was tested in four different specialty and primary care clinics. The aggregation of open time slots for HCPs that resulted from the implementation of the process was utilized in various ways, including the addition of new patient appointments in the open blocks of time.

Improving the Health Care of Older Adults

Older adults bear a higher burden of illness and frailty, and may transition frequently between healthcare systems, leading to both increased economic costs and physical risk. More than 125 million Americans had at least one chronic disease diagnosis in 2000, and this number is expected to grow to 157 million by the year 2020 (Wu & Green, 2000). A disproportionately large number of older adults are dealing with chronic illnesses. Potentially avoidable hospitalizations in older adult clients often result in poor outcomes, which are unnecessary and create excessive expenditures. By improving communication across systems, clinical informatics may assist HCPs in meeting the challenges of caring for older adults. For example, the Regenstrief Medical Record System (RMRS), housed at the University of Indiana and serving the Indianapolis area, contains records from more than 1.3 million patients. As early as 1974, the RMRS began to deliver automatic reminders in the form of paper reports, creating reminders for preventive services such as fecal occult blood testing, mammography, and vaccinations—topics pertinent to the care of older adults. In a 2-year randomized trial involving 130 providers and more than 12,000 patients, investigators found that older adult patients of physicians who received reminders for influenza vaccinations were twice as likely to receive the vaccination as patients of physicians who did not receive electronically generated reminders (Weiner et al., 2003).

Challenges in Clinical Informatics

Clinical informatics technologies have multiple purposes—to improve health of people, aggregates, communities, and populations. However, several barriers must be overcome if technology can really improve the U.S. healthcare system. The first and biggest barrier is the lack of system interoperability, which restricts the flow of data from one information system to others (Thede, 2012). There are many reasons for the interoperability problem, including the purchase of "best of breed" systems for specialty practices, the use of legacy systems that cost too much to upgrade, and integration processes that are too difficult to implement. Poor usability of health IT is the second barrier (Thede, 2012). When nurses and other HCPs are burdened with technology rather than helped by it, the health IT has been improperly designed for the user experience and for the workflow. A related and important third barrier is the failure to design health IT for human factors to prevent errors (Thede, 2012). The interaction of humans with technology is studied in other fields and applied in the design of technology and processes. In clinical informatics, attention to human factors is emerging and will become more prominent as a strategy to improve patient safety.

The Role of the Nurse

Nurses will play key roles in the redesign of healthcare delivery systems, with expanded roles, knowledge, and skill sets, to address problems facing the health IT world, such as lack of interoperability. The challenges of working with specific populations, complex comorbidities, and multiple healthcare systems, along with the increasing need to incorporate evidence-based practice make it necessary for nurses at all levels of educational preparation to master essential informatics competencies. In addition to familiarity with basic computer skills, nurses will need proficiency with patient-care technologies and "an attitude of openness to innovation and continual learning, as information systems and patient care technologies are constantly changing" (American Association of the Colleges of Nursing, 2008, p. 19).

Bridging the Gap Between Development and Clinical Use

With their experience in multiple aspects of patient care, nurses have the capacity to be far more than end users. Participating in the design, testing, and launch of informatics technologies can help to increase the accuracy, ease of use, and adoption of valuable tools, such as the EHR. Previous studies have reported an 83% increase in the success of entry of history of present illness and review of systems data into an electronic chart when the task was assigned to a nurse (EHR Intelligence, 2012). Nurses have often found themselves serving as translators for patients, families, and other healthcare professionals. Many nurses will find a natural extension of this talent in their work with assisting other HCPs to efficiently use health IT technologies.

▶ Summary

HCPs recognized the impact of informatics to improve outcomes for patients more than 100 years ago. New applications for informatics-based tools continue to emerge, offering nurses and other HCPs a valuable mechanism of improving delivery and outcomes of care for patients. While not every nurse will require more formal education in informatics, every nurse must realize that health IT technology is simply another tool to be used in nursing care. As nursing students acquire familiarity with technically complex tasks such as gaining intravenous access or inserting Foley catheters, it is reasonable to include the attainment

© nednapa/Shutterstock

of familiarity with health IT technologies as an expectation. Understanding informatics concepts, which is the basis for development of sophisticated health IT tools, will provide a groundwork for nurses to develop their skills in a growing aspect of health care.

References

Altarum Institute (2017). *Health sector economic indicators: Insights from monthly national health spending data through December 2016.* Retrieved from http://altarum .org/sites/default/files/uploaded-related-files/CSHS -Spending-Brief_February_2017.pdf

American Association of the Colleges of Nursing. (2008). *The essentials of baccalaureate nursing education for professional nursing practice.* Retrieved from http:// www.aacn.nche.edu/education-resources/BaccEssentials 08.pdf

American Medical Informatics Association. (n.d.). *Video Library 1: Nursing informatics pioneers.* Retrieved from http://www.amia.org/programs/working-groups /nursing-informatics/history-project/video-library-1

Bourgeois, F. C., Olson, K. L., & Mandl, K. D. (2010). Patients treated at multiple acute health care facilities: Quantifying information fragmentation. *Annals of Internal Medicine, 170*(22), 1989–1995.

Centers for Disease Control and Prevention. (2013). *2013 Recommended immunizations for children from birth through 6 years old.* Retrieved from http://www.cdc.gov /vaccines/parents/downloads/parent-ver-sch-0-6yrs.pdf

Centers for Medicare and Medicaid Services, Office of the Actuary, National Health Statistics Group. (2015). *National health expenditures 2015 highlights.* Retrieved from https://www.cms.gov/Research-Statistics-Data-and-Systems /Statistics-Trends-and-Reports/NationalHealthExpend Data/downloads/highlights.pdf

The Commonwealth Fund. (2014). *U.S. health system ranks last among eleven countries on measures of access, equity, quality, efficiency, and healthy lives.* Retrieved from http://www.commonwealthfund.org/publications /press-releases/2014/jun/us-health-system-ranks-last

Davis, M. M., Devoe, M., Kansagara, D., Nicolaidis, C., & Englander, H. (2012). "Did I do as best as the system would let me?" Healthcare professionals' views on hospital to home care transitions. (2012). *Journal of General Internal Medicine, 27*(12), 1649–1656.

EHR Intelligence. (2012). *Adoption and Implementation News. Nurse involvement, acceptance is critical to successful EHR use.* Retrieved from https://ehrintelligence.com/news /nurse-involvement-acceptance-is-critical-to-successful-ehr-use/

Graves, J., & Corcoran, S. (1989). The study of nursing informatics. *Journal of Nursing Scholarship, 21*(4), 227–231.

The Great Idea Finder. (1997–2007). *Ada Lovelace*. Retrieved from http://www.ideafinder.com/history/inventors/lovelace.htm

Hyman, A. (1982). *Charles Babbage: Pioneer of the Computer*. Princeton, NJ: Princeton University Press.

Institute of Medicine. (2011). *Health IT and patient safety: Building safer systems for better care*. Washington, DC: Committee on Patient Safety and Health Information Technology, Board on Health Care Services.

International Medical Informatics Association, Nursing Informatics Special Interest Group. (2009). *Definition*. Retrieved from http://imia-medinfo.org/ni/node/28

Lian, J., Distefano, K., Shields, S. D., Heinichen, C., Giampietri, M., & Wang, L. (2010). Clinical appointment process: Improvement through schedule defragmentation. *IEEE Engineering in Medicine and Biology Magazine, 29*(2), 127–134. doi: 10.1109/MEMB.2009.935718

Liu, C. W., Einstadter, D., & Cebul, R. D. (2010). Care fragmentation and emergency department use among complex patients with diabetes. *American Journal of Managed Care, 16*(6), 413–420.

McGonigle, D., & Mastrian, K. G. (2012). *Nursing informatics and the foundation of knowledge* (2nd ed.). Burlington, MA: Jones & Bartlett Learning.

McKinney, M. (2013). *Study: EHRs underutilized by preventionists*. Retrieved from http://www.modernhealthcare.com/article/20130225/NEWS/302259955

Merriam-Webster. (2013). *Computer*. Retrieved from http://www.merriam-webster.com/dictionary/computer

Ozbolt, J. G., & Saba, V. K. (2008). A brief history of nursing informatics in the United States. *Nursing Outlook, 56*, 199–205.

San Diego Computer Science Center. (1997). *Ada Byron, Countess of Lovelace*. Retrieved from http://www.sdsc.edu/ScienceWomen/lovelace.html

Thede, L. (2012). Informatics: Where is it? *OJIN: The Online Journal of Issues in Nursing, 17*(1). Retrieved from http://www.nursingworld.org/MainMenuCategories/ANAMarketplace/ANAPeriodicals/OJIN/Columns/Informatics/Informatics-Where-Is-It.html

U.S. Census Bureau. (n.d.). *UNIVAC I*. Retrieved from http://www.census.gov/history/www/innovations/technology/univac_i.html

Weiner, M., Callahan, C. M., Tierney, W. M., Overhage, M., Mamlin, B., Dexter, P. R., & McDonald, C. J. (2003). Using information technology to improve the health care of older adults. *Annals of Internal Medicine, 139*, 430–436.

Wu, S., & Green, A. (2000). *Projection of chronic illness prevalence and cost inflation*. Santa Monica, CA: RAND Corporation.

Yusuf, H., Adams, M., Rodewald, L., Pengjun, L., Rosenthal, J., Legum, S., & Santoli, J. (2002). Fragmentation of immunization history among providers and parents of children in selected underserved areas. *American Journal of Preventive Medicine, 23*(2), 106–112.

CHAPTER 2

Information Needs for the Healthcare Professional of the 21st Century

Haley Hoy, PhD, ACNP

Susan Alexander, DNP, ANP-BC, ADM-BC

Gennifer Baker, DNP, RN, CCNS

LEARNING OBJECTIVES

1. Describe the importance of informatics related to the nurse's role in clinical guidelines, protocols, procedures, and accessibility for all clinicians.
2. Recognize the importance of clinical informatics to achieve efficient quality improvement techniques within a complex healthcare system.
3. Discuss the application of clinical informatics in optimizing the nurse's role in interprofessional collaboration and practice workflow through nursing leadership in information technology.
4. Describe the importance of clinical informatics in nursing curricula and continuing education.

KEY TERMS

Clinical guidelines
Continuing education
Continuous quality improvement (CQI)

Fast healthcare interoperability resources (FHIR)
Health information exchange (HIE)

Interprofessional collaboration
Procedures
Protocols

▶ Chapter Overview

Clinical informatics is evident throughout the healthcare system. Nurses are expected to enter the field with a baseline knowledge of clinical informatics as well as an understanding of its application to clinical guidelines, protocols, and procedures. Moreover, many quality improvement (QI) techniques aimed at preventing medical errors involve informatics and are necessary to achieve cost reduction as well as patient and clinician satisfaction. The role of the nurse in informatics related to interprofessional practice, practice workflow, and leadership in information technology (IT) will be discussed in this chapter. Finally, nursing education curricula and their alignment with the expectations of a complex healthcare system related to clinical informatics will be described.

▶ Accessibility to Guidelines, Protocols, and Procedures

Clinical informatics as it applies to clinical guidelines, protocols, and procedures may be the most easily understood application for nurses. A struggle for clinicians prior to the 21st century was maintaining awareness of current guidelines as many of these groups update their guidelines every few years as new evidence evolves. Through clinical informatics, and the advent of handheld devices, the most up-to-date **clinical guidelines** are at every clinicians' fingertips.

Handheld devices and applications make readily available the most current guidelines and clinical protocols (see **FIGURE 2-1**; Moorman, 2002). Guidelines, primarily evidence-based recommendations, are usually generated from an authority group consisting of experts in the field and are published regularly. A well-known example is the set of guidelines published annually by the American Diabetes Association (2017). A council of experts assesses, critiques, and updates the clinician guidelines for care of the patient with diabetes. In years past, clinicians who regularly care for patients with diabetes would carry these guidelines in their lab coat for easy reference. Today, these guidelines are updated with new recommendations to safeguard patients with regard to the physical and psychological health of people with diabetes. Clinicians now have the ability to access these updated guidelines because of the work in the field of informatics. Other common clinical

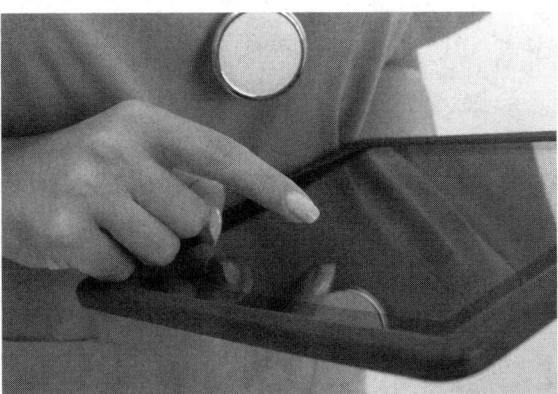

FIGURE 2-1 Today's nurses must possess competence in patient care, communication, and data management.
© hocus-focus/iStockphoto.com

guidelines are the National Heart, Lung, and Blood Institute (NHBLI) for the management of asthma and hypertension published by the Joint National Committee (JNC) and colorectal screening guidelines released periodically by the U.S. Preventive Services Task Force (**TABLE 2-1**).

Protocols are usually evidence-based but tend to be team-based approaches to practices in a locale or region. Through shared drives and web-based applications, teams of clinicians can share and access protocols to improve uniformity and best practices germane to a particular practice. Common protocols encountered by nurses are treatment protocols and procedure protocols. **Procedures** are commonly performed skills in practice setting. These procedures can be accessed, shared, and easily updated with the emergence of new evidence with the use of clinical informatics. The application of clinical informatics allows the nurse to review procedures prior to performing them and also adds to the uniformity of procedures performed within a given practice. Common medical applications, such as Epocrates and UpToDate, offer a centralized repository of many guidelines, protocols, and procedures and are discussed further in a later chapter.

▶ Quality Improvement Techniques and Nursing Informatics

QI and patient safety are intimately related to clinical informatics in health care. Healthcare

TABLE 2-1　Examples of Commonly Used Clinical Resources

Topic	Release Date	URL	Reference
Colorectal Cancer Screening	2016	http://jamanetwork.com /journals/jama/fullarticle /2529486	U.S. Preventive Services Task Force et al. (2016)
Diabetes	2017	https://professional .diabetes.org/sites /professional.diabetes.org /files/media/dc_40_s1 _final.pdf	American Diabetes Association (2017)
Hypertension	2014	http://jamanetwork.com /journals/jama /fullarticle/1791497	*2014 Evidence-Based Guideline for the Management of High Blood Pressure in Adults: Report from the Panel Members Appointed to the Eighth Joint National Committee*
Asthma	2007	http://www.nhlbi.nih .gov/guidelines/asthma /asthgdln.pdf	*National Heart, Lung, and Blood Institute, National Asthma Education and Prevention Program, Expert Panel Report 3: Guidelines for the Diagnosis and Management of Asthma, Full Report, 2007*

organizations and practice settings create data from detailed records of patient histories, diagnoses, treatments, and the outcomes of treatments. With the help of health IT, the data can be used to create a wealth of knowledge that improves the quality and efficiency of care.

The transformation of data into knowledge and wisdom is the foundation of informatics. It is a continuous process that requires the tools provided by IT and the expertise and interpretive skills of the healthcare provider (HCP). The efficacy of knowledge is directly related to the breadth of the data from which it is derived. As time progresses and the adoption of technologies such as the electronic health record (EHR) continues, this process will become more important and more efficacious, and the skills required for knowledge creation will become more and more integral to the nursing practice.

The National Academy of Medicine, formerly the Institute of Medicine, highlights six main aims of HCPs: effectiveness, safety, efficiency, patient-centeredness, timeliness, and equitability (Agency for Healthcare Research and Quality [AHRQ], 2016). The QI system, then, must develop measures of quality that reflect these aims. Because of the complex and unpredictable nature of health care, measuring quality can be difficult; it is particularly hard to attribute the outcomes of treatment to any one particular cause. Another factor contributing to the complexity of QI is that errors and adverse events should be rare, exceptional events (Hughes, 2008). Several groups have attempted to address this issue by researching, vetting, and endorsing measures of quality that are valid and reliable and more proximal to the actual care provided rather than a long-term measurement. AHRQ is the primary provider of these vetted quality measures, and a breakdown of these measures can be found on its National Quality Measures Clearinghouse website (http://www.qualitymeasures.ahrq.gov).

Using clinical guidelines, HCPs can begin to assess quality through benchmarking. With internal benchmarking, HCPs compare their current performance to their past performance. This benchmarking is helpful in identifying best practices within an organization. In external benchmarking, performance is compared to other HCPs outside the organization. External benchmarking is important to ensure that HCPs and organizations are not isolated and have quality equivalent to others regardless of geographic location. Sources for comparative data for external benchmarking include the AHRQ's annual *National Healthcare Quality Report* and *National Healthcare Disparities Report.* There are also other more nursing-specific sources, such as the American Nurses Association (ANA)'s National Database of Nursing Quality Indicators (Hughes, 2008).

Quantitative measures of quality are useful, but they do not provide the entire picture. In order to use them to their fullest potential, a thorough understanding of the structures and processes that make up the workflow of the organization and an open and collaborative team approach to QI are vital. This is where **continuous quality improvement (CQI)** systems come in. With CQI systems, the belief is that there is always room for improvement in every aspect of the process. Organizations that use CQI set up holistic systems that focus on every aspect of an organization and strive to make improvement the primary purpose of the organization. This holistic approach includes defining processes, honing organizational management, working in teams, gathering and assessing data, and translating those assessments into changes in the function of the practice (Hughes, 2008). The continuous nature of these types of systems means constantly reevaluating and assessing the changes made in the past. These systems are some of the most team-oriented, requiring a large commitment from the organization's leadership and its constituents, but they can produce amazing results if implemented by a willing and committed staff. A detailed list of QI strategies and tools can be found at the AHRQ's website

(https://innovations.ahrq.gov/qualitytools
/quality-improvement-quality-toolbox).

▶ Interprofessional Collaboration and Practice Workflow

Clinical informatics impact the ability of professionals to interact and build upon one another's contribution to patient care. In years past, **interprofessional collaboration** was limited to verbal encounters, phone calls, and facsimiles. With the application of clinical informatics, clinicians now routinely collaborate through portals and electronic medical records (EMRs), review and attest one another's patient notes, and make referrals conveying critical information to other clinicians through informatics (Oyler & Vinci, 2008). In fact, in 2017, **fast healthcare interoperability resources (FHIR)**, a standard for electronically sharing healthcare information, released an update and will soon move from a trial version to its final version. The primary goals of FHIR are to improve interoperability among healthcare systems through **health information exchanges (HIEs)** and improve access to healthcare information on multiple devices including computers, tablets, and cell phones (Munro, 2014). HIEs are high-level systems that are designed to promote the rapid sharing of data across facilities. Although technological factors are certainly essential in the success of an HIE, understanding how the HIE impacts users is also important. Unertl, Johnson, and Lorenzi (2012) conducted a 9-month qualitative, ethnographic study, gathering data from six emergency departments (EDs) and eight ambulatory clinics in the Southeastern United States. They found that HIEs were incorporated into the workflow in user-specific roles; for example, nurses reported frequent access of HIEs to confirm patients' reports of care at other facilities within the exchange (Unertl, Johnson, & Lorenzi, 2012). Additional positive impacts of HIEs on workflow were noted by participants in other ways, such as how they assist in medical decision making by supplying essential information when laypersons were unable to do so and facilitate referrals and transfers to other facilities.

▶ Nursing Workflow

Health IT has a profound effect on the way that nurses provide care for patients, regardless of the location of that care. In many cases the effects may be negative, by reducing the efficiency of nursing care processes, also called nursing workflow. Because workflow issues are so important, an entire chapter is devoted to the topic later in the book. However, a short description is warranted here to emphasize the role that nurses have when using health IT.

Quantitative research methods are often used to evaluate the implementation of informatics tools in nursing workflow because these methods can describe details such as cost, time, and other factors that are often associated with health IT use in organizations. However, a more comprehensive understanding of the scope of health IT implementation in nursing workflow requires an assessment of the attitudes and perceptions of the nurses who will work directly with the technology (see **FIGURE 2-2**). This type of information may be better captured with the use of qualitative research methods. In complex bedside procedures, such as the administration of intensive insulin therapy (IIT) in the patient with diabetes who is experiencing a hyperglycemic crisis, the use of a computer-assisted clinical decision-support system may be helpful. In a qualitative ethnographic study of 49 instances of nurses who used such a system embedded in a provider order-entry system to administer IIT to patients, researchers found that nurses felt that the documentation associated with the use of the system presented a hindrance to patient care, but valued its ability to recommend insulin dosages based on their data input (Campion, Waitman, Lorenzi, May, & Gadd, 2011).

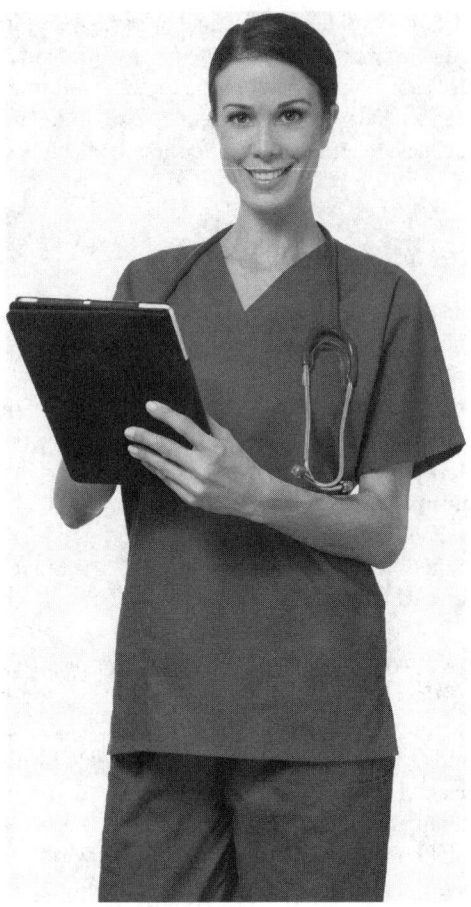

FIGURE 2-2 Describing the impact of health IT implementation on nursing workflow necessitates assessment of nurses' attitudes and perceptions about the use of technology in patient-care settings.

© EricHood/iStockphoto.com

Due to the importance of clinical informatics related to QI, interprofessional collaboration, and nursing workflow, it is imperative that nurses remain leaders in health IT (see case study in **BOX 2-1**). Chief Nursing Officer (CNO) must understand informatics concepts and the needs of the nursing staff to engage successfully with the Chief Information Officer (CIO) of the organization (American Organization of Nurse Executives, [AONE], 2015). Too often lack of communication between the CNO and CIO leads to poor

technology selection or flowed implementation. Lack of this critical relationship can lead to an implementation of health IT solutions that is met with resistance or fails to address specific needs of the nursing discipline. Introduction of clinical informatics early in nursing curricula is a first step in creating nurses who are prepared to be leaders in IT.

▶ Nursing Curricula and Continuing Education

The American Association of Colleges of Nursing (AACN, 2008), in *The Essentials of Baccalaureate Education for Professional Nursing Practice,* summarizes the need for informatics content in curricula: "Knowledge and skills in information management and patient care technologies are critical in the delivery of quality patient care" (p. 4). **TABLE 2-2** lists the specific competencies that nurses should possess when they graduate from any Bachelor of Science in Nursing program.

Nursing education programs are working to implement health informatics education into present curricula, but this can be a difficult process. Time constraints and a shortage of nursing faculty with health informatics expertise have been cited as barriers to the full integration of health informatics content in programs of study in the United States and abroad (Bartholomew, 2011). In a study of 186 students enrolled in healthcare professions in the United Kingdom, 61% reported that they desired more training in the use of clinical information systems (Bartholomew, 2011). It is essential that students understand that working with health IT tools is a meaningful component of the professional nurse's skill set. Exposure to an academic EHR and repeat opportunities to develop competency in the use of the EHR have been cited as important throughout the curricula. These exposures may be important approaches in assisting nursing students to meet the evolving health IT expectations in healthcare settings (Gardner & Jones, 2012).

BOX 2-1 Case Study: Establishment and Utilization of the IT/Nursing Workflow Group

When change is inevitable for an organization such as in a product, process, or pathway, it is in the best interests of the organization to include in the process of change those who would be defined as end users. The end user is someone who actually touches or uses whatever is being addressed in an ongoing basis. Involvement of end users assists in streamlining changes and creates an environment of appreciation and ownership that yields a greater volume of interest and increased morale. In turn, the EHR would become end-user friendly and have the possibility to decrease time and effort in charting workflow and allowing for more direct patient care.

Shannon's hospital is planning to upgrade the EHR admission assessment and charting workflow for nurses, and he is charged with getting direct care nurses involved in the process. Collaborative communication with a senior IT applications analyst resulted in a formal meeting for direct care nurses, held in a location away from the nursing units. Shannon schedules monthly meetings, allotting 4–5 hours for each, in order to provide an opportunity for the direct care nurses to voice concerns with the current charting, make suggestions to streamline electronic workflow, and help make decisions regarding desired upgrades.

Several months before the scheduled upgrade, Shannon requested the nursing directors to ask each nursing manager to recruit a staff nurse to participate in the monthly meeting. The goal was to have an adequate representation of nursing staff who delivered direct care to patients representing multiple disease processes, range of acuity, and throughout the life span. Desired participants were described as direct care nurses who would be willing to speak up in a group of their peers and give honest input. Each would need to be proficient with EHR charting.

Each month the senior applications analyst worked with Shannon to establish an agenda for the meeting to coincide with the upgrade timeline. It was imperative that this group remained on task in order to meet the overall goal for the organization. Participation flourished in the beginning as workflow was redefined.

During the meetings prior to the upgrade, Shannon and the direct care nurses validated there were several ways in which to chart multiple data elements. Identification of these multiple elements became a high priority, along with streamlining charting by nursing within the EHR. Duplication and cumbersome charting in the EHR were identified as nursing dissatisfiers, and as such, became of high importance to nursing and hospital administration. The direct care nurses were glad to see their concerns were heard and that they were trusted to work toward problem resolution.

Over the period of 9 months, Shannon was able to lead the direct care nursing workflow group in offering invaluable input into how the nursing staff charts in the EHR. They minimized and streamlined charting pathways and gave input on the training materials for the upgrade roll out. Over time, staff nurse participation decreased, and those who persisted brought vital worth to the project. These individuals also stepped up to assist in facilitating the education of their peers throughout the organization. This well-organized group created an improved charting path that was embraced by other bedside nurses throughout the hospital.

▶ Ongoing Education and Nursing Informatics

Continuing education is required for all nurses to stay current in practice, meet their state-mandated continuing education units (CEUs), and fulfill requirements for certification/recertification in specialty practice. For example, 30 states in the United States require CEUs for renewal of the registered nurse (RN) license. Some states have special requirements for CEUs including education on human immunodeficiency virus/acquired immune deficiency syndrome, professional practice, pain management, bioterrorism, domestic violence, and reporting

TABLE 2-2 AACN Essentials of Baccalaureate Education for Professional Nursing Practice. Essential IV: Information Management and Application of Patient-Care Technology

Demonstrate skills in using patient-care technologies, information systems, and communication devices that support safe nursing practice.

Use telecommunication technologies to assist in effective communication in a variety of healthcare settings.

Apply safeguards and decision-making support tools embedded in patient-care technologies and information systems to support a safe practice environment for patients and healthcare workers.

Understand the use of clinical information systems to document interventions related to achieving nurse-sensitive outcomes.

Use standardized terminology in a care environment that reflects nursing's unique contribution to patient outcomes.

Evaluate data from all relevant sources, including technology, to inform the delivery of care.

Recognize the role of information technology in improving patient-care outcomes and creating a safe care environment.

Uphold ethical standards related to data security, regulatory requirements, confidentiality, and patients' right to privacy.

Apply patient-care technologies as appropriate to address the needs of a diverse patient population.

Recognize that redesign of workflow and care processes should precede implementation of care technology to facilitate nursing practice.

Participate in evaluation of information systems in practice settings through policy and procedure development.

Reproduced from American Association of Colleges of Nursing. (2008). *The Essentials of Baccalaureate Education for Professional Nursing Practice*. Retrieved from http://www.aacn.nche.edu/education-resources/baccessentials08.pdf

to public health authorities (ANA, 2013). For nurses with national certification in specialized nursing areas or in advanced practice roles, CEU requirements are more extensive and vary by the certification. As clinical evidence rapidly evolves, an efficient means to gain access to education is available through online programs offering CEUs (see **TABLE 2-3**).

Many professional nursing organizations, for-profit companies, and universities offer quality educational material online (see the companion website to this text for resources). Nurses who wish to take CEUs by using online resources need to make sure that the CEUs will meet the requirements of state licensure or certification.

Online CEU offerings can take different forms: text documents with examination questions returned to the CEU provider by email, fax, or U.S. mail; asynchronous webinars with embedded examination questions that upload to CEU providers; synchronous webinars with question-and-answer sessions; and interactive tutorials with embedded questions that upload to a CEU provider. The ANA hosts Twitter chats occasionally found at #ANAChat; nurses who tweet can participate in the discussion and earn free CEUs. Podcasts are also methods by which nurses can obtain CEUs.

Even complete certificate programs are available online from organizations such as the Institute for Healthcare Improvement's (2012)

TABLE 2-3 Resources	
Resource	**Internet Address**
Agency for Healthcare Research and Quality: Quality Measures Website	http://www.qualitymeasures.ahrq.gov
Agency for Healthcare Research and Quality: Patient Safety Website	http://www.patientsafety.gov
American Library Association Information Literacy Competency Standards for Higher Education	http://www.ala.org/ala/mgrps/divs/acrl /standards/informationliteracycompetency.cfm
American Nurses Association States Which Require Continuing Education for RN Licensure	http://nursingworld.org/MainMenuCategories /Policy-Advocacy/State/Legislative-Agenda-Reports /NursingEducation/CE-Licensure-Chart.pdf
ECDL Foundation, which is an international organization whose mission is to raise digital competence in the workforce, education, and society (European Computer Driving License Qualifications, 2013)	http://www.ecdl.org/programmes/ecdl_icdl
Technology Informatics Guiding Education Reform(TIGER) Initiative (Health Information and Management Systems Society, 2017)	http://www.himss.org/professionaldevelopment /tiger-initiative

Open School. Completion of a series of asynchronous tutorials in patient safety and QI provide, at the time of this writing, 26 hours of continuing education with a certificate of completion for nurses and other HCPs. Certainly, universities offer certificate programs online such as post-master's certificates in nursing education, nursing informatics, and geriatrics.

Other methods of professional development may not provide CEUs, but they can help clinicians stay abreast of developments in their areas of interest. For example, web-conferencing or voice over Internet with Skype or other methods can connect nurses to specialists in their areas of interest. With smartphones and/or Internet access, nurses can follow Twitter feeds from universities, federal agencies, and well-respected healthcare organizations. From this simplest form to more complex adaptations, IT will remain an important means for nursing collaboration and maintaining continuing education.

▶ Summary

Nurses and other HCPs use health IT in all aspects of providing patient care. There is no choice about being competent with basic computer skills and with information management skills. Nursing informatics competencies are identified in *The Essentials of Baccalaureate Education for Professional Nursing Practice,* by the TIGER Initiative, and the *Nursing Informatics: Scope and Standards of Practice* (2nd ed.). Informatics competencies are required to improve nursing workflow and care delivery processes. Nurses who are competent users of technology can also keep themselves abreast of changes in practice by engaging in continuing education using interactive Internet- or mobile-based education.

References

Agency for Healthcare Research and Quality. (2016). *The six domains of health care quality*. Retrieved July 23, 2017, from https://www.ahrq.gov/professionals/quality -patient-safety/talkingquality/create/sixdomains .html

American Association of Colleges of Nursing. (2008). *The essentials of baccalaureate education for professional nursing practice*. Retrieved from http://www.aacn.nche .edu/education-resources/baccessentials08.pdf

American Diabetes Association (2017). Standards of medical care in diabetes 2017. *Diabetes Care: The Journal of Clinical and Applied Research and Education, 1,* (supplement).

American Nurses Association. (2013). *States which require continuing education for RN licensure*. Retrieved from http://nursingworld.org/MainMenuCategories /Policy-Advocacy/State/Legislative-Agenda-Reports /NursingEducation/CE-Licensure-Chart.pdf

American Organization of Nurse Executives. (2015). AONE Nurse Executive Competencies. Chicago, IL: Author. Retrieved from http://www.aone.org/resources/nurse -leader-competencies.shtml

Bartholomew, N. (2011). Is higher education ready for the information revolution? *International Journal of Therapy and Rehabilitation, 18*(10), 558–566.

Campion, J. R., Waitman, L. R., Lorenzi, N. M., May, A. K., & Gadd, C. S. (2011). Barriers and facilitators to the use of computer-based intensive insulin therapy. *Journal of International Medical Informatics, 80,* 863–871.

European Computer Driving License Qualifications. (2013). *About ECDL Foundation*. Retrieved from http://www .ecdl.org/index.jsp?p=93&n=94&a=3235

Gardner, C. L., & Jones, S. J. (2012). Utilization of academic electronic medical record in undergraduate nursing education. *Online Journal of Nursing Informatics (OJNI), 16*(2). Retrieved from http://ojni.org/issues/?/p=1702

Health Information and Management Systems Society. (2017). The TIGER initiative. Retrieved from http://www .himss.org/professionaldevelopment/tiger-initiative.

Hughes, R. G. (2008). Tools and strategies for quality improvement and patient safety. In R. G. Hughes (Ed.), *Patient safety and quality: An evidence-based handbook for nurses*. Rockville, MD: Agency for Healthcare Research and Quality. Retrieved from http://www.ahrq.gov /professionals/clinicians-providers/resources/nursing /resources/nurseshdbk/nurseshdbk.pdf

Institute for Healthcare Improvement. (2012). *How to improve*. Retrieved from http://www.ihi.org/knowledge /Pages/HowtoImprove/default.aspx

Moorman, L. P. (2010, January). Nurse leaders discuss the nurse's role in driving technology decisions. *American Nurse Today*. Retrieved from https://www.american nursetoday.com/nurse-leaders-discuss-the-nurses -role-in-driving-technology-decisions/

Munro, D. (2014, March 30). Setting healthcare interop on fire. *Forbes*. Retrieved from https://www.forbes .com/sites/danmunro/2014/03/30/setting-healthcare -interop-on-fire/#23585d40f2ba

Oyler, J., & Vinci, L. (2008). Teaching internal medicine residents quality improvement techniques using the ABIM's practice improvement modules. *Journal of General Internal Medicine, 23*(7), 927–930.

Unertl, K. M., Johnson, K. B., & Lorenzi, N. M. (2012). Health information exchange technology on the frontline of healthcare: Workflow factors and patterns of use. *Journal of the American Medical Informatics Association, 19,* 392–400. doi:10.1136/amiajnl-2011-0004

U.S. Preventive Services Task Force, Bibbins-Domingo, K., Grossman, D. C., Curry, S. J., Davidson, K. W., Epling J. W. Jr., . . ., Siu. A. L. (2016). Screening for colorectal cancer: US Preventive Services Task Force recommendation statement. *JAMA, 315*(23), 2564.

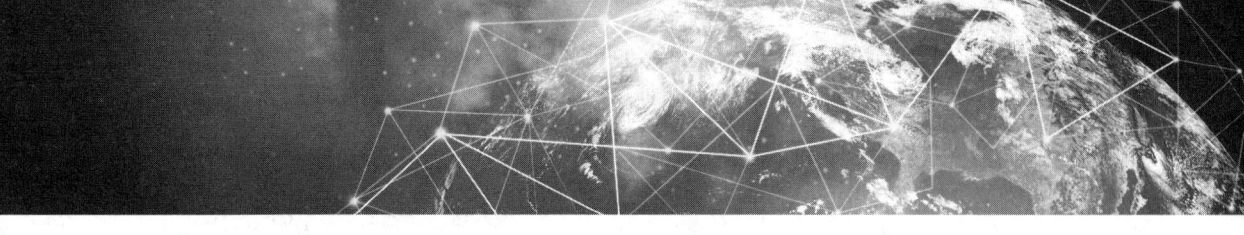

CHAPTER 3

Informatics and Evidence-Based Practice

Janie T. Best, DNP, RN, ACNS-BC, CNL

Karen H. Frith, PhD, RN, NEA-BC

Ron Schwertfeger, MLIS

LEARNING OBJECTIVES

1. Distinguish between the hardware and software components of computer systems.
2. Search electronic resources for evidence-based practice (EBP), including databases, journals, and professional organizations, efficiently to find current nursing research, systematic reviews, and clinical practice guidelines.
3. Discuss methods of integrating EBP into electronic health records or other health information technology.
4. Apply knowledge of EBP to patient care.
5. Discuss the role of health information technology standards in EBP.

KEY TERMS

Agency for Healthcare Research and Quality (AHRQ)
Boolean operators
Centers for Disease Control and Prevention (CDC)
Clinical decision-support systems (CDSS)
Cochrane Databases
Cumulative Index to Nursing and Allied Health Literature (CINAHL)
Directory of Open Access Journals (DOAJ)
Evidence-based practice (EBP)
Google Scholar
Interlibrary loan
Literature search
Medical Subject Headings (MeSH)
National Center for Biotechnology Information (NCBI)

National Guideline
  Clearinghouse
National Library of Medicine
  (NLM)
Open access

Plan-Do-Study-Act (PDSA)
PubMed
PubMed Advanced Search
  Builder
PubMed Clinical Queries

PubMed LinkOut
PubMed sidebar filters
Rich Site Summary (RSS feeds)
Zotero

▶ Chapter Overview

Since the passage of the Affordable Care Act in 2009, and with the opportunity to capture incentive monies from the Centers for Medicare and Medicaid Services (CMS), the use of technology has exploded as healthcare organizations have accepted the challenge to convert their paper records to an electronic health record (EHR) (Duffy, 2015). Gugerty and Delaney (2009) describe how the Technology Informatics Guiding Education Reform (TIGER) initiative addressed this explosion of technology in health care and the need for nurses to be prepared to effectively use technology to provide evidence-based care. TIGER competencies include: (a) basic computer proficiency; (b) the ability to identify a clinical question, find, evaluate, and apply information on the question (information literacy); and (c) the ability to appropriately collect, process, and communicate data (information management). The TIGER report encourages inclusion of all three areas in nursing programs as these are key skills of evidence-based practice (Cheeseman, 2012; Gugerty & Delaney, 2009).

Successful use of technology by nurses to implement evidence-based practice and thus to improve patient care requires a basic understanding of computer architecture, computer terminology, and data and file management (Cheeseman, 2012). Developing the skill of finding and appraising current evidence from research, systematic reviews of literature, and clinical practice guidelines may be difficult as the nurse moves from the academic to practice settings. However, **evidence-based practice (EBP)** is a core skill necessary to improve nursing care and enhance the safety of patients. This chapter provides basic computer information, a synopsis

of EBP, describes the major steps associated with EBP, and supplies readers with resources to conduct literature searches for evidence. Finally, this chapter gives an overview of health information management technology standards as they apply to clinical practice.

▶ Introduction to Information and Computer Science

Computer Architecture

Computers are used to find, manipulate, and store data in an electronic format. In recent years, computers have become more complex and mobile, and they are increasingly essential to individuals in their personal and professional lives (Kaminski, 2015). Desktop devices, laptops, tablets, cell or smartphones, and a wide variety of medical and household equipment use computer software to perform their functions (Dainow, 2016). A basic understanding of how computers operate provides the nurse with the first step to exploring the evidence as it relates to clinical practice (Cheeseman, 2012).

A computer system has four main functions: collection, processing, storage, and retrieval of data (Cheeseman, 2011), and consists of input devices, the central processing unit (CPU), memory, and output devices. Two main components of a computer are its hardware (physical components) and software (applications). Physical components include the casing (desktop, laptop, or mobile) and the internal mechanisms (CPU, motherboard, power supply, hard disc, and memory). External hardware includes touch screens, keyboards, a mouse to control screen position, and a monitor that displays information on a screen. Additional hardware is available to help the user print information or enhance listening (Kaminski, 2015).

Computers are further categorized on the basis of size and use. Supercomputers are large and only run a few programs at a high processing speed. Their specific uses range from animations and simulations, or training to weather forecasting. Mainframe computers have large memory capacity, work at a high speed, and have the ability for many users to operate the computer system at the same time. Healthcare and university computer systems are examples of mainframe computers. The smallest computers, microcomputers or personal computers, are designed for single users, can be connected as a network, and are small and affordable to most individuals (Cheeseman, 2011).

Data Organization, Representation and Structure

A computer's work begins with input of information via an external or touch-screen keyboard to a CPU where a processor chip collects data and makes decisions based on the software's program code (instructions). The memory of a computer is divided into random-access (RAM) and read-only (ROM). RAM provides temporary storage of data during the creation of work before it is stored in a more permanent location, either in the computer's hard drive or other storage location. Unless saved to a more permanent location, RAM storage is lost when the program is closed or the computer is turned off. ROM is located in the motherboard (circuit boards) and saves data in a more permanent way after the computer is turned off. During work, data are uploaded in the RAM and, when directed by the user, stored in ROM on the hard drive, on a USB flash drive, or in other external locations. (Cheeseman, 2011; Kaminiski, 2015).

The ability to store information is based on the capacity of the device. The basic (smallest) unit of memory is a bit; a byte consists of eight bits of data. From these small units, storage can be expanded in increments of 1,000 to kilobytes (KB), megabytes (MB), gigabytes (GB), and terabytes (TB). Decisions about the amount of storage needed in a computer system is based on the amount of data to be processed and stored, and on estimated storage time. Data can be collected, organized, and stored in a database where it can be retrieved easily and in a way that is meaningful to the user. Commonly used databases in health care include electronic medical records, databases that support mobile applications, and many more, which are described in chapters that follow. In academic settings, bibliographic and citation databases are commonly used. Synthesized databases allow the user to search for information from practice guidelines, systematic reviews, and meta-analysis documents (Cheeseman, 2011). Directions for how to conduct a literature search using large databases are discussed later in this chapter.

Software applications are internal programs that can be modified without changes to the external hardware of the computer (Dainow, 2016). These applications are categorized as productivity, creative, or communication programs. Productivity software includes a variety of programs including databases, email, presentations, spreadsheets, and word processing applications to support a wide variety of information processing needs. Creative software can be used to create drawings, music, or digital photography/videos. Communication software includes email programs, Internet browsers, instant messaging, and a variety of conferencing programs (Dainow, 2016; Kaminski, 2015).

Networking and Data Communication

Computer networks are formed when two or more computers are linked in a way that allows them to share information. A local area network (LAN) is confined to a single site, a metropolitan area network (MAN) connects regional areas, and a wide area network (WAN) reaches far beyond the single location to connect many LANs together. Connections to the Internet are available through cable or digital subscriber lines (DSL) or through dial-up telephone services (Cheeseman, 2011; Dainow, 2016). To connect to the Internet, the computer has to be connected to an Internet service provider (ISP) through a modem and a unique Internet protocol (IP) address (Dainow, 2016). Each website is identified by a unique uniform resource locator (URL) protocol. Two types of URL addresses are commonly used to reach web resources: hypertext transfer protocol (HTTP) or hypertext transfer protocol—secure (HTTPS). There are also URL addresses for email and file transfers (FTP) (Cheeseman, 2011; Dainow, 2016; TechTarget, 2016).

Computer networks allow knowledge to be shared in multiple ways. The World Wide Web (www) is a network program that is familiar to most Internet users. A collection of documents, images, and web pages, the World Wide Web makes it possible to gather information from many resources, as well as to share information around the globe. Smartphones add another layer of information gathering and storage via telephone and global positioning system (GPS) technology, preserving the ability to access and disseminate information, no matter where we are, 24 hours a day (Cheeseman, 2011; Dainow, 2016; Kaminiski, 2015).

Another use of the Internet is to store large amounts of information in a *cloud*. This method of storage allows an organization to achieve cost savings in many areas (maintenance, infrastructure, use of less expensive computers). For an organization that requires fast and consistent access to the *cloud* storage, loss of, or a slow, Internet service connection will be a disadvantage of this method of data storage (Cheeseman, 2011).

Health care has benefited from recent computer advances in software programming, including educational packages for online instruction through courses, simulation experiences (avatars, high-fidelity mannequins, and online student resources), artificial intelligence/robotics to improve life for individuals with disabilities, and research (e.g., the Human Genome Project to map DNA). Social networking applications (also known as social media) are software programs that encourage communication with others. Individuals can set up blogs or join social networks like Facebook or Twitter to share information with friends, family, or others with similar health conditions (Dainow, 2016). Social media has become a way that patients, families, and caregivers gain information and support from one another, particularly with chronic illnesses or life-limiting illnesses (Rupert et al., 2016).

Basic Terminology of Computing

Understanding basic computer terminology is the first step to effective computer use. Many Internet sites have compiled comprehensive lists of computer terms and definitions that can be easily accessed and used for teaching and learning basic computer language. One list, created specifically for the older population, has been developed by the National Institute on Aging and can be found at https://nihseniorhealth.gov /toolkit/toolkitfiles/pdf/Glossary.pdf.

Having a common terminology is essential to the effective use of retrieved computer data to improve patient care and outcomes. Nurses must be able to capture their work in a way that is meaningful and allows for evaluation of the effectiveness of nursing interventions (Rutherford, 2008). The American Nurses Association (2012) published 12 approved standardized terminologies that support nursing work. The International Council of Nurses (2015) developed a framework for nursing practice that allows for inclusion of different terminologies that support the work of nurses. The goals of these two documents are similar and support the use of common nursing language to raise awareness of nursing work, communication within the healthcare team, ease of data retrieval and analysis for evaluation of nursing work, and increased ability to incorporate and adhere to evidence-based standards of care (Rutherford, 2008). Use of standard terminologies ensures that communications are understood and interpreted in the same way by all members of the healthcare team (Halley, Sensmeier, & Brokel, 2009).

▶ Integrating Evidence-Based Practice

Introduction

EBP is a process that has developed from a need to improve the quality and manage the economics of healthcare delivery (Salmond, 2007). The components of EBP include a systematic and critical evaluation of the current literature, the nurse's clinical expertise and available resources, and patients' values and preferences. This information is used to make deliberate clinical decisions based on theory and relevant research that guide patient care (Ahrens & Johnson, 2013; Ingersoll, 2000; Melnyk & Fineout-Overholt, 2011). The expected results of these carefully considered decisions are improved outcomes for patients, efficiency, and cost-effective care delivery for organizations (Melnyk & Fineout-Overholt, 2011; Salmond, 2007).

Cultivating a Spirit of Inquiry

The process of EBP is best learned in sequence with distinct steps. The preliminary step, *cultivating a spirit of inquiry* (Melnyk, Fineout-Overholt, Stillwell, & Williamson, 2010, p. 51), means to be curious about the effectiveness of nursing interventions, to take interest in changing nursing practice or questioning practice, and to try new approaches. Nurses with a spirit of inquiry understand EBP as a way of thinking, not an additional burden to their practice. Nurses who are passionate about EBP will likely become informal leaders, or be promoted to leadership positions, and can influence others to grow support for EBP. Those who have a spirit of inquiry will have questions and a desire to find the best evidence to support their practice (Melnyk, Fineout-Overholt, Stillwell, & Williamson, 2009).

Writing the Question

Nurses who use the steps of EBP to formalize their questions about practice should use the PICOT format (Lawson, 2005; Melnyk & Fineout-Overholt, 2011). The term PICOT identifies the patient or population (P), issue or intervention (I), what will be compared (C), the expected outcome (O), and the time (T) that it will take to achieve and evaluate the outcome (Melnyk & Fineout-Overholt, 2011). The PICOT format is a systematic method of question writing and helps decrease the time and effort it takes to find evidence specific to the topic being investigated. Consistently using a set format to write the question ensures that all components of the question are addressed before the **literature search** begins (Stillwell, Fineout-Overholt, Melnyk, & Williamson, 2010).

It takes time and practice to learn how to write questions in the PICOT format. Melnyk and Fineout-Overholt (2011) suggest that it takes "practice, practice, practice" to become proficient in writing PICOT questions (p. 31). Questions may be written following a template and may focus on interventions, predictions or prognosis of outcomes for a specific patient population, comparison of diagnosis or diagnostic tests, etiology and associated risk factors for a specific condition, or meaning within a situation (Melnyk & Fineout-Overholt, 2011; Stillwell et al., 2010).

Nurses who embrace EBP may find support in forming groups interested in certain topics. Lawson (2005) suggests that getting other nurses involved helps to clarify clinical issues and to write clear and specific clinical questions. Once a group is assembled and the individuals are comfortable in identifying issues and writing questions, the second step, searching for evidence, can begin.

Finding the Evidence Using Library Sources

In order to use evidence in EBP, a nurse must locate and review the evidence found in research articles as published in reliable sources. This process begins with using appropriate electronic databases and performing effective online searches. Using appropriate databases can be easier for nursing students during their coursework and for nurses at university-affiliated hospitals and clinics, with their many research database subscriptions, but other options are available.

Nurses should use databases and websites that have valid and reliable information. **PubMed** and **Cumulative Index to Nursing and Allied Health Literature (CINAHL)** are two databases that index a comprehensive body of healthcare literature. The **Cochrane Databases** and the **National Guideline Clearinghouse** support EBP by including systematic reviews and current practice guidelines. Government sources for reliable information include the **Centers for Disease Control and Prevention (CDC)** and the **Agency for Healthcare Research and Quality (AHRQ)**. Many professional organizations have their journals and evidence-based guidelines available electronically for members or individuals who have subscribed online (Fineout-Overholt, Berryman, Hofstetter, & Sollenberger, 2011; Hoss & Hanson, 2008). Information about additional resources is addressed later in this chapter.

Searching for Evidence in Research Literature

Searching the literature may seem like a daunting task, and overwhelming to those who have not had experience with electronic databases. While lack of access to an onsite library or computer database applications can be a major barrier to conducting a search for evidence, the inability of a nurse to effectively use the computer to search the literature adds an additional barrier to embracing EBP (Hoss & Hanson, 2008; Wells, Free, & Adams, 2007). Nurses without computer skills or experience in data searches can seek assistance from a university or hospital librarian, or other experienced professionals (Fain, 2009). Time spent with a librarian who loves to teach others how to find these treasure troves of information is priceless, and will return a lifetime of information power. Links to tutorials and videos for using commonly accessed databases can be found in the companion website for this book.

One of the greatest skills that nurses learn in their academic program is the ability to find relevant research on clinical topics. To begin the search in one of these research databases, nurses should select key terms from the PICOT question. These terms are entered using **Boolean operators** (*and, or, not*) to combine multiple search terms. In addition, many databases allow the use of quotation marks to search for phrases of multiple words. A good search technique is to set limits on the search, to narrow down the results to articles that are more suitable. For example, limiting a search to English-language, peer-reviewed journals and articles published within the last 5 years can help in the selection of valid findings that may be applicable to the topic (Hoss & Hanson, 2008; Melnyk & Fineout-Overholt, 2011).

Systematic Reviews and Clinical Practice Guidelines

Systematic reviews are literature reviews that follow a certain methodology to standardize the critique of research findings. Two excellent sources of systematic reviews are McMaster Plus Nursing[+] and the Cochrane Collaboration. McMaster Plus has three functions: (1) it serves as a database of peer-reviewed articles that have been rated by nursing professionals, (2) it contains an email alert system for selected topics of interest, and (3) it provides links to abstracts of systematic reviews of research literature. The Cochrane Collaboration is a library built by healthcare professionals who author Cochrane Reviews, which are the gold standard for preappraised research evidence. Only a few Cochrane reviews are free; most are contained in the Cochrane Database of Systematic Reviews and available with a subscription. Nurses can join the Cochrane Journal Club and other electronic notifications of systematic reviews and clinical practice guidelines at no cost. **TABLE 3-1** provides a list of resources and Internet addresses for these sites.

TABLE 3-1 Resources to Learn About EBP	
Tutorials	**Internet Address**
Appraising the Evidence	http://nursingworld.org/MainMenuCategories/The PracticeofProfessionalNursing/Improving-Your-Practice /Research-Toolkit/Appraising-the-Evidence
American Nurses Association (ANA) list of online tutorials about EBP	http://ana.nursingworld.org/research-toolkit/Education
University of North Carolina EBP tutorials	http://www.hsl.unc.edu/Services/Tutorials/EBM /welcome.htm
Academic Center for Evidence-Based Practice at the University of Texas Health Science Center at San Antonio	
Basic Modules	http://acestar.uthscsa.edu/modules/Basic.htm
Intermediate Modules	http://acestar.uthscsa.edu/modules/Intermediate.htm

Clinical guidelines are valuable because they contain preappraised research. Authors of clinical practice guidelines rate the research for the quality of evidence and the strength of making a recommendation for change based on the findings. The federal government provides at least three sources of free clinical practice guidelines at the Agency for Healthcare Quality and Research, the National Guidelines Clearing House, and the **PubMed Clinical Queries**. **TABLE 3-2** provides the Internet addresses for the free resources for clinical practice guidelines.

Using Free Resources

After students leave their colleges and universities, access to subscription databases, such as CINAHL, depends on resources available in their places of employment. For those in academic medical centers, access to databases may be assured; those in community hospitals or ambulatory settings will likely find themselves disconnected from the very lifeline of evidence-based practice—a library.

There are ways to access libraries free or at low costs for individual nurses. The best place to start is PubMed, which is freely available online. Some of the research journals published online are available as open access journals— if those journals are indexed in PubMed, then those results will link to the article. Google Scholar can also be a useful tool.

PubMed

As a service of the **National Center for Biotechnology Information (NCBI)** at the U.S. **National Library of Medicine (NLM)**, PubMed is an extensive index of published medical literature with over 22 million citations. Nursing literature is indexed in this service too. However, unlike CINAHL and other subscription databases, it does not provide full-text access to those articles. While articles can be accessed with the LinkOut functionality, they may not be housed within the PubMed database.

PubMed offers several noteworthy features. Rather than using keywords, the most effective

TABLE 3-2 PubMed Tutorials and Videos: Learn How to Search Efficiently for Articles

Tutorials	Internet Address
PubMed Tutorial	http://www.nlm.nih.gov/bsd/disted/pubmedtutorial/
Medical Subject Headings (MeSH) in MEDLINE/PubMed: A Tutorial	http://www.nlm.nih.gov/bsd/disted/meshtutorial/introduction/index.html
Branching Out: The MeSH Vocabulary	http://www.nlm.nih.gov/bsd/disted/video/
Videos	
My NCBI—National Center for Biotechnology Information	http://www.youtube.com/watch?v=ks46w3mNAQE
PubMed Simple Subject Search	http://www.nlm.nih.gov/bsd/viewlet/search/subject/subject.html
PubMed Author Search	http://www.nlm.nih.gov/bsd/viewlet/search/author/author.html
Getting Full-text Articles from PubMed	http://www.youtube.com/watch?v=V0NYKFSphKY
Using Sidebar Filters to Limit Results	http://www.youtube.com/watch?v=696R9GbOyvA&feature=youtu.be
Advanced PubMed Search Builder	http://www.youtube.com/watch?v=dncRQ1cobdc&feature=relmfu
Save Search Results in Collections, Including Favorites	http://www.youtube.com/watch?v=iXSttEKntCE
Searching by Using the MeSH Database	http://www.youtube.com/watch?v=uyF8uQY9wys
Search for Journal in PubMed	http://www.nlm.nih.gov/bsd/viewlet/search/journal/journal.html
Retrieving Citations from a Journal Issue	http://www.nlm.nih.gov/bsd/viewlet/search/scm/scmissue.html
Selecting Outside Tool Preference	http://www.nlm.nih.gov/bsd/viewlet/myncbi/pref_otool.html

way to search in PubMed is by using **Medical Subject Headings (MeSH)**. MeSH is a thesaurus of controlled-vocabulary terms. Once MeSH terms are found for the topic, a more fruitful yield will result from searches of PubMed. **FIGURE 3-1** shows a MeSH tree for obstructive sleep apnea. Other features of PubMed are the PubMed Advanced Search Builder, sidebar filters, LinkOut, and My NCBI.

The MeSH terms selected are entered into the **PubMed Advanced Search Builder**, the open boxes in PubMed. The drop-down menus are then set to MeSH terms, and Boolean operators (*and, or, not*) should be used as needed. If the yield is too high for a reasonable review of articles, then the **sidebar filters** can be added including article types (clinical trials, systematic reviews, practice guidelines, to name a few), text availability (abstract available, free full text available, or full text available), and publication dates. The filters will limit the search to a number that is more manageable. When the desired articles are selected, some full-text articles may be freely available using the **LinkOut** service.

Previous Indexing:

- Apnea (1966-1979)
- Sleep (1966-1979)
- Sleep Apnea Syndromes (1980-1999)

All MeSH Categories

 Diseases Category

  Respiratory Tract Diseases

   Respiration Disorders

    Apnea

     Sleep Apnea Syndromes

      Sleep Apnea, Obstructive

       Obesity Hypoventilation Syndrome

All MeSH Categories

 Diseases Category

  Nervous System Diseases

   Sleep Disorders

    Dyssomnias

     Sleep Disorders, Intrinsic

      Sleep Apnea Syndromes

       Sleep Apnea, Obstructive

        Obesity Hypoventilation Syndrome

FIGURE 3-1 MeSH tree of obstructive sleep apnea produced from a search of PubMed.

Courtesy of National Center for Biotechnology Information. Available at http://www.ncbi.nlm.nih.gov/pubmed

LinkOut is found in the upper right-hand corner of the screen. To find the desired reference material, the LinkOut icon should be clicked. Icons change depending on the source of the reference material. If full text is not available, nurses can order the articles from their hospitals or from public libraries using **interlibrary loan** services. Typically, a public library will have a nominal charge for an interlibrary loan.

Searches of PubMed should be managed such that the MeSH terms and the yields from searches can be retrieved if needed. PubMed provides a cloud-based folder called *My NCBI* (My National Center for Biotechnology Information) for searching and storing the history of searches. Up to 6 months of search histories can be stored in My NCBI. Registration and use is free. Written tutorials and short videos provide excellent help for nurses who are new to PubMed. Some of the most helpful tutorials and videos are listed in **TABLE 3-3**.

Google Scholar

Google Scholar is a web-based search engine for scholarly literature across a broad range of disciplines. Its index includes literature from both free and paid repositories, professional societies, academic publishers, and other sources across the web. The primary focus is to index all academic papers on the web (Google). While there is no doubt of the value of the service for researchers of all kinds, it also has its shortcomings. Google takes articles from everywhere it can access on the web, and users must be careful to vet the articles they find using Google Scholar, because the articles may or may not be peer reviewed. One particularly celebrated and useful feature of Google Scholar is the "cited by" feature. The "cited by" feature allows users to view a list of later works that have cited the original paper. This ability to connect literature through citations has historically only been available through paid services. A particularly pervasive shortcoming of the service is that it strengthens the Matthew Effect, a term coined by sociologist Robert Merton to refer to the way in which starting advantages tend to build on themselves (Rigney, 2010). With Google Scholar this is seen in the way that articles with more citations are more likely to be at the top of the search results, and newer articles with fewer citations are more likely to be lower on the page

TABLE 3-3 Electronic Alerts for Systematic Reviews and Clinical Practice Guidelines	
Resource	**Internet Address**
McMaster Plus, *British Medical Journal* Updates	https://plus.mcmaster.ca/EvidenceAlerts/
PubMed	https://www.ncbi.nlm.nih.gov/pubmed/
Knowledge Finder from the National Library of Medicine	http://www.kfinder.com/kfinder/Default.htm
Cochrane Library Journal Club Scroll to bottom to find sign-up form	http://www.cochranejournalclub.com/self-monitoring-and-self-management-oral-anticoagulation-clinical/default.asp?moreinfo-1#moreinformation
National Guideline Clearinghouse Email Alerts	http://www.guideline.gov/subscribe.aspx

and thus less likely to be read and used (Beel & Gipp, 2009). Google Scholar is a valuable resource for researchers of all kinds, but, as is true with all research tools, it is the responsibility of researchers to verify the veracity of any sources they use.

Open Access Journals

Freely available articles are provided by publishers who offer **open access**. The rationale for providing free, online access to scholarly articles and research is to advance scientific thought, particularly for individuals in developing countries who cannot afford the high prices of journal subscriptions (Carroll, 2011). The cost of publication is shifted to the authors, rather than the readers. While this makes research available, nurses must ensure that they are selecting articles from peer-reviewed journals. Journals that are open access can be found by searching online for the **Directory of Open Access Journals (DOAJ)**. A particular advantage of the DOAJ is that it gives smaller publications a way to expand their reach. Nurses should always be vigilant about the quality of their sources, but they should not neglect open access journals, as they often have research from more varied sources and in smaller research niches.

Analyzing the Literature

Not all evidence is equal; nor will all evidence be applicable to a particular clinical setting. When searching for evidence, it is prudent to look for clinical practice guidelines, systematic reviews, meta-analyses of evidence, or randomized controlled trials relevant to the particular clinical question. Single studies or case studies can be used to demonstrate how evidence is put into practice, and textbooks can be used as resources for information on a particular condition. Most nursing research and evidence-based practice textbooks will have guides to help evaluate the quality of quantitative and qualitative research studies (Levin, 2013; Fineout-Overholt et al., 2011). The American Nurses Association has developed a list of resources to help nurses

evaluate the quality of research studies. These tools address the validity of the study, reliability of the results, and the applicability to the particular patient care setting (see Table 3-1).

Putting the EBP Process into Practice

Once the literature is analyzed using a systematic approach, nurses working on an EBP project will need to decide if a change in practice is needed. If so, then creating enthusiasm for the project and soliciting input from all stakeholders early in the planning stages will be critical. Early and frequent communication by email or other innovative strategies such as Twitter, Facebook, or blogging can keep stakeholders involved.

As with any change, a plan needs to be prepared. A theoretical model or process, such as **Plan-Do-Study-Act (PDSA)**, can be used as a framework to plan and implement the project. A timeline for the project is essential to keep it on track. Even strategies to overcome barriers to the planned change need to be included. Selecting an evaluation strategy as part of the initial project plan is also necessary (Melnyk & Fineout-Overholt, 2011). The plan must address any ethical issues and protected health information issues by seeking Institutional Review Board approval for the project (Levin, 2013). The project plan can be made using an Excel spreadsheet or using specific software for project planning such as Microsoft Project. Following the timeline and sharing the project results during implementation will help other nurses and stakeholders remain engaged in the practice change (Lawson, 2005).

Communicating the Findings

Once the practice change is stable, the final step of EBP is to share the results with others. Failure to share the outcomes of EBP projects may lead to unwarranted duplication and delay in getting evidence into practice throughout the practice setting and beyond. Results can be disseminated in the organization at staff meetings, in a nursing newsletter, as a blog posting, or as a poster presentation. Findings should be presented at local specialty group meetings or at regional or national conferences (Melnyk et al., 2010). Nurses can also partner with local schools or colleges of nursing to create an Evidence-Based Practice Day, in which nurses from various clinical settings can share the results of their projects.

Evaluating EBP

Standardized computer terminology and databases provide the opportunity to evaluate EBP. Outcome data are available from the EHR, disease-specific registries, and other quality care databases. In order for these data to be useful, they must be entered correctly, processed in a meaningful way, and retrieved and analyzed using appropriate statistical tools (Tymkow, 2016).

Finding More About EBP Online

Because this chapter provides a brief overview of EBP, Internet-based resources can be used to supplement knowledge of EBP. The American Nurses Association (ANA) provides a list of online tutorials that can assist nurses in learning more about EBP, and the University of North Carolina also has free EBP tutorials available for nurses who seek information about the EBP process. These resources can be found in the companion website for this book.

Using Reference Manager Software to Store and Use Sources

Nurses who plan to carry out formal EBP projects need to learn how to manage the results of their searches using software. This is particularly critical if the nurse plans to communicate findings in poster sessions or in published articles. Without software, the research articles, systematic reviews of literature, and clinical practice guidelines can become stacks of paper with little or no organization. Fortunately, there are free software

solutions: Zotero and Mendeley, among others. Each of these citation management programs (sometimes called citation managers or reference managers) has different computer requirements and installation instructions.

As one example, **Zotero** can be installed either as a plug-in for the Mozilla Firefox Internet browser or as a standalone desktop program. (If the standalone desktop program is installed, a browser plug-in for Google Chrome, Apple Safari, and/or Firefox should also be installed.) Once Zotero is installed, databases such as PubMed, CINAHL, or Google Scholar can be searched as normal. Any relevant search results can easily be saved into the Zotero library on the computer. Researchers can also create a free online account with Zotero, in order to save their desktop/laptop citation library online (in order to have access to their library when working at another computer). In addition to storing references, many citation managers (including Zotero) can be integrated into Microsoft Word (or other word-processing programs). This add-in feature is the real magic of reference software. When a reference is selected in the Zotero library, with the click of one icon the reference is cited in the narrative and added to a reference list in the word-processing document. Any changes are automatically reflected in the in-text citations and reference list. Finally, references in Zotero can be shared with other Zotero users; this feature is helpful for teams of nurses focused on EBP.

There are multiple choices for reference managers, in addition to Zotero. (Mendeley works in a similar manner, is fully compatible with Windows and Mac operating systems, and can work with any Internet browser.) In most cases, a researcher will only need to select and use one reference manager (e.g., Zotero or Mendeley, but not necessarily both). In selecting which reference manager to use, it may help to check with colleagues. (If sharing a citation library with colleagues, it is helpful for all the team members to use the same reference manager.) Note that free programs like Zotero and Mendeley provide users with the option to pay for upgraded levels

TABLE 3-4 Repositories of Clinical Practice Guidelines	
Resource	**Internet Address**
Agency for Healthcare Research and Quality (AHRQ)	http://www.ahrq.gov/clinic/cpgsix.htm
AHRQ Innovations Exchange	https://innovations.ahrq.gov/
National Guideline Clearinghouse	http://www.guideline.gov/
PubMed Clinical Queries	https://www.ncbi.nlm.nih.gov/pubmed/clinical
National Institute for Health and Care Excellence (NICE) Organization	http://www.nice.org.uk/
McMaster Plus Nursing[+]	http://plus.mcmaster.ca/np/Default.aspx

of online cloud storage. On the other hand, EndNote is an example of a reference manager with an up-front cost, but which includes greater levels of online storage and free online training (along with other resources).

▶ Staying Current in Nursing Practice and Specialty Areas

Email Notifications

It is impossible to read enough journals to stay current with the short shelf-life of most research. Using technology to stay current is a smart decision. With registration at journal publisher websites, email notifications will be sent when new content is available. Publishers send a table of contents with every issue of the journal. Links from the table of contents often provide an abstract. If an interesting journal article is in the table of contents, then the nurse can order the article using interlibrary loan if it is not available from other sources. **TABLE 3-5**

lists journal publishers who provide free email notifications.

Rich Site Summary

Rich Site Summaries (RSS), often called **RSS feeds**, are simplified summaries of the information provided on whole websites. For example, an RSS feed of the CNN website would show a list of all the stories on the page. RSS feeds provide a clear and easy way of tracking information from a large number of sources, and nurses should be aware of the wealth of information available to them through RSS feeds. Some notable sources of feeds include the National Institutes of Health, the Food and Drug Administration, the CDC, and the AHRQ. The U.S. government web portal provides a large index of these feeds on their website (https://www.usa.gov).

Social Media

Social media includes Facebook, Twitter, LinkedIn, and all the other similar services. In health care, social media has not been a widely used tool, but that may be changing. Social media services help people to connect, share their

TABLE 3-5 Electronic Subscriptions to Journal Email Notifications

Resource	Internet Address
RSS Feeds for Nursing Journals	http://journals.lww.com/ajnonline/_layouts/15/oaks.journals/feeds.aspx
Mobile CINAHL	https://health.ebsco.com/products/the-cinahl-database
Lippincott Williams & Wilkins Email Alerts	http://journals.lww.com/pages/login.aspx?ContextUrl=%2fsecure%2fpages%2fmyaccount.aspx
Sage Publishers Email Alerts	http://www.sagepub.com/emailAlerts.sp?_DARGS=/common/components/extras_big.jsp.1_A&_DAV=Dummy&_dynSess-Conf=19947590846134099176
Springer Publishing Email Alerts	http://www.springerpub.com/products/Journals/Nursing#.UdjEufnVCQo

experiences, develop groups, and communicate more effectively. For a healthcare provider (HCP) that might mean instant-messaging services between patients and nurses or doctors, or video-conference-based appointments. It could also mean social networks specific to nurses and doctors where opportunities, research, and wisdom could be shared. A free EHR system called Hello Health is used by a Brooklyn-based practice that provides a model for this type of integration (Hawn, 2009). The practice has developed a patient management platform where patients can communicate with their HCP via private instant messaging, schedule video-chat appointments, renew prescriptions, and access their own personal health record (Hawn). As the landscape continues to develop and these tools evolve, nurses must adapt. By focusing on the improved communication enabled by social media, nurses will be able to build communities and share their experiences and wisdom.

Webinars and Teleconferences

Communication technology, particularly Internet-based communications, have opened up

new ways for nurses to engage with one another to learn about the best practices in patient care. Technologies such as Skype, Google Hangouts, and join.me offer low-cost or free services to connect multiple people with audio, video, and desktop sharing. When used as continuing education or webinars, nurses can participate with experts on clinical topics anywhere Internet service is available. Sortedahl (2012) developed an online journal club for school nurses and assessed nurses' satisfaction with the method after 3 months. Sortedahl found that the nurses valued three key elements: having well-informed knowledgeable moderators, getting research articles in advance, and discussing the application of findings to nursing practice. The researcher also found that using Internet-based technology allowed the journal club to invite the author of a research article to the club meeting, which benefited the researcher and nurses. There were issues with slow Internet connections, firewalls and other security measures, and operating system incompatibilities. Despite the technical issues, the nurses liked the method and wanted even more interaction with each other between journal club meetings (Sortedahl).

▶ Evidence-Based Practice Integrated in Clinical Decision-Support Systems

The most efficient means for integrating EBP in clinical processes is to have **clinical decision-support system (CDSS)** embedded in health information technology (health IT). Clinical decision-support systems are computer systems designed to impact clinical decision making about individual patients at the moment those decisions are made (Berner & La Jande, 2007) by presenting contextually appropriate information. CDSSs bring the available, applicable knowledge and research together into systems that clinicians can use throughout the decision-making process. The key aspect is that the usefulness comes from the interaction of the human and the computer. Modern CDSSs are not designed as black boxes that interpret information and deliver concrete answers, but as tools that provide the clinician with the best possible evidence relevant to the patient's assessment data and laboratory results to ensure the patient receives the best possible care (Berner & La Jande, 2007).

Most CDSSs are made up of three essential components: the knowledge base, the reasoning engine, and a mechanism to communicate with the user (Berner & La Jande, 2007). The knowledge base contains all the relevant knowledge expressed as if-then rules. The reasoning engine contains a set of instructions that tell the computer how to apply the rules to real patient data. The communication mechanism provides the means for patient data to be entered into the system and for any pertinent findings to be relayed to the user. Many CDSSs rely on the user to input data manually, but the continued acceptance of EHRs and improved interoperability among systems will enable more systems to input data automatically from multidisciplinary team members (Berner & La Jande, 2007).

Commercially available EHRs typically have CDSSs, but the system may need to be customized for use in the particular healthcare setting. Nurses and other HCPs need to be involved in the development of the CDSS because the system should reflect the best *clinical* decisions, and HCPs are equipped to translate clinical research into clinical processes through a reasoning engine in the EHR (Brokel, 2009). In a very basic way, order sets and nursing plans of care in EHRs represent clinical decision support because the predetermined orders are used to simplify the cognitive processes necessary for planning care. When order sets and nursing plans of care are developed, nurses can influence the process by serving on a task force to develop the CDSS by bringing research evidence and clinical practice guidelines to this decision-making group. In this way, nurses contribute to the implementation of evidence-based practice (Brokel, 2009).

Health Information Technology and EBP

Health information includes all the information related to the interactions of patients, HCPs, and the health information management (HIM) team. Beginning with the registration process, health information is captured, categorized, stored, and retrieved to use in making decisions related to the delivery of health care. Managing health information through the life span of EHRs is the responsibility of HIM professionals (ITI Planning Committee, 2015).

As outlined in the ITI Planning Committee white paper (2015), responsibilities and requirements for HIM professionals include ensuring the integrity, protection, and availability of health information. HIM professionals work in a variety of roles to capture, validate, maintain, and analyze data as well as providing decision support for health professionals. HIM practice by these professionals support the life cycle of health information from capture or input of data into the computer system to the disposal of health information data. Principles governing health information have been developed by the

BOX 3-1 Case Study: Searching for, Evaluating, and Managing Research Articles

Beth works at the OB/GYN clinic in a medium-sized hospital. She has noticed that many of her patients develop diabetes during their pregnancy, even though they do not have a previous history of diabetes. Beth wants to use EBP to help improve the care these patients receive.

As her first step, Beth wants to look in a reputable online resource for evidence-based research in medicine and nursing. She decides to use PubMed.

When Beth begins her research in PubMed, she searches for "diabetes," but she finds a lot of the results do not seem relevant; many of the research articles describe older patients, or teenagers, or males. In order to perform a more effective search for evidence-based research on her topic, Beth uses the MeSH database option within PubMed. When she searches in the MeSH database for diabetes and pregnancy, she finds the term "Diabetes, Gestational."

When Beth adds the MeSH term "Diabetes, Gestational" to her search in PubMed, she finds thousands of articles that are specific to diabetes during pregnancy. After beginning to scan through the articles in this list, she uses filters to narrow down her search to articles from the last 5 years that are about clinical trials. She still finds hundreds of articles, so she starts reading the following article:

Karamali, M., Heidarzadeh, Z., Seifati, S. M., Samimi, M., Tabassi, Z., Hajijafari, M., . . . Esmaillzadeh, A. (2015). Zinc supplementation and the effects on metabolic status in gestational diabetes: A randomized, double-blind, placebo-controlled trial. *J Diabetes Complications, 29*(8), 1314–1319.

Beth decided to start with this article, because the citation indicates that this research article is relevant to her area of research, it is recent, and it reports on clinical trials with human patients. After she reviews this article and saves it, she continues looking for other similar articles.

As Beth continues her research for recent articles about clinical trials with human patients, she begins to save the article citations into a personal "library." In order to easily review these articles, she begins to use Zotero, saving her articles on her laptop and online. This has several added benefits: she can save citations from PubMed as well as articles that she finds in other research databases, she can access those citations from other computers, she can share her library of references with her colleagues, and she can build a bibliography from these articles, if she wants to document the EBP at her clinic.

Check Your Understanding

1. When Beth starts her research, she decided to start in PubMed. For what possible reasons might she have started in PubMed (over another medical database, such as CINAHL)? What advantages would PubMed have over another resource, such as Google Scholar?

2. In Beth's first PubMed search, she found a lot of results for older patients or males. What benefits does she gain from using a MeSH term?

3. In the results that Beth found, she started with the 2015 article "Zinc supplementation and the effects on metabolic status in gestational diabetes." Why would she choose this article? What information in this citation indicates that it might meet her needs?

4. When Beth starts to save a personal library of her references, she has several reasons to use Zotero. How can a citation manager like Zotero (or Mendeley, or EndNote, etc.) help you with your research?

American Health Information Management Association (AHIMA) and are focused on integrity, protection, transparency, accountability, compliance, and the timely availability, retention, and disposition of health information (ITI Planning Committee, 2015). Standards governing the use of health information are focused on the interoperability of information technology systems to support distribution of patient information by authorized users (Halley et al., 2009). Incorporation of clinical practice guidelines and nursing terminology into the EHR provides a common language and interventions that support data collection and evaluation of clinical outcomes (Barey, Mastrian, & McGonigle, 2016).

The use of sophisticated CDSS, developed by multidisciplinary teams, is an efficient way to translate research evidence into everyday practice. However, the steps involved in the appraisal of evidence cannot be missed. It would be irresponsible to take current practice and automate the clinical decisions based on status quo. Likewise, it would be imprudent to base care on a single research article. Nurses and other HCPs need to take the time to examine their current practices with respect to best practices when EHRs or other health IT are implemented.

▶ Summary

While moving from academia to nursing practice based on evidence may seem daunting, nurses should transform traditional practices into ones supported by the best scientific evidence. Nurses can get access to primary research, systematic reviews, and clinical practice guidelines by using information technology effectively. Information management strategies are essential including subscribing to RSS feeds, registering for email alerts from journal publishers and from government resources, and purchasing subscriptions to services that provide EBP support. Finally, nurses should advocate for the selection of health information technology that has best practices as an integrated feature. Technology can make the practice of EBP more seamless for nurses and fulfill the need to improve patient care.

References

Ahrens, S., & Johnson, C. S. (2013). Finding the way to evidence-based practice. *Nursing Management, 44*(5), 23–27. doi: 10.1097/01.NUMA.0000429009.93011.ea

Alexander, S., Hoy, H., Maskey, M., Conover, H., Gamble, J., & Fraley, A.M. (2013). Initiating collaboration among organ transplant professionals through web portals and mobile applications. *Online Journal of Issues in Nursing, 18*(3). doi: 10.3912/OJIN.Vol18No02PPT03

American Nurses Association. (2012). *ANA recognized terminologies that support nursing practice.* Retrieved from: http://www.nursingworld.org/npii/terminologies.htm

Barey, E. B., Mastrian, K., & McGonigle, D. (2016). The electronic health record and clinical informatics. In S. M. DeNisco & A. M. Barker (Eds.), *Advanced practice nursing: Essential knowledge for the profession* (3rd ed., pp. 349–367). Burlington, MA: Jones & Bartlett Learning.

Beel, J., & Gipp, B. (2009). Google Scholar's ranking algorithm: An introductory overview. In B. Larse & J. Leta (Eds.), *Proceedings of the 12th International Conference on Scientometrics and Informetrics (ISSI '09), 1,* 230–241, Rio De Janeiro (Brazil). International Society for Scientometrics and Informetrics. Retrieved from http://www.sciplore.org/publications/2009-Google_Scholar%27s_Ranking_Algorithm_--_An_Introductory_Overview_--_preprint.pdf

Berner, E., & La Jande, T. (2007). Overview of clinical decision support systems. In E. Berner (Ed.), *Clinical decision support systems: Theory and practice* (2nd ed., pp. 4–18) New York: Springer.

Best, J., Frith, K., Anderson, F., Rapp, C. G., Rioux, L., & Ciccarello, C. (2011). Implementation of an evidence-based order set to impact initial antibiotic time intervals in adult febrile neutropenia. *Oncology Nursing Forum, 38*(6), 661–668. doi:10.1188/11.ONF.661-668

Brokel, J. M. (2009). Infusing clinical decision support interventions into electronic health records. *Urologic Nursing, 29*(5), 345–353.

Carroll, M. W. (2011). Why full open access matters. *PLoS Biol, 9*(11), e1001210. doi:10.1371/journal.pbio.1001210

Centers for Disease Control and Prevention. (2016). *Meaningful use.* Retrieved from http://www.cdc.gov/ehrmeaningfuluse/introduction.html

Cheeseman, S. E. (2011). Mastering basic computer competencies one byte at a time. *Neonatal Network, 30*(6), 413–419.

Cheeseman, S. E. (2012). Information literacy: Using computers to connect practice to evidence. *Neonatal Network, 31*(4), 253–258.

Dainow, E. (2016). *Understanding computers, smartphones and the Internet.* Retrieved from https://www.smashwords.com/books/view/630245

Duffy, M. (2015). Nurses and the migration to electronic health records. *American Journal of Nursing, 115*(12), 61–66.

Fain, J. A. (2009). *Reading, understanding, and applying nursing research* (4th ed.). Philadelphia: FA Davis.

Fineout-Overholt, E., Berryman, D. R., Hofstetter, S., & Sollenberger, J. (2011). Finding relevant evidence to answer clinical questions. In: B. M. Melnyk & E. Finout-Overholt, (Eds.), *Evidence-based practice in nursing & healthcare: A guide to best practice.* (2nd ed.). Philadelphia: Lippincott Williams & Wilkins.

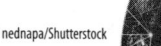

Google Scholar. *About.* Retrieved from http://scholar.google.com/intl/en/scholar/about.html

Gugerty, B., & Delaney, C. (2009). *Technology Informatics Guiding Educational Reform (TIGER). TIGER Informatics Competencies Collaborative (TICC) final report.* Retrieved from http://tigercompetencies.pbworks.com/f/TICC_Final.pdf

Halley, E. C., Sensmeier, J., & Brokel, J. M. (2009). Nurses exchanging information: Understanding electronic health record standards and interoperability. *Urologic Nursing, 29*(5), 305314.

Hawn, C. (2009). Take two aspirin and tweet me in the morning: How Twitter, Facebook, and other social media are reshaping healthcare. *Health Affairs, 28*(2), 361–368. Retrieved from http://content.healthaffairs.org/content/28/2/361.full#sec-6

Health RSS Feeds. USA Government Web Portal. Retrieved from http://www.usa.gov/Topics/Reference-Shelf/Libraries/RSS-Library/Health.shtml

Hello Health Patient Information. *Hello Health.* Retrieved from https://hellohealth.com/telemedicine/overview/

Hoss, B., & Hanson, D. (2008). Evaluating the evidence: Web sites. *AORN Journal, 87*(1), 124–141.

Ingersoll, G. L. (2000). Evidence-based nursing: What it is and what it isn't. *Nursing Outlook, 48*(4), 151–152. doi:10.1067/mno.2000.107690

ITI Planning Committee. (2015). *Integrating the health care infrastructure white paper: Health IT standards for 10 health information management practices.* Retrieved from http://ihe.net/uploadedFiles/Documents/ITI/IHE_ITI_WP_HITStdsforHIMPratices_Rev1.1_2015-09-18.pdf

International Council of Nurses. (2015). *International classification for nursing practice (ICNP) information sheet.* Retrieved from http://www.icn.ch/images/stories/documents/pillars/Practice/icnp/ICNP_FAQs.pdf

Kaminski, J. (2015). Computer science and the foundation of knowledge model. In D. McGonigle & K. G. Mastrian (Eds.), *Nursing informatics and the foundation of knowledge* (2nd ed., pp. 33–56). Burlington, MA: Jones & Bartlett Learning.

Karamali, M., Heidarzadeh, Z., Seifati, S. M., Samimi, M., Tabassi, Z., Hajijafari, M., . . . Esmaillzadeh, A. (2015). Zinc supplementation and the effects of metabolic status in gestational diabetes: A randomized, double-blind placebo-controlled trial. *Journal of Diabetes Complications, 29*(3), 1314–1319.

Lawson, P. (2005). How to bring evidence-based practice to the bedside. *Nursing 2005, 35*(1), 18–19.

Levin, R. F. (2013). Searching the sea of evidence: It takes a library. In: R. F. Levin & H. R. Feldman (Eds.), *Teaching evidence-based practice in nursing* (2nd ed., pp. 103–118). New York: Springer.

Melnyk, B. M., & Fineout-Overholt, E. (2011). *Evidence-based practice in nursing & healthcare: A guide to best practice* (2nd ed.). Philadelphia: Lippincott Williams & Wilkins.

Melnyk, B. M., Fineout-Overholt, E., Stillwell, S. B., & Williamson, K. M. (2010). The seven steps of evidence-based practice. *American Journal of Nursing, 10*(1), 51–53.

Rigney, D. (2010). What is the Matthew Effect? *The Matthew Effect: How advantage begets further advantage.* New York: Columbia University Press. Retrieved from http://cup.columbia.edu/book/978-0-231-14948-8/the-matthew-effect/excerpt

Rupert, D. J., Gard Read, J., Amoozegar, J. B., Moultrie, R. R., Taylor, O. M., O'Donoghue, A. C., . . . O'Donoghue, A. C. (2016). Peer-generated health information: The role of online communities in patient and caregiver health decisions. *Journal of Health Communication, 21*(11), 1187–1197. doi:10.1080/10810730.2016.1237592

Rutherford, M. (2008). Standardized nursing language: What does it mean for nursing practice? *OJIN: The Online Journal of Issues in Nursing, 13*(1). doi: 10.3912/OJIN.Vol13No01PPT05

Salmond, S. W. (2007). Advancing evidence-based practice: A primer. *Orthopaedic Nursing, 26*(2), 114–123.

Sortedahl, C. (2012). Effect of online journal club on evidence-based practice knowledge, intent, and utilization in school nurses. *Worldviews on Evidence-Based Nursing, 9*(2), 117–125. doi: 10.1111/j.1741-6787.2012.00249.x

Stillwell, S. B., Fineout-Overholt, E., Melnyk, B. M., & Williamson, K. M. (2010). Asking the clinical question: A key step in evidence-based practice. *American Journal of Nursing, 110*(3), 58–61.

TechTarget. (2016). *URL.* Retrieved from http://searchnetworking.techtarget.com/definition/URL

Tymkow, C. (2016). Clinical scholarship and evidence-based practice. In S. M. DeNisco & A. M. Barker (Eds.), *Advanced practice nursing: Essential knowledge for the profession* (3rd ed., pp. 495–552). Burlington, MA: Jones & Bartlett Learning.

Wells, N., Free, M., & Adams, R. (2007). Nursing research internship: Enhancing evidence-based practice among staff nurses. *Journal of Nursing Administration, 37*(3), 135–143.

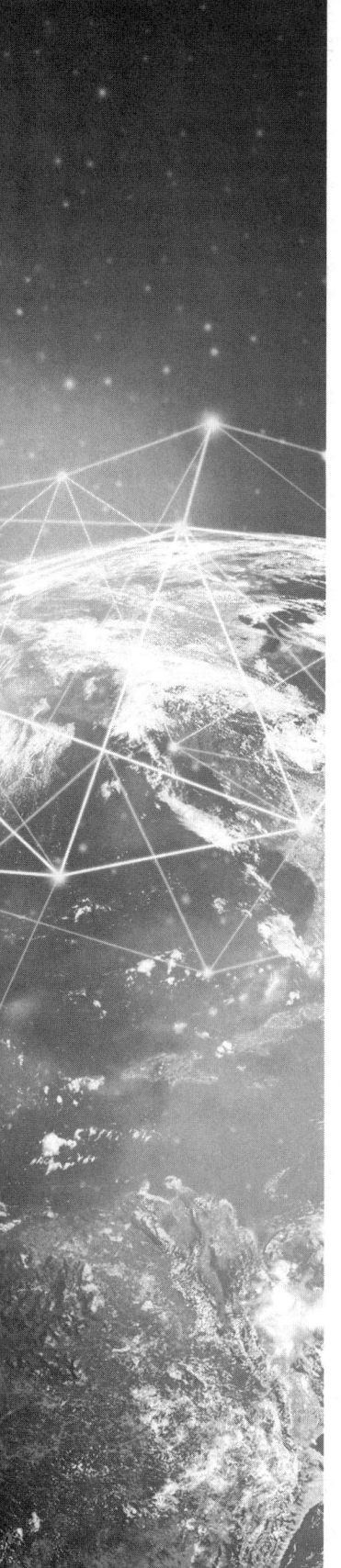

SECTION II

Use of Clinical Informatics in Care Support Roles

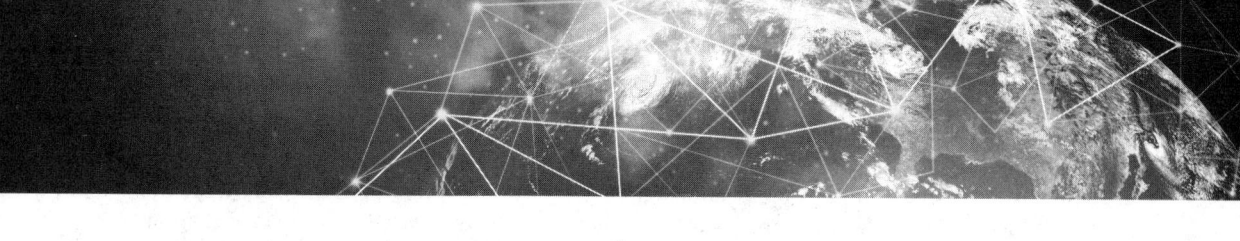

CHAPTER 4

Human Factors in Computing

Steffi Kreuzfeld, Dr. med.

Regina Stoll, Dr. med. habil.

LEARNING OBJECTIVES

1. Define ergonomics and associated concepts as applied in healthcare settings.
2. Describe the importance of understanding human factors in healthcare settings.
3. Know the key International Organization for Standardization (ISO) standards for ergonomic principles and design of work settings.
4. Comprehend the influence of work systems on the nurses' physical and psychological health.
5. Analyze information systems and computer applications with regard to human–computer interactions.

KEY TERMS

Anthropometry
Dialogue
Ergonomics
Graphical user interface (GUI)
Hardware ergonomics
Human–computer interaction (HCI)

Information processing
Interactivity
International Organization for Standardization (ISO)
Natural user interfaces
Selective attention
Software ergonomics

Task design
User interface
Visual display terminal (VDT)
Voice user interfaces
Work systems

▶ Chapter Overview

Computer systems and computer applications are used in all areas of life, from leisure to work. The systems range from computer workstations, notebooks, and smartphones, to networked household appliances and medical devices. To allow humans to comfortably interact with the various applications in a safe and efficient manner, ergonomic principles must be applied. This chapter describes the physiological, psychological, and social aspects of human interaction with computer systems and the effects of computer technology on people at work, particularly in healthcare settings.

▶ Introduction

Humans and computers form a complex socio-technical **work system**. If they are to distribute their workloads in a meaningful manner, the different qualities and abilities of human and machine must be considered. The human recognizes problems and can draw on wide-ranging general and specific knowledge in various areas to combine knowledge with experience to creatively apply them to problem solving. The human is capable of complex decisions and accepting the resulting responsibility. For example, nurses have knowledge, skills, and values developed by completing collegiate education in nursing, participating in continuing education, and by practicing in work settings. Nurses, equipped with education and experience, make complex decisions in noisy, fast-paced work environments that have consequences for the safety of patients in their care.

In contrast, computer systems can process huge amounts of data quickly and error free, repeat similar tasks multiple times without fatigue, extract important information, and exclude irrelevant data. Computers can function under extreme conditions and endure factors that would be detrimental to human health (Dul & Weerdenmeester, 2008).

The conditions under which humans work constitute significant factors that influence

health and wellbeing, as well as productivity and successful outcomes of work. The individual performance of the human is determined, on one hand, by external performance-shaping factors such as work environment, assigned task, technical feasibilities, time constraints, and modes of cooperation. On the other hand, it is also influenced by internal performance-shaping factors, such as physical and psychological states of the human. Computer applications that are well suited to humans can ease and enrich human performance. Standards, laws, and recommendations can be used to create a framework to prevent humans from sustaining lasting harm by their work.

▶ Human Factors/ Ergonomics (HFE)

In 2000, the International Ergonomics Association (IEA, 2000) defined **ergonomics** as follows:

> Ergonomics (or human factors) is the scientific discipline concerned with the understanding of the interactions among humans and other elements of a system, and the profession that applies theory, principles, data and methods to design in order to optimize human well-being and overall system performance. Practitioners of ergonomics and ergonomists contribute to the design and evaluation of tasks, jobs, products, environments and systems in order to make them compatible with the needs, abilities and limitations of people.

The term *ergonomics* derives from the Greek words *ergon* (work) and *nomos* (law) and describes the systematic study of all aspects of human activity as it relates to work. Ergonomics is a dynamic, interdisciplinary field of study that continuously evolves through new insights into the interaction between humans and work (Wilson, 2000). It differentiates itself from other fields of study through its direct applicability.

Ergonomics is central to safety programs in many different fields including manufacturing, aerospace, and health care. The application of ergonomics in health care is gaining attention in the United States as a result of reports by the Institute of Medicine (IOM, 1999, 2004, 2011).

As new knowledge is applied, it should lead to greater humanization of work. This implies that the human is at the center and that the work is being adapted to human needs, not the other way around. Besides increased safety, health, and comfort for the worker, there are also economic considerations included among the target parameters of applied ergonomics. Productivity, quality, and efficiency can be improved by applying ergonomic production processes, and costs can be lowered by decreasing work-related illnesses and illness-related absences from work (Dul et al., 2012). For example, in the United States, the economic influence of properly applied ergonomics can result in better reimbursement from the Centers for Medicare and Medicaid Services (CMS) because adverse events, many of which are caused by the mismatch of technology to human factors, can be reduced (Amarasingham, Plantinga, Diener-West, Gaskin, & Powe, 2009; CMS, 2008).

The second part of the IEA definition of ergonomics indicates the breadth of the spectrum of research in ergonomics: It spans from capturing work content and organizational aspects of work, to environmental factors, to consideration of physical and psychological factors and limitations that humans face as they interact with various work equipment. Ergonomics requires specialized education. The disciplines involved are primarily occupational science, human and social sciences, the humanities, computer and design science, and industrial engineering. In the United States, a subspecialty called human factors engineering contributes to knowledge generation through research and improvements in work environments by application of research to healthcare settings.

There are different areas of ergonomics, each with its own focus. For example, in physical ergonomics, the health consequences of working posture and repetitive motions are studied as the origins of musculoskeletal disorders. Organizational ergonomics deals with the optimization of work processes and structures, such as time management, teamwork, communication within an organization, telecommuting, and quality control. In contrast, the area of cognitive ergonomics focuses on such issues as cognitive and memory processes in the human brain, decision making, recognition and elimination of work-related stress, reliability of human actions, and **human–computer interactions (HCIs)**.

▶ Standards, Laws, Recommendations, and Style Guides

A part of the ergonomic knowledge has been summarized and recorded by way of standards, laws, and recommendations. International standards are issued by the **International Organization for Standardization (ISO)**. They are based on firmly established scientific principles and are determined on an international level, frequently in lengthy discussions, and adopted by majority decision. They form the lowest common denominator on which representatives from politics, economics, and science can agree and constitute a framework for their practical application and careful "should do" recommendations. The disadvantage of such generally accepted standards is that they are frequently too nonspecific and new scientific findings are often not considered.

Likewise, laws are frequently nonspecific and provide only minimal standards for occupational safety. They also do not adapt well to the current state of knowledge in the short term. In contrast, recommendations in books or publications incorporate current findings more easily and promote more concrete applications. However, they may be open to interpretation, and extensive prior knowledge may be required of the user. Style guides are guidelines for standardizing designs of user interfaces. Generally, they are published by the manufacturer as part of the documentation for computer operating systems (e.g., Microsoft Windows). They frequently are based on the principles of software ergonomics. **BOX 4-1** lists pertinent international ISO standards on ergonomics.

ISO 6385: Ergonomic Principles in the Design of Work Systems

This international standard contains the significant findings and definitions in ergonomics; it explains relevant basic terms and provides an occupational science framework for all specialists who are involved in the wide-ranging design of work systems. Technical, economic, organizational, and social aspects must all be considered. The standard also applies to the design of products that are not associated with work.

A work system provides a super structure for the cooperation of individuals or groups of employees (or users) that allows them to complete their tasks using their tools and equipment within their occupational domain. To create a work system based on ergonomic principles and ISO standards, the following subcategories of the system must be considered: organization of work, task design, design of activity, design of work environment, design of tools and equipment, and design of workplace and work station.

ISO 9241: The Ergonomics of Human System Interaction

ISO 9241 is a multipart international standard that initially consisted of 17 parts making demands on office work ("Ergonomic requirements for office work with visual display terminals"). Meanwhile, these recommendations do not only apply to office work. Thus, the 2006 standard has been given the more general title "Ergonomics of human system interaction." It has been revised and extended since then. Three chapters of the original ISO 9241 structure remain (part 1, 2, and 11), while the rest will be rearranged in series, structured in "hundreds," in order to facilitate the standard's handling and readability. Chapter 20 has been added. An overview of the thematic priorities of ISO 9241 can be found in **BOX 4-2**.

The comprehensive collection of recommendations regarding the design of the workplace, hardware, and software aims at reducing health risks caused by display-based work and facilitating the user's job demands. ISO 9241 is used particularly by those who work on planning, design, and usability of office workstations, office layouts, information/communication technology equipment, the development of software platforms, software applications, and display technologies, or the evaluation of usability goals of a computer system.

Organization of Work

Organization of work is defined as the systematic organization and design of workflow under consideration of task-specific, content-specific, and time-specific aspects. It is important to analyze how individual workplaces and activities within a work system (e.g., a hospital), depend on or limit each other, or work synergistically or antagonize

---

BOX 4-1 Examples of International ISO Standards on Ergonomics

ISO 6385:	Ergonomic principles in the design of work systems
ISO 9241:	The ergonomics of human system interaction
ISO 9355-2:	Ergonomic requirements for the design of displays and control actuators— Part 2: Displays
ISO/TR 16982:	Ergonomics of human–system interaction—Usability methods supporting human-centered design
ISO 10075-3:	Ergonomic principles related to mental workload

BOX 4-2 ISO 9241, Old and New Parts

Ergonomic requirements for office work with visual display terminals (VDTs)

Part 1:   General introduction
Part 2:   Guidance on task requirements
Part 5:   Workstation layout and postural requirements
Part 6:   Guidance on the work environments
Part 11:   Guidance on usability
Part 12:   Presentation of information
Part 13:   User guidance
Part 14:   Menu dialogues
Part 15:   Command dialogues
Part 16:   Direct manipulation dialogues
Part 17:   Form-filling dialogues

Ergonomics of human–system interaction

Part 20:   Accessibility guidelines for ICT equipment and services
100 series: Software ergonomics
200 series: Human–system interaction processes
300 series: Displays and display-related hardware
400 series: Physical input devices—ergonomics principles
500 series: Workplace ergonomics
600 series: Environment ergonomics
700 series: Application domains—control rooms
900 series: Tactile and haptic interactions

ICT = Information/Communication Technology

Data from ISO. (2010). ISO 9241-210: 2010(en). Ergonomics of human-system interaction: Part 210: Human-centred design for interactive systems. Retrieved from https://www.iso.org/obp/ui/#iso:std:iso:9241:-210:ed-1:v1:en

each other. A typical organization in an acute care hospital in the United States has functional departments, such as nursing, respiratory therapy, physical therapy, laboratory, radiology, surgery, dietary, housekeeping, and administration. However, employees in the distinct departments must work cooperatively to move patients through an inpatient experience. For example, a patient seen in an emergency department is evaluated by a healthcare provider, treated by nurses and other ancillary providers, and admitted for inpatient treatment. Movement of the patient to a hospital room (task-specific aspects) depends on availability of transfer equipment and personnel, communication between the healthcare providers in the two different treatment areas, and transfer of health information from one area to another (content-specific aspects). The transfer may also be dependent on the availability of a receiving nurse, which can be delayed during shift changes or when nurses have urgent tasks to complete for other patients (time-specific aspects). The overall workflow in an organization can be improved when ergonomic principles are applied to technologies and the humans who use them.

Contemporary information and telecommunication technologies support and promote cooperation between workers and computers (machines) in different work settings. They guide workers through typical task sequences, monitor error-free completion of work segments, and log outcomes. Frequently, the results achieved by one worker become the basis for additional tasks by other workers.

Task Design

The design of tasks is the second subcategory of ergonomic design of work systems. Important guidelines on **task design** are listed in Part 2 of ISO 9241. In general, well-designed tasks include the following features:

- They make use of the experience and abilities of the workers.
- They allow the workers to develop their skills and competencies.
- They comprise steps from planning to execution.
- They allow the worker to feel invested in the whole process.
- They afford the worker a certain measure of decision making and autonomy.
- They provide sufficient feedback about the completion of the task.
- They make use of existing abilities and promote development of new skills.

To have an adequate degree of autonomy, the worker should be able to determine such factors as the sequence of tasks, the speed, and manner in which they are executed. The IOM's report, *Keeping Patients Safe: Transforming the Work Environment of Nurses*, called for direct-care nurses to have input into nursing work and work-space design or redesign to improve patient safety (IOM, 2004). Despite the clear recommendation by the IOM, the autonomy of nurses over their own work is not universal. For nurses who work in hospitals that have earned the designation of Magnet hospital, perceived autonomy is higher than it is for nurses who work in non-Magnet hospitals (Hess, DesRoches, Donelan, Norman, & Buerhaus, 2011).

When jobs require a high degree of concentration, it is important to make available time segments without interruption. In addition, the work pace varies among workers but also within the same person depending on time of day and current physical state. Rigid workplace rules in regard to work pace or which impose significant restriction of autonomy and excessive dependency on technical systems can create stress and undermine wellbeing. Several research reports illustrate the chaotic and time-pressured nature of nursing work (Cornell et al., 2010; Cornell, Riordan, Townsend-Gervis, & Mobley, 2011; Halbesleben, Savage, Wakefield, & Wakefield, 2010). For example, Cornell and colleagues (2010) reported that 75% of tasks in 98 hours of observations lasted 30 seconds or less. The researchers noted that nurses were constantly shifting between tasks because of time pressures and interruptions. Time pressure is perceived as a stressor by many workers today. Chronic time pressure can promote mental illness, feelings of reduced vitality, and emotional exhaustion (Escribà-Agüir & Pérez-Hoyos, 2007).

The requirement for sufficient feedback regarding the completion of a job includes feedback via software, but also feedback from coworkers and supervisors. Feedback via software needs to be clear and unambiguous. For example, if a nurse enters data outside of acceptable values in an electronic health record (EHR), the software should provide feedback to the user (the nurse) to check the entry to validate the data. Other types of helpful feedback are guided steps for tasks, alerts from clinical decision support, or error messages. Feedback about the quality of the work from supervisors or colleagues is a form of social support. If the feedback is immediate, it can be an effective tool for stress reduction, because the workers receive an affirmation that problems are handled jointly. A prerequisite for well-designed workplaces is the opportunity for social interaction along with a cooperative and communicative office environment (Squires, Tourangeau, Laschinger, & Doran, 2010; Welp & Manser 2016). Others have described the "culture of safety" as a work environment that encourages all employees to speak up about work conditions that might put the safety of patients or employees at risk (Squires et al., 2010). To have a culture of safety requires supervisors to build relationships with employees by listening, relating, and responding to concerns (Squires et al.).

Design of Activity

Activities should be designed so that they provide an optimal workload for the employee, physically and mentally. In ergonomics, the term *workload* has a neutral connotation (ISO 6385) as opposed to its meaning in common usage. Workload includes all external influences acting on humans. This means that degree of task difficulty must be considered in addition to the environmental conditions under which the task is being executed.

The total workload can stimulate and challenge workers, promote learning, or fatigue workers. The effect of the workload depends on many factors such as individual preconditions, experience, attitudes, and opinions. The workload that is optimal provides neither too much nor too little challenge. Important elements in avoiding either are appropriate rest periods, job rotation, and job enhancement and job enrichment by assigning multiple sequential tasks rather than repetitive single tasks.

The workload of nurses is measured by counting the number of patients per nurse for inpatient care and the number of patient visits per day in ambulatory settings. There is a body of literature showing that the number of patients per nurse is a significant predictor of inpatient length of stay, medication errors, hospital-acquired conditions, falls, and other adverse outcomes (Frith et al., 2010; Frith, Anderson, Tseng, & Fong, 2012; Kane, Shamliyan, Mueller, Duval, & Wilt, 2007). Technology as a factor in nurse workload has been rarely studied as a predictor of patient outcomes.

Design of the Work Environment

The environment of a workplace includes such external conditions as temperature, lighting, and noise level. Guidelines are listed in ISO 9241 Part 6: environmental requirements. Related to the renumbering process of ISO 9241, this part will be replaced by the ISO 9241-600 subseries (Travis, 2014). The ambient conditions are determined by temperature, humidity, air circulation, and heat radiation. What constitutes comfortable ambient conditions is dependent on the individual worker. Surveys of employees show that they are more satisfied when they can choose their ambient conditions. In general, an air temperature of 68–72°F is recommended for visual display terminal workplaces. Drafty conditions or circulating cold air should be avoided because they can promote neck and back pain.

The lighting at a computer terminal workstation must be adapted to the vision of the worker and the specific task to be accomplished. Indirect lighting from the ceiling in combination with adjustable desk lighting is considered optimal. The illumination in the immediate work area should be at least 500 lux. Illumination of 500–1000 lux increases visual acuity and reading becomes more effortless, especially for older workers. The lighting should be even throughout the room so that eyes do not have to continually adjust. To avoid extreme contrasts, glare, and reflections, computer screens should be positioned upright and parallel to the window. If that is not possible, blinds can attenuate incoming sunlight. Evidence-based design of healthcare environments is beginning to appear in the medical and nursing literature. Findings show that patients have better outcomes with natural light from windows with shades or blinds and adjustable lighting levels that patients can control (Bazuin & Cardon, 2011).

Similarly, noise perception and tolerance are very individual. Noises that are substantially below the danger threshold can still be perceived as annoying. In addition to the volume (noise level measured in decibels), the individual task at hand also influences noise perception. Sound levels are closely monitored using measurements describing continuous and maximal sound pressure levels for specified periods of time. The equivalent continuous A-weight sound pressure level measured over a period of time, such as a 10-hour shift, is termed equivalent sound levels (LAeq). The maximum sound pressure level measured is also monitored (LAmax). For work requiring intellectual effort and concentration, the ISO 9241 recommends LAeq up to 45 decibels (dBA); for simple administrative work requiring communication, it recommends up to 60 dBA. According to the World Health Organization's (WHO) guidelines for community noise for hospitals, the continuous sound pressure level should not exceed 35 dBA in the patient's room, and 40 dBA for a maximum sound event (LAmax) during the night, respectively (Berglund, Lindvall, & Schwela, 1999).

When the ambient noise becomes too loud, errors may increase (e.g., chart entry of patient data) or important signals may be missed. Studies have shown that higher than recommended levels of noise are common in hospitals (McLaren & Maxwell-Armstrong, 2008; Pope, 2010; Zborowsky, Bunker-Hellmich, Morelli, & O'Neill, 2010). For patients who are treated in hospitals, noise can interrupt sleep, lead to delirium, and raise the risk for falls (Tzeng, Hu, & Yin, 2011). Tests with sound acoustic panels installed on vertical walls and ceilings of hospital floors show that they can decrease the mean level of background or ambient noise. When installing these sound acoustic panels, however, hospital standards of hygiene and safety have to be taken into account. Also, the patient flow should not be restricted (Farrehi, Nallamothu, & Navvab, 2016).

Beside the undesirable effects, such as elevating stress and disturbing sleep, sound in clinical settings might fulfill other roles: "sound can also be soothing, reassuring and a rich source of information about the environment as well. It may be used to secure a degree of privacy for oneself, to exclude others or a source of solidarity among friends and colleagues. The challenge then is to understand the work that sound does in its ecological context in health care settings" (Brown, Rutherford, & Crawford, 2015).

We should point out that there are comprehensive, interdisciplinary studies on the effects of different sounds, soundscapes, and music in hospital settings. Whether a sound is perceived as pleasant or annoying depends on individual preferences as much as physical condition and present chronic complaints (e.g., hearing loss and tinnitus). Naturalistic sounds as those of birds, ocean waves, or rain showers are perceived as relaxing by patients as well as staff. Therefore, sounds should be applied purposely under controlled conditions in the hospital spaces, particularly with regard to possible safety implications (communication difficulties during surgical operations, ignoring acoustic signals).

Those who wish to get more information on this topic will find a good overview of the current scientific knowledge by Iyendo (2016). Some positive impacts of music in terms of medical treatment are summarized in **BOX 4-3**.

Design of Work Equipment (Hardware and Software Ergonomics)

The user-friendly design of computer systems must include elements of hardware and software ergonomics. **Hardware ergonomics** supplies

---

BOX 4-3 Selected Positive Impacts of Music in Terms of Medical Treatment

- Reduce stress symptoms
- Enhance emotion
- Decrease depression
- Lower blood pressure and heart rate
- Boost immune function
- Decrease pain
- Stimulate relaxation

Data from Iyendo, T. O. (2016). Exploring the effect of sound and music on health in hospital settings: A narrative review. *International Journal of Nursing Studies, 63*, 82–100. doi: 10.1016/j.ijnurstu.2016.08.008

the technical framework and sets the conditions for optimal HCI. Input devices (e.g., keyboard or mouse) are differentiated from output devices (e.g., screen, loudspeaker, or printer). Both constitute the operational platform of a computer system and, combined with the software, become the **user interface**.

Software ergonomics deals with the analysis, evaluation, and optimization of user interfaces. By applying various strategies, either the needs of the user can be emphasized or the display of information—the interaction between information and subsequent operations—can be improved. This interaction between display of information and operation is called **dialogue** (refer to the dialogue principles section later in this chapter).

There are various types of user interfaces. The **graphical user interface (GUI)** constitutes a complex platform that allows users to interact with the computer through electronic devices or the computer mouse. Interaction is facilitated by visual elements such as icons (symbols, pictograms). Most modern computers, including laptops and tablets, have GUIs. EHRs typically look more structured in table formats, and providers use tab keys or the mouse to move from input field to field. **Voice user interfaces** make human–machine interactions possible through a voice or synthesized speech platform. Input requires a speech recognition system. Voice user interface can be used with EHRs and is commonly called voice recognition (VR) software. In a study of implementation of VR software in a military hospital's on-site and 12 outlying clinics, Hoyt and Yoshihashi (2010) found that the majority of providers persisted in the use of VR. "Compared to clinicians that continued VR, discontinuers generally rated it much lower in helpfulness, accuracy, minutes saved per day, improvement in the quality of EHR notes, and the ability to close the encounter in one day" (Hoyt & Yoshihashi). **Natural user interfaces** avail themselves of the natural finger and hand movements of the user on a touch screen. They allow intuitive use of the interactive devices.

Interactivity is a key component of computer applications. Depending on user input or given parameters, the flow of information in computer-based applications leads to an output as directed by the application software. Software ergonomics is also dedicated to the question of how to design interactive processes for user friendliness. The usability of systems is determined by the incorporated ergonomic principles. Evaluation methods and design standards have been created to establish the usability of computer-based applications.

Design of the Workplace and Workstation

Anthropometry plays an important role in the design of the workplace in that it allows the worker to assume a comfortable working posture and promotes safety and efficiency as tasks are carried out. The workplace design optimizes visual and tactile human interaction with equipment, allows freedom of leg movement, and promotes support (e.g., seat or auxiliary technical equipment) and optimal arrangement of displays.

The design of the workplace takes into consideration aspects of mobility and stability of posture, sensory requirements and the limits of human perception (e.g., visual or auditory capabilities), and the variation in individual body dimensions. The working height of a table may be ergonomically suitable for an average American male but unsuitable for a small woman. An important characteristic of a well-designed workplace is its capacity to adjust to individual physical requirements, such as the adjustment in table height in the previous example.

When constructing workstations, equipment planners take into consideration the average body size of the population. At intervals the population of a country is measured; various body dimensions are determined for each gender and representative average values (percentiles) are calculated. Generally, an adjustable design is created so that it can serve more than 90% of the population. This range covers body dimensions from the fifth percentile of females (only 5% of women are smaller = small operator) to the 95th percentile of males (only 5% of men are larger = large operator) (Helander, 2006). The 50th percentile represents the population average for a selected physical feature.

For **visual display terminals (VDTs)** clear guidelines have been established because of the demands on the musculoskeletal system and the eyes, which take into consideration the dimensions of the workstation and the arrangement of the individual elements (e.g., table, chair, and computer). Guidelines are listed in ISO 9241—Part 5. According to the International Standard Association's plans, this part will be within the ISO 9241-500 subseries in the future.

The most important elements are summarized in **FIGURE 4-1**.

Table and chair height have an impact on the correct posture and must, therefore, be adjustable according to body height. The seat height should be adjusted so that the feet rest on the floor. A footrest may be helpful for short persons. Chairs should pivot and roll to reduce the need of axial body movements. The height of the back support should also be adjustable, and its convex shape should mirror the curvature of the lower back. Correct table height results in an angle of 70 to 90 degrees between upper and lower arms. The height of the keyboard also needs to be considered. Elbow rests of chairs should also be adjustable in height and be short enough to avoid contact with the table. There must be enough room in front of the keyboard to allow support for the wrists. Wrist cushions are optional. There must be sufficient space to allow for changes in working posture and motions. Musculoskeletal problems are frequently the result of prolonged sitting (especially in neck

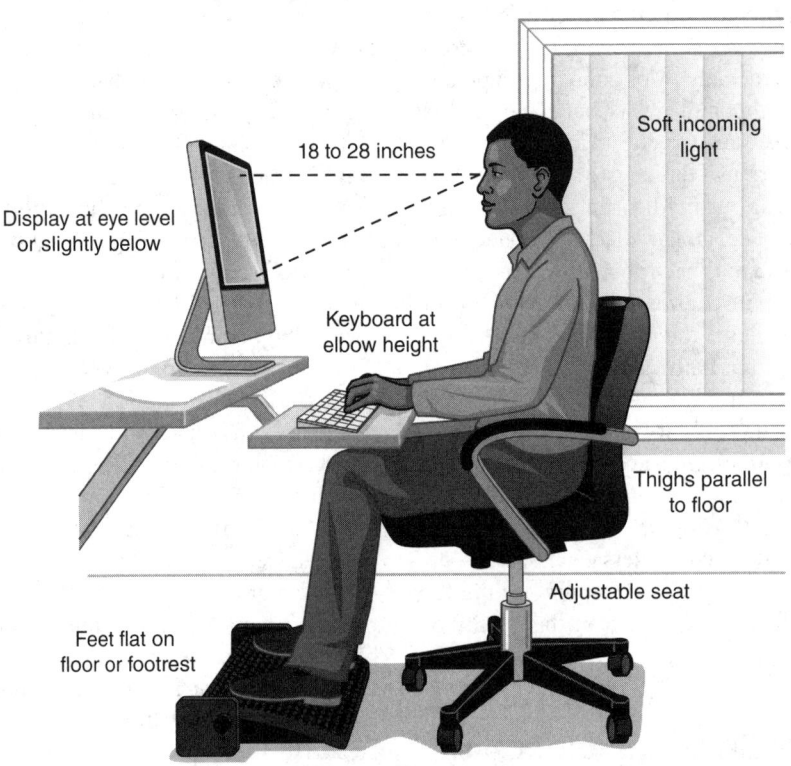

FIGURE 4-1 Posture recommended for visual display terminals (VDTs).

and lower back regions); therefore, standing up at regular intervals is recommended. The creation of workstations that combine sitting and standing tasks is ideal.

The natural head posture results in a gaze that angles down. Therefore, the computer screen should be oriented in such a way that its center is 25–35 degrees below the horizontal visual axis. This position eliminates the need to raise the head while reading and decreases stress on the neck and shoulder musculature. The distance from the eye to the screen should be approximately 50 cm (50–80 cm), depending on screen size. When prescribing appropriate bifocal or multifocal lenses, the exact distance to the screen should be known.

The area that can be seen when the gaze is fixed and the head is held still is called the field of vision. In the horizontal dimension, the field of vision stretches over approximately 180–200 degrees, and in the vertical dimension the field of vision is approximately 130 degrees. Even though humans perceive that everything is in

focus within this field, the ability to see details is in reality limited to a small cone (vertex angle 1 degree) around the visual axis (Grandjean, 1979). This is due to the uneven distribution of photo receptors in the retina of the eye. Because the fovea centralis has the greatest number of photo receptors, the visual acuity is greatest there. If one assumes an eye-screen distance of 50 cm, the area of focus is approximately 17 mm in diameter. This equates to a field of about 10 letters that can be visualized simultaneously (Preim & Dachselt, 2010). The eye must continually shift while reading. Toward the periphery, the visual acuity decreases markedly. In the field enclosed in 1–40 degrees around the visual axis, the detection of high contrasts and movements is possible despite the lack of focus. Due to rapid eye movements between discrete objects, the visual perception seems unaffected. In the outer portion of the field of vision (vertex angle between 40 and 70 degrees), movements are still detectable. **FIGURE 4-2** illustrates the visual fields of a person as he views computer screens.

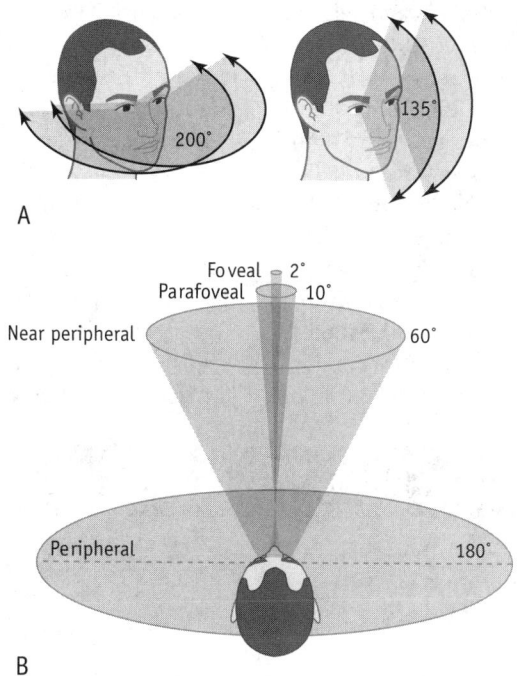

FIGURE 4-2 Field of vision.

Requirements of Visual Displays. Displays must be designed in such a way that information can be acquired quickly, error free, and with little effort. Important factors that influence the acquisition of information are the size of the screen, the quality of the screen, and the recognizability of characters. The following discussion of particulars not only applies to computer screens, but also to monitors and other displays of medical devices.

The size of the screen must conform to the task. For office work, the accepted size today is 19–21 inches (diagonal measurement of the screen 48–53 cm). The recommended eye-screen distance is approximately 70–80 cm. The greater the distance, the larger the characters need to be for ease of recognition. At the distance of 70 cm, uppercase letters must be at least 4.5 mm in height; at a distance of 60 cm, 3.9 mm in height. At a distance of 50 cm (e.g., 15-inch notebooks), a minimum height of 3.2 mm is recommended (ISO 9241-303). **BOX 4-4** shows the calculation of letter height.

Notebooks and tablet PCs intended for mobile applications are lightweight and reduced in size. To increase the ease of work and data acquisition, the addition of external keyboards and accessory screens of suitable size is recommended. Data acquisition is influenced not only by screen size but also by screen quality. As opposed to the old cathode ray tube (CRT) monitors, the liquid crystal display (LCD) and thin-film transistor (TFT) screens or e-book readers do not flicker and do not have any distortions. Ease of reading is improved by brightness and contrast. A 5:1 ratio of light-dark contrast is required along with crisp edge definition of the characters. The size and number of the pixels determine how well defined the characters are. The smaller the pixels and the denser they are, the more well defined are the characters. The definition is also influenced by the screen resolution, which is variable and, in turn, depends on screen size and the particular application.

Glare and reflections can decrease the quality of the screen image. This can be largely eliminated by matte or antiglare finishes (see classification of types of reflections). Even for computer housings, matte finishes and light or neutral colors are recommended.

Colors can influence how information is categorized and ranked and how pieces of information relate to each other. Colors can focus the attention of the observer on certain aspects or promote recognition. Colors can negatively influence character recognition; therefore, color is used sparingly in electronic displays.

The human eye perceives color through a type of light-sensitive receptor called the cone, which is located in the retina. These receptors respond to various wavelengths. Some cones are sensitive to red, green, or blue. When light of a certain wavelength enters the eye, different types and numbers of cones are activated to create a subjective color perception after processing by optical neurons. Because there are fewer blue-sensitive cones than red- and green-sensitive cones, the eye perceives blue colors as less intense and cannot distinguish well among shades of blue (Eysel, 2005). In computer applications and electronic displays, this implies that pure blue colors should be avoided for use in text, thin lines, and small formats.

Hue, saturation, and brightness are important factors in the perception of colors. From a

---

BOX 4-4 Calculation of Letter Height

Assignment: Calculate and verify the height of the characters on your computer screen or monitor of a medical device with the following formula:

Minimum uppercase letter height (e.g., E, B, H, M, N) in mm = eye-screen distance/155

Modified from ISO. (2011). ISO 9241-303: 2011. Ergonomics of human-system interaction—Part 303: Requirements for electronic visual displays. Retrieved from https://www.iso.org/standard/57992.html

psycho-physiological perspective, humans can distinguish about 200 shades of color. Saturation describes how a pure color changes with the addition of gray. Colors with low saturation do not display much color content. Colors with high saturation are similar to pure colors. There are 20 degrees of saturation and 500 degrees of brightness (Eysel, 2005). Saturated colors command our attention and should be used sparingly in software design. They must have a high contrast to be easily distinguishable. **FIGURE 4-3** shows the low contrast between background and letters, which can lead to an error.

The highest contrast is created by dark characters on a light background (positive display). However, one cannot easily distinguish among darker colors. The best contrast on a light background is created by black and dark green, red, and magenta.

Certain colors convey specific meanings (ISO 9241-125). Red means imminent danger, stop, or no permission. Yellow signifies alert or caution. Green is linked to safety or lack of danger. Emergency and aid stations and escape routes are symbolized by green. Color coding needs to consider the conventional meaning of color. Hospital executives and department managers often use dashboard or scorecards that use color to signal performance (Belden, Grayson, & Barnes, 2009).

A typical example is the display of medical devices. Through the use of different colors, various states can be indicated such as normal operation (green) or malfunction (red). Optical alerts must be quickly and easily recognizable from a greater distance (4 m). Their luminance should be a minimum of six times greater than the immediate surroundings (ISO 61310-1). Additionally, an indicator for dangerous conditions that require immediate action should flash at a frequency of 1–3 Hz (ISO 9241-303).

Requirements of Acoustic Signal Devices.
Acoustic signals and alarms are used as adjuncts when important events take place while executing visual tasks, or when certain conditions occur that require immediate action. However, acoustic signals should be used sparingly because they interrupt the workflow. If several acoustic signals sound simultaneously, a conflict is created for the worker on how to prioritize necessary responses.

For acoustic signals to be recognized with certainty, they need to fulfill certain requirements (ISO 60601-1-8): The sound pressure level (volume) should be at least 5 dBA above the background noise level. Consideration must be given to the environment in which the medical device is used. For warning and alarm signals, 15 dBA above the background noise level are recommended. The minimum recommended sound pressure level for acoustic signal devices is 65 dBA.

In health care, the high number of false-positive alarm signals has been a problem for years. Varpio, Kuziemsky, MacDonald, and King (2012) conducted 49 hours of observations and found that an alarm sounded every 7 seconds. Even though critical states are identified with great certainty, this comes at the cost of a high number of alarms lacking clinical relevancy (Chambrin, 2001; Konkani, Oakley, & Bauld, 2012). These low-priority alarms deluge healthcare providers, causing high stress levels in personnel and patients. Beyond the strain caused by the flood of acoustic signals, people pay less attention and become desensitized to alarms. Varpio and colleagues (2012)

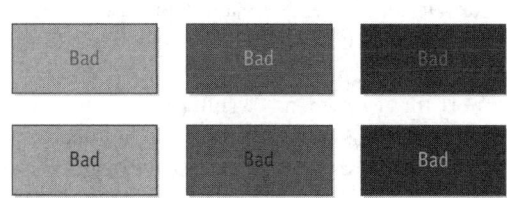

FIGURE 4-3 Low contrast between background and letters can lead to errors.

found that 70% of the time, no response to alarms was made. Even more troubling was the finding that 40% of life-threatening alarms were ignored. Conversely, problems arise when alarms fail to sound or are accidentally deactivated in situations requiring action. Critical or life-threatening situations might be overlooked. These and many other studies show that human factor issues such as audibility, identification, and urgency mapping of alarms are important fields for more research and technical improvements (Konkani, 2012). Individualization of default medical alarm settings (Graham & Cvach 2010), the use of artificial intelligence combining information from several vital signs (smart alarms), or third-party alarm notification systems provide manifold opportunities to enhance the health and safety of patients.

Dialogue Principles (ISO 9241-Part 110)

A dialogue is the interaction between a user and an interactive system to achieve a goal that is based on the actions of the user (input) and the reactions of the interactive system (output) (ISO 9241-110). The most common types of health information technology using dialogue are clinical decision support, computerized provider order entry (CPOE), and barcode medication administration systems as stand-alone systems or integrated into EHRs. Well-planned dialogues significantly add to the usability of a product. The dialogue is designed to eliminate typical user problems that cause unnecessary difficulties. These include insufficient or confusing information, unnecessary operational steps, unexpected responses of the interactive system, or the inefficient correction of errors.

Dialogues need to provide relevant, context-specific information for tasks, eliminate the user to search manuals or other external sources of user information, and support the user when learning to navigate the system. Dialogues should conform to generally expected standards and be consistent and predictable to users based on

their experience with a system. Even though dialogues may appear automatically, the dialogues should be designed so that users can control the direction or speed of dialogues until the task is completed (ISO 9241-110).

▶ Information Processing

At the core of HCI are information input, information processing, decision making, and information storage. The starting point is the perception of stimuli from the environment. Of greatest importance in HCI are visual, acoustic, and tactile stimuli.

Rasmussen (1986) assumes that a large part of human **information processing** happens below the threshold of consciousness. Perceived information is subconsciously compared with an inner, dynamic perspective and used to initiate motor processes. This allows automatic actions, such as the automatic limb coordination while walking, or the shifting of gears by an experienced driver. From the plethora of perceived information, only few messages emerge into consciousness—those that are needed for conscious action. For example, in a traffic situation, this information would pertain to the current traffic flow, traffic lights, traffic signs, and so on. The ability to concentrate on relevant stimuli and ignore irrelevant information is termed **selective attention**. For an example of this phenomenon, watch Daniel J. Simons's (1999) famous YouTube video (freely available), which has generated millions of views. It can be found using the search terms "selective attention" or "selective awareness." Informational content that otherwise would be ignored can surface into consciousness, especially when mismatches or ambiguities are detected in familiar actions, such as a pedestrian stumbling on uneven pavement or a car not shifting into gear. Such events cause a shift from unconscious to conscious information processing. Human information processing relies on two strategies that, in principle, can also be useful in error avoidance: the focus on essential information and the conscious perception of deviations from the norm.

How much attention is paid to information depends on the manner in which it is presented, on the time available to assimilate the information, and on competing environmental stimuli. Attention is also the key to memory. Perception is the interpretation of certain stimuli (visual, auditory, etc.). Perception aids in the fast grasp of words or sounds, but it can also cause humans to make errors when they "see" what they "expect to see." Medications that have similar spellings or similar sounding names are particularly problematic. A nurse working on a medical unit that specializes in the treatment of respiratory problems might read the brand name drug Advicor (niacin and lovastatin) as Advair (fluticasone and salmeterol) and make a medication error. Attention can be negatively affected by stress, heavy workload, lack of sleep, and interruptions. Added to the stress, poor design of CPOE systems can set up the circumstances for a prescribing order error.

In general, memory is defined as the ability of the human nervous system to retain, arrange, and retrieve information. To describe the cognitive processes that enable us to memorize certain information to a greater or lesser extent, sometimes for life, scientists have developed models that show certain similarities to data storage in computers. They greatly simplify the complicated neuronal processes. The multistore model developed by Atkinson and Shiffrin (1968, 1971) proposes three structures of memory: sensory memory, short-term or working memory, and long-term memory.

The sensory memory acquires stimuli via the sensory organs (e.g., eyes, ears) and retains them in the short-term memory. Visual information is already lost after 0.2 second. Acoustic stimuli can be retained significantly longer (up to 2 seconds). Consciousness and attention play a major role as these data are transferred into the working or long-term memory (Proctor & Vu, 2012).

The expressions *short-term* and *working* memory are used synonymously for memory of limited capacity, where "chunks" of information can be retained for a short duration. Repetition

can significantly increase and competing stimuli can significantly decrease retention time. Chunks are units of information like numbers, abbreviations, pictograms, words, or complex ideas (e.g., the idea of a person as a whole). Miller (1956) assumed that the short-term memory can store seven chunks. More recent studies point to a storage capacity of three to four chunks (Cowan, 1991). Chunks can be artificially created by grouping information, which allows optimal use of the working memory.

Rouder, a psychologist at the University of Missouri, gave an example in a newspaper interview about how the grouping of information can aid short-term memory. It may be difficult for a person to memorize a sequence of nine letters. However, when the same person is asked to memorize the letters grouped into three acronyms (e.g., IBM-CIA-FBI), the task becomes much easier, and the working memory will need only three slots to retain the information (University of Missouri–Columbia, 2008).

From 1993 to 2003, Baddeley extended and refined the concepts of how working memory functions (Baddeley, 1993, 2002, 2003). It is assumed that the short-term memory is not a single storage unit but a complex aggregate of interacting subsystems that are partially associated with the long-term memory. The data are processed in these subsystems according to their content (e.g., spatial/visual, language).

After processing, storage of information takes place in the long-term memory. Current knowledge seems to indicate that the long-term memory has unlimited storage capacity and duration. The decrease in the ability to memorize new information with increasing age seems to relate less to problems with storage capacity and more to the inability to integrate new information into the long-term memory in a suitable manner to be able to network new with existing information (Herczeg, 2009). Through these associations, various information units are linked, which makes generalizations and comparisons possible, and correlations are established. The counterpoint to the retrieval of information from an arbitrarily distant past is the phenomenon of forgetting. Forgetting, however, is not so much a loss of information as it is a lack of access to the requested information. Linked to this are the entities recall and recognition. Recognition happens much easier than direct access to information by way of association (Herczeg, 2009).

Important conclusions can be drawn about HCIs from knowledge of information-processing theory:

1. Selective grouping of information facilitates retention by the user (Preim & Dachselt, 2010) and assists in the learning process.
2. Tasks should not be too complex due to the limited capacity of the working memory. If the degree of difficulty is high and there is a decision-making requirement, the error rate and the processing time can increase (Jacko & Ward, 1996). Too many possible solutions burden the working memory unnecessarily due to the need for decision making.
3. Due to rapid loss of information from the working memory, complex tasks can be solved only when feedback is received at regular intervals about the status of completion and the attained interim goal, so the next action can be planned (Herczeg, 2009).

A case study demonstrating human factors in complex healthcare settings using health information technology is presented in **BOX 4-5**.

BOX 4-5 Case Study in Human Factors in a Complex Sociotechnical Work System

An important concern for managing patients with complex medical needs in intensive care units (ICUs) is blood glucose control in order to avoid the development of infections and to reduce the chance of longer lengths of stay in ICU. Glucommander, a health information technology (health IT) used in many ICUs, helps physicians make insulin dosing orders through decision support. Glucommander is interactive: It tracks the patient's glucose levels and guides nurses to change intravenous or subcutaneous insulin doses consistent with the physicians' orders.

In an ideal ICU environment, the only persons to interact with the Glucommander are the registered nurses who have been trained on the software and insulin protocol. However, in ICUs with a limited number of computers, other healthcare providers such as occupational therapists, physical therapists, physicians, respiratory therapists, dieticians, unit secretaries, and nurse techs/aids use computers where Glucommander software is running. With so many providers using the same computer, the Glucommander software occasionally gets accidentally closed without the nurse's knowledge. This leads to a potential medication error in the insulin infusion rate, an incorrect lapse of time between blood glucose checks, and a potential loss of the insulin rate infusion history.

The physical environment in the ICU is often hectic and noisy with multiple interruptions from other staff, alarms, other medical devices, portable pagers, telephones, overhead pages, patients' needs, and family members. The computers are located outside of each patient's room in a cubby area that is shared with all providers involved in the patient's care. No defense against the Glucommander's being closed accidentally is present except one confirmation box. A registered nurse, caring for two to three critical patients at various locations in the ICU, may not know if the Glucommander has been turned off. Long lapses can occur before the nurse knows the software is off.

Check Your Understanding
1. What conditions create the potential for medication errors in this situation?
2. What can a registered nurse do to protect patients who are on the Glucommander protocol?
3. What responsibility does a registered nurse have if the software is stopped by accident?
4. What are possible solutions to prevent accidental closing of the software?

▶ Summary

The successful use of interactive systems strongly depends on the physiologic state of the workers in addition to their needs and expectations, which must be matched to the technical capabilities of modern computer technologies. Due to the present extensive knowledge in the area of ergonomics, improper workload can be avoided by the user. Likewise, errors made by users and errors in the execution of tasks can be averted to prevent harm to patients. The changing work environment demands that the organizational framework consider such factors as increasing workload, time pressure, and personnel management.

References

Amarasingham, R., Plantinga, L., Diener-West, M., Gaskin, D. J., & Powe, N. R. (2009). Clinical information technologies and inpatient outcomes: A multiple hospital study. *Archives of Internal Medicine, 169*(2), 108–114.

Atkinson, R. C., & Shiffrin, R. (1968). Human memory: A proposed system and its control processes. In K. W. Spence & J. T. Spence (Eds.), *The psychology of learning and motivation: Advances in research and memory* (Vol. 2). New York: Academic Press.

Atkinson, R. C., & Shiffrin, R. (1971). The control of short-term memory. *Scientific American, 225*(2), 82–90.

Baddeley, A. D. (1993). *Working memory, thought and action.* Oxford, UK: Oxford University Press.

Baddeley, A. D. (2002). Is working memory still working? *European Psychologist, 7*, 85–97.

Baddeley, A. D. (2003). Working memory. Looking back and looking forward. *Nature Reviews Neuroscience, 4*, 829–839.

Bazuin, D., & Cardon, K. (2011). Creating healing intensive care unit environments: Physical and psychological considerations in designing critical care areas. *Critical Care Nursing Quarterly, 34*(4), 259–267.

Belden, J., Grayson, R., & Barnes, J. (2009). *Defining and testing EMR usability: Principles and proposed methods of EMR usability evaluation and rating.* Retrieved from http://www.himss.org/files/HIMSSorg/content/files/himss_definingandtestingemrusability.pdf

Berglund, B., Lindvall, T., Schwela, D. (1999). *Guidelines for community noise.* World Health Organization. Retrieved from http://www.who.int/docstore/peh/noise/guidelines2.html

Brown, B., Rutherford, P., & Crawford, P. (2015). The role of noise in clinical environments with particular reference to mental health care: A narrative review. *International Journal of Nursing Studies, 52*, 1514–1524. doi: 10.1016/j.ijnurstu.2015.04.020

Centers for Medicare and Medicaid Services (CMS). (2008). *Hospital-acquired conditions.* Retrieved from http://www.cms.hhs.gov/HospitalAcqCond/06_Hospital-Acquired_Conditions.asp

Chambrin, M. C. (2001). Alarms in the intensive care unit: How can the number of false alarms be reduced? *Critical Care, 5*, 184–185.

Cornell, P., Herrin-Griffith, D., Keim, C., Petschonek, S., Sanders, A. M., D'Mello, S., . . . Shepherd, G. (2010). Transforming nursing workflow, part 1: The chaotic nature of nurse activities. *Journal of Nursing Administration, 40*(9), 366–373. doi: 10.1097/NNA.0b013e3181ee4261

Cornell, P., Riordan, M., Townsend-Gervis, M., & Mobley, R. (2011). Barriers to critical thinking workflow interruptions and task switching among nurses. *Journal of Nursing Administration, 41*(10), 407–414. doi: 10.1097/NNA.0b013e31822edd42

Cowan, N. (1991). The magical number 4 in short-term memory: A reconsideration of mental storage capacity. *Behavioral and Brain Sciences, 24*, 87–114.

Dul, J., Bruder, R., Buckle, P., Carayon, P., Falzon, P., Marras, W. S., . . . van der Doelen, B. (2012). A strategy for human factors/ergonomics: Developing the discipline and profession. *Ergonomics, 55*(4), 377–395.

Dul, J., & Weerdenmeester, B. (2008). *Ergonomics for beginners: A quick reference guide.* Boca Raton, FL: CRC Press, Taylor & Francis Group.

Escribà-Agüir, V., & Pérez-Hoyos, S. (2007). Psychological well-being and psychosocial work environment characteristics among emergency medical and nursing staff. *Stress & Health: Journal of the International Society for the Investigation of Stress, 23*(3), 153–160.

Eysel, U. (2005). Visual organ. In R. Klinke, H.-C. Pape, & S. Silbernagl (Eds.), *Physiology* (pp. 685–712). New York: Thieme.

Farrehi, P. M., Nallamothu, B. K., & Navvab, M. (2016). Reducing hospital noise with sound acoustic panels and diffusion: A controlled study. *BMJ Quality & Safety, 25*, 644–646. doi: 10.1136/bmjqs-2015-004205

Frith, K. H., Anderson, E. F., Caspers, B., Tseng, F., Sanford, K., Hoyt, N. G., & Moore, K. (2010). Effects of nurse staffing on hospital-acquired conditions and length of stay in community hospitals. *Quality Management in Health Care, 19*(2), 147–155.

Frith, K. H., Anderson, E. F., Tseng, F., & Fong, E. A. (2012). Nurse staffing is an important strategy to prevent medication error in community hospitals. *Nursing Economics, 30*(5), 288–294.

Grandjean, E. (1979). *Physiological work design* (3rd ed.). Thun, Switzerland: Ott.

Graham, K. C., & Cvach, M. (2010). Monitor alarm fatigue: Standardizing use of physiological monitors

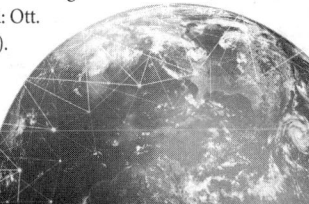

and decreasing nuisance alarms. *American Journal of Critical Care, 19*(1), 28–34, doi: 10.4037/ajcc2010651

Halbesleben, J. R., Savage, G. T., Wakefield, D. S., & Wakefield, B. J. (2010). Rework and workarounds in nurse medication administration process: Implications for work processes and patient safety. *Health Care Management Review, 35*(2), 124–133. doi: 10.1097/HMR.0b013e3 181d116c200004010-201004000-00004 [pii]

Helander, M. (2006). *A guide to human factors and ergonomics* (2nd ed.). Boca Raton, FL: Taylor & Francis Group.

Herczeg, M. (2009). *Software-ergonomics. Theories, models and criteria for usable interactive computer systems.* München, Germany: Oldenbourg.

Hess, R., DesRoches, C., Donelan, K., Norman, L., & Buerhaus, P. I. (2011). Perceptions of nurses in Magnet hospitals, non-Magnet hospitals, and hospitals pursuing Magnet status. *Journal of Nursing Administration, 41*(7/8), 315–323. doi: 10.1097/NNA.0b013e31822509e2

Hoyt, R., & Yoshihashi, A. (2010). Lessons learned from implementation of voice recognition for documentation. *Perspectives in Health Information Management, 7.*

Institute of Medicine (IOM). (1999). *To err is human: Building a safer health system.* Washington, DC: National Academies Press.

Institute of Medicine (IOM). (2004). *Keeping patients safe: Transforming the work environment of nurses.* Washington, DC: National Academies Press.

Institute of Medicine (IOM). (2011). *Health IT and patient safety: Building safer systems for better care.* Washington, DC: Committee on Patient Safety and Health Information Technology, Board on Health Care Services.

International Ergonomics Association (IEA). (2000). Definition of ergonomics. Retrieved from http:// www.iea .cc/01_what/WhatisErgonomics.html

Iyendo, T. O. (2016). Exploring the effect of sound and music on health in hospital settings: A narrative review. *International Journal of Nursing Studies, 63,* 82–100. doi: 10.1016/j.ijnurstu.2016.08.008

Jacko, J. A., & Ward, K. G. (1996). Towards establishing a link between psychomotor task complexity and human information processing. *Computers and Industrial Engineering, 31*(1–2), 533–536.

Kane, R., Shamliyan, T., Mueller, C., Duval, S., & Wilt, T. (2007). The association of registered nurse staffing levels and patient outcomes: Systematic review and meta-analysis. *Medical Care, 45*(12), 1195–1204.

Konkani, A., Oakley, B., & Bauld, T. J. (2012). Reducing hospital noise: A review of medical device alarm management. *Biomedical Instrumentation & Technology,* 478-487.

McLaren, E., & Maxwell-Armstrong, C. (2008). Noise pollution on an acute surgical ward. *Annals of the Royal College of Surgeons of England, 90*(2), 136–139. doi: 10.1308/003588408x261582

Miller, G. A. (1956). The magical number seven, plus or minus two: Some limits on our capacity for processing information. *Psychological Review, 63,* 81–97.

Pope, D. (2010). Decibel levels and noise generators on four medical/surgical nursing units. *Journal of Clinical Nursing, 19*(17–18), 2463–2470. doi: 10.1111/j.1365 -2702.2010.03263.x

Preim, B., & Dachselt, R. (2010). *Interactive systems. Volume 1: Basics, graphical user interfaces, visualization of information.* New York: Springer.

Proctor, R. W., & Vu, K.-P. L. (2012). Human information processing: An overview for human-computer interaction. In J. A. Jacko (Ed.), *The human-computer interaction handbook. Fundamentals, evolving technologies, and emerging applications* (3rd ed., pp. 21–40). Boca Raton, FL: Taylor & Francis Group.

Rasmussen, J. (1986). *Information processing and human-machine interaction, an approach to cognitive engineering* (pp. 74–83). New York: North-Holland.

Simons, D. J. (1999). Selective attention test. Retrieved from http://www.youtube.com/ watch?v5vJG698U2Mvo

Squires, M., Tourangeau, A., Laschinger, H. K. S., & Doran, D. (2010). The link between leadership and safety outcomes in hospitals. *Journal of Nursing Management, 18*(8), 914–925. doi: 10.1111/j.1365-2834.2010.01181.x

Travis, D. (2014). *Bluffers' guide to ISO 9241* (9th ed.). London, UK: Userfocus Ltd.

Tzeng, H.-M., Hu, H. M., & Yin, C.-Y. (2011). The relationship of the hospital-acquired injurious fall rates with the quality profile of a hospital's care delivery and nursing staff patterns. *Nursing Economics, 29*(6), 299–316.

University of Missouri–Columbia. (2008, April 24). Psychologists demonstrate simplicity of working memory. *Science Daily.* Retrieved from 080423171519.htm

Varpio, L., Kuziemsky, C., MacDonald, C., & King, W. J. (2012). The helpful or hindering effects of in-hospital patient monitor alarms on nurses: A qualitative analysis. *Computers, Informatics, Nursing, 30*(4), 210–217. doi: 10.1097/NCN.0b013e31823eb581

Welp, A., & Manser, T. (2016). Integrating teamwork, clinician occupational well-being and patient safety-development of a conceptual framework based on a systematic review. *BMC Health Services Research, 16*(1), 281. doi: 10.1186/s12913-016-1535-y

Wilson, J. R. (2000). Fundamentals of ergonomics in theory and practice. *Applied Ergonomics, 31*(6), 557–567.

Zborowsky, T., Bunker-Hellmich, L., Morelli, A., & O'Neill, M. (2010). Centralized vs. decentralized nursing stations: Effects on nurses' functional use of space and work environment. *HERD, 3*(4), 19–42.

CHAPTER 5

Usability in Health Information Technology

Karen H. Frith, PhD, RN, NEA-BC

LEARNING OBJECTIVES

1. Define user-centered design.
2. Identify the importance of usability testing in health care.
3. Describe the iterative process of design and testing health information technologies.
4. Select among different methods of usability testing.

KEY TERMS

Effectiveness
Efficiency
Health information technology
  (health IT)
Human–computer interaction

Iterative
Qualitative method
Quantitative method
Satisfaction
System development life cycle

Usability testing
User experience (UX)
User-centered design (UCD)

▶ Chapter Overview

The focus of this chapter is to understand a nurse's role in planning and implementing usability tests to study the effects of computer-based technology on the people who use it. Simply put, computers change the way people interact with others at

work and with **health information technology (health IT)**. Whether computers are carried in pockets, embedded in medical equipment, or positioned on desks, these systems can lead to fundamental changes in workflow. It is this interaction between humans and computers that is central to usability and **usability testing**.

▶ Introduction

Usability has many definitions and attributes (Shultz & Hand, 2015). Most of the definitions of usability concern the interaction of health IT with users (nurses, physicians, patients, family members) in terms of ease of learning to use health IT (learnability), consistency of interface (memorability), effectiveness and efficiency to accomplish the goals of a task (productivity) and the satisfaction with the health IT (Shultz & Hand, 2015). Usability testing is concerned with functionality of health IT: It measures users' perceptions about the **effectiveness** and **efficiency** of the product, users' **satisfaction** with the product, and the tendency for errors with the product ("Usability Evaluation Basics," 2013). To illustrate usability, consider two common devices used to control traffic in the United States: traffic lights and four-way stop signs. A traffic light is a device that has three colors—green, yellow, and red. The colors are arranged either from top to bottom or left to right in the same order. Drivers know that green means go, yellow means prepare to stop, and red means stop. Traffic lights work because they are easy for people to understand, are used in a consistent manner, and are effective in controlling traffic. In contrast, four-way stop signs used at intersecting roads are not as effective, because drivers have to make decisions based on the context. Drivers must always stop at the intersection, look at traffic on the other three roads, and go *if they have the right of way*. The right of way is determined by who arrives at the intersection first. The rule is easy if only one car is at the intersection, but if multiple cars arrive at the same time, the car farthermost to the right leaves the intersection first. Using this illustration, usability testing can show that both types of traffic signals are effective—drivers follow consistent rules for stopping at intersections. However, drivers likely find that four-way stop signs are not as efficient, satisfying, or error free as traffic lights because of the multiple decisions about crossing the intersection.

Every piece of technology can be evaluated for its usability and compared to other similar technologies. The goal of usability testing in health care is to develop or purchase electronic health records (EHRs), medical devices, and other health IT that meet users' needs, improve productivity, and safeguard against errors.

The need for usability testing is significant because EHRs and other health IT have been shown to slow workflow, impair performance, and introduce new error-prone processes (Jones, Heaton, Rudin, & Schneider, 2012). Participants at the Institute of Medicine's (IOM) workshop on comparative user experiences for health IT called for public reporting of the usability of EHRs (IOM, 2011; Sinsky, Hess, Karsh, Keller, & Koppel, 2012). A panel of experts commissioned by the IOM called for public reporting, similar to reviews by *Consumer Reports* of other products to provide essential information to potential purchasers and lead to improvements made by vendors (Sinsky et al., 2012). They further proposed that usability testing of EHRs and other health IT should provide information about cognitive workload, accuracy of decision making, time required to perform tasks, and implementation experience, because these characteristics profoundly affect any healthcare provider's (HCP's) ability to deliver safe patient care. The federal government has a high stake in improving usability of all health IT. The Office of the National Coordinator (ONC) for Health IT in its Federal Strategic Plan for 2015–2020 (ONC, n.d.) lists "increase access to and usability of high-quality electronic health information and services" as a high priority objective to achieve *Goal 5*, which is to "advance research, scientific knowledge, and innovation" in health IT ("Federal Health IT Strategic Plan 2015–2020," n.d.)

▶ Importance of Usability Testing

The ideal way to develop EHRs and health IT is to test usability as part of the design project plan. For vendors of EHRs and health IT, usability testing implemented from the beginning of product development is less costly than later changes requiring major revision to the code (Shenoy, 2008). Even teamwork is hurt by late usability testing. Any computer programmer will agree that resistance to reworking code is "directly proportional to the number of lines of code that has already been written" (Shenoy, 2008). Usability testing is important enough that the National Institute of Standards and Technology, an agency of the U.S. Department of Commerce, issued a report outlining an EHR usability protocol for vendors to follow in the design of their products (Lowry et al., 2012).

Poor **user experience (UX)** with health IT occurs when the technology is mismatched to the needs of the user. Poor UX is frustrating, dissatisfying, and unlikely to get better without significant redesign of the health IT. Systems with poor UX are costly in terms of dollars, personnel turnover, and unnecessary medical errors. With most EHR systems priced in the range of millions of dollars, selection of a system with poor usability often cannot be undone. In other words, once a system has been purchased, the healthcare organization cannot return it for a better system, so the organization is burdened with poor usability for the life of that system. Even admirable efforts to customize the system are typically inadequate to overcome damage to workflow and the reduced productivity of HCPs. Providers can become so frustrated and dissatisfied that they leave the organization (Kjeldskov, Skov, & Stage, 2010). Poor usability can lead to medical errors and leave the potential for efficiencies and safety as unrealized goals (Horsky et al., 2010).

▶ The Role of Nurses in Usability

Nurses are the frontline providers in most healthcare settings—they interact with many different and complex health IT every day (Smallheer, 2015). The quality of nurses'

experiences with health IT varies greatly depending on the design of the software and hardware of each system. For example, Cho, Kim, Choi, and Staggers (2016) evaluated the usability of six different EHRs focused on nursing documentation. They found that navigation patterns were different among the six systems, with two systems requiring multiple, complex interactions between nurses and the documentation system. These two systems had the lowest usability scores, as measured by the System Usability Scale, and the lowest nurse satisfaction scores (Cho et al., 2016). Network problems or interruptions in WiFi or Bluetooth connectivity cause dropped sessions during medication administration (Staggers & Sengstack, 2015). Hardware issues, such as small fonts on medical devices, poor illumination in darkened rooms, and handheld devices teetered with cords too short to reach patients, create usability problems for nurses (Staggers & Sengstack, 2015). However, the most prevalent usability problem is the misalignment of the health IT with nurses' cognitive and workflow processes (Siwicki, n.d.). Staggers, Iribarren, Guo, and Weir (2015) conducted usability testing on the electronic medication administration record (e-MAR) that is used by the Veterans Administration (VA) hospitals. They found 99 issues of usability with 15 being classified as catastrophic, which were due, in part, to interoperability problems between systems at the VA (Staggers et al., 2015).

Because nurses must use health IT to get their work done, they must also participate in the entire life cycle for health IT by being knowledgeable end users in user-centered design of health IT (described in the next section). Nurses must also speak up when usability problems exist and demand changes (Staggers & Sengstack, 2015). Nurses have power in numbers that can be manifest by submitting usability issues to the help desk, keeping logs of issues that could contribute to errors, and by reporting when workarounds are more expedient than the system as it was designed. Nurses should not just accept health IT with usability problems, but should be the leading voice for change in their organization (Staggers, 2012).

Nurses can influence future purchases by participating in vendor demonstrations and thinking about the health IT in terms of usability. For example, a hospital plans to purchase new smart infusion pumps for all units and specialty areas. Nurses can provide informed feedback about the functions in the infusion pump as compared to needs in their area of practice. For nurses who work on general medical–surgical floors, an infusion pump with complex settings may not be perceived as an effective technology because only a few setting options would be needed for their work. On the other hand, nurses who work in an emergency department, surgery center, or intensive care unit might need more functions. Nurses could make purchase recommendations based on the functions of the infusion pump compared with the work functions in order to get the most usable infusion pump.

Nurse informaticists should be members of every design team to select or develop usability testing plans. Because the nurse informaticists understand clinical work, they can select usability methods that are most likely to uncover usability problems. Selection should also be guided by the need for user feedback in each step of user-centered design (UCD): planning, designing, testing, and deploying. For example, in the testing phase, a nurse informaticist could develop several case studies to simulate patient care and HCPs' interaction with the target health IT. The case studies could require provider interactions, such as finding lab results, documenting interventions, and responding to alerts. Knowledge of the health IT and the nature of clinical work make nurse informaticists essential members of the design team in all phases of usability testing.

Nurses and nurse informaticists who use the language of usability will be able to harness power when participating with vendors, and purchasing departments in healthcare agencies. It is imperative to make the cognitive work of nurses visible and the focus of purchasing decisions so that health IT supports rather than hinders the nurses' work. To that end, the next sections on UCD and usability testing provide an introduction to the concepts and process of each.

▶ User-Centered Design

User-centered design (UCD) is a method for assessing usability throughout the **system development life cycle** (HHS, 2012). UCD means that the users' needs, desires, and limitations are the driving factors for design, not the capabilities of the technology. In other words, UCD would require a development team to create features valuable to end users and omit those of little importance, even if the features were technologically challenging or cool to the development team. UCD requires developers to understand **human–computer interaction** and to design a natural way for users to interact with the system that satisfies, rather than frustrates, them.

The design of health IT is beyond the scope of this chapter, but readers are encouraged to refer to McGonigle & Mastrian (2012) for a discussion of the system development life cycle. Smart design teams employ UCD and usability testing with HCPs throughout the system development life cycle. When conducted only by health IT designers, testing frequently will fail to uncover usability issues. When UCD and usability are intertwined and **iterative**, each step informs the next, resulting in health IT that is suited to the needs of HCPs. **FIGURE 5-1** illustrates the iterative design-test-redesign process. Even after health IT has been implemented, usability testing can uncover problems and frustrations experienced by HCPs that result in potentially unsafe workarounds. When health IT is found to have usability problems, it should be redesigned or retired. Subsequent sections of this chapter present different frameworks for and methods of usability testing.

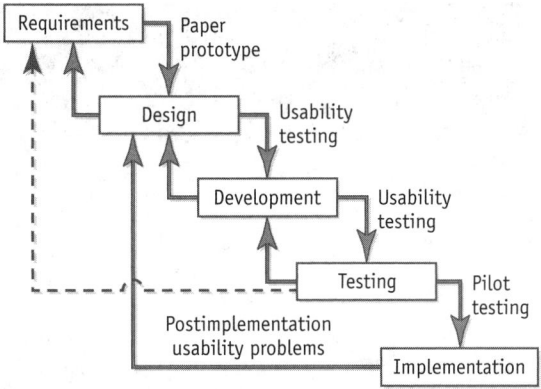

FIGURE 5-1 User-centered design: Iterative process of usability testing and design in the system development life cycle.

▶ Dimensions of Usability

The dimensions examined in most usability tests are effectiveness, efficiency, and satisfaction. The International Organization for Standardization (ISO, 1998) defines effectiveness as the "accuracy and completeness with which users achieve specified goals," efficiency as the "resources expended in relation to the accuracy and completeness with which users achieve goals," and satisfaction as the "freedom from discomfort and positive attitudes toward the user of the product" (p. 2).

Measures of the Three Dimensions of Usability

Since the 1990s, published usability studies and systematic reviews have provided numerous measures appropriate to include in usability evaluations (Hornbæk, 2006; Horsky et al., 2010; Jaspers, 2009; Khajouei, Hasman, & Jaspers, 2011; Kushniruk & Patel, 2004; Park & Hwan Lim, 1999; Zhang & Walji, 2011). Measures can overlap, but most are associated with a particular usability dimension.

Effectiveness

Measures that assess the health IT's fit with the work to be done are typically used in the effectiveness dimension (**TABLE 5-1**). Work domain saturation refers to the number of work functions available in the health IT compared to the number of work functions in a job. For example, HCPs could use an information system to manage immunizations. The information system might have functions for documentation, alerts for missed immunizations, a quick reference guide for the immunization schedule, inventory management with alerts, and printable immunization cards. If the HCP only needs to document, use the reference, and print immunization cards, the information system has more functions than are needed by the user. Sometimes the mismatch of the information system to the work results in a more complicated system that reduces the efficiency and satisfaction of users. Other measures in the effectiveness domain are task completion, accuracy, recall, and quality of outcomes. Task completion and accuracy measure the users' interaction with health IT's features to complete work functions. Recall of the interface is also an effectiveness measure, because when users recall the layout or content, the interface can be a good fit with the work domain. The final measures of effectiveness are quality of outcomes. Effective health IT helps users meet their work goals in an acceptable manner.

TABLE 5-1 Effectiveness Measures Used in Usability Studies

Measures	Definitions
Work domain saturation	Ratio of work functions in software to work functions in domain
Task completion	Percentage of tasks completed during a defined session
Accuracy	Percentage of errors in a task
Recall	User's memory of design and content in interface
Quality of outcome	The extent to which software meets the user's goals
Expert assessment	Usability expert's evaluation of quality of outcomes

Efficiency

Measures in the efficiency dimension are designed to assess how easy health IT is to learn and use (**TABLE 5-2**). Using specified tasks, the number of trials to completion, time on task, and input rate can be quantified. Success on tasks in short periods of time indicates an efficient system. Efficiency can be assessed by users' mental efforts to interact with health IT; systems that require little thinking to complete tasks are considered efficient. Patterns and numbers of features used in the system can indicate resources users need to complete tasks. Usage patterns that deviate from ideal patterns or pathways can indicate inefficiencies in the interface. System errors reduce the efficiency of health IT. Measures include the incidence of errors and the percentage of time required by the system to recover from errors. Experts use heuristics or rules of thumb to assess the design of a system's interface. A well-known set of heuristic assessment of a system was developed by Nielsen (1995) and can be found on the companion website to this text.

Satisfaction

Satisfaction, the third dimension of usability, is a subjective measure of the user's approval of health IT. Satisfaction is most commonly assessed with questionnaires (Bangor, Kortum, & Miller, 2008; Chin, Diehl, & Norman, 1988; Davis, 1989; Lewis, 1993; Lund, 2001). These tools can query users on the perceived ease of use, usefulness, ease of learning, satisfaction with work completed, and overall satisfaction. Some satisfaction measures ask for user preference by asking them to rank the choice of features or functions. Others ask opinions about the content, features, outcome or interactions with software, or an overall experience rating (Hornbæk, 2006). Most satisfaction questionnaires use a Likert rating scale with five or seven answer options. Semantic differential scales are also used and have a line with bipolar adjectives at each end. Users mark how close they feel with respect to one of the two opposite adjectives (see **FIGURE 5-2**). Readers who wish to locate satisfaction questionnaires should refer to the references in this chapter.

Research Methods for Examining Usability

Usability studies often employ mixed research methods to understand the effectiveness, efficiency, and satisfaction of users with health IT. **Quantitative methods** produce numbers such

TABLE 5-2 Efficiency Measures in Usability Studies

Measures	Definitions
Learnability	Number of trials to reach a performance level
Time	Time on task
Input rate	Rate to add data with a mouse, keyboard, or other input device
Mental effort	User's cognitive function in software used
Usage patterns	Count of how much a function in software is used
Error prevention	Error occurrence rate or error recovery rate
Expert assessment	Usability expert's evaluation of efficiency using heuristics

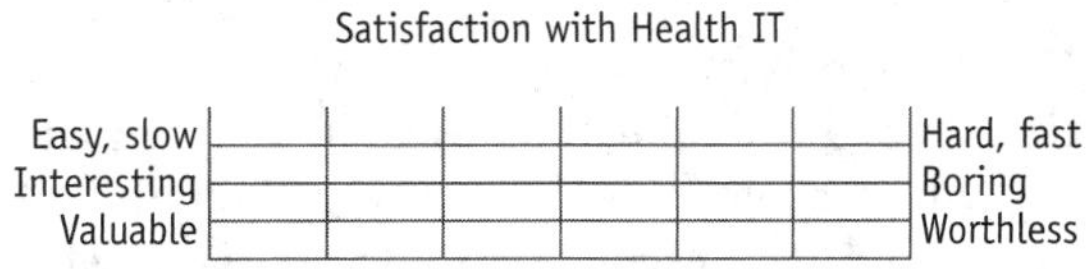

Satisfaction with Health IT

Easy, slow						Hard, fast
Interesting						Boring
Valuable						Worthless

FIGURE 5-2 Example of semantic differential scale.

as counts, frequencies, and ratios. Quantitative methods might include assessments of tasks, surveys, usage logs, and error logs. **Qualitative methods** produce text, video, or audio. Sometimes qualitative data can be converted to quantitative data by counting, for example, instances of users having difficulty finding information on a website. Qualitative methods can include interviews, focus groups, direct or video-recorded observation, "think-aloud" techniques, and task analysis. In simple terms, quantitative methods can show how many usability problems exist, whereas qualitative methods can uncover why usability problems exist and sometimes how to fix them. Because of the complementary nature of the methods, the combination is found to be more successful in the design-redesign cycle (Horsky et al., 2010).

▶ Planning Usability Testing

Planning for usability testing is done at the beginning of a project, not after health IT has been fully developed. In fact, it is an iterative process of development-testing-redesign so that results from usability testing serve as feedback for the next steps of development. Most experts advocate for no more than five users in a round of usability testing, because 85% of usability problems can be found with five and having more users simply takes longer and costs more money (Krug, 2010; Nielsen, 2000). Usability testing should be conducted regularly; monthly half-day testing with users is recommended (Krug, 2010). A guide with 234 tips for finding and recruiting participants for usability testing is available for free on the companion website to this text (Sova & Nielsen, 2003).

The design team creates a detailed plan for development and testing, using Gantt charts, flowcharts, and other management tools. The plan includes tasks, start and end dates, milestones, and resources allocated to the various tasks. Because the plan is detailed and shared among team members, specialized project management software is used. Project software can also automate email reminders, calculations of costs associated with tasks, and revisions to the timeline, if milestones are missed. **FIGURE 5-3** illustrates a typical Gantt chart that design teams use to manage the system development life cycle, including plans for usability testing.

Phases of Usability Testing

Planning

In the early stages of UCD, usability is focused on analysis of users' needs and tasks before any design discussions begin. Methods appropriate in the analysis phase to understand users' needs include focus groups, individual interviews, and contextual interviews (HHS, 2012). **BOX 5-1**

provides a list of questions that the design team could use to develop specific questions for focus groups and interviews. Two other methods used to understand tasks to be implemented in the proposed health IT are task analysis and card sorting (UsabilityNet, 2006).

Designing

In the design phase, the development team changes focus from understanding needs to brainstorming ideas for the health IT solution. Usability experts advocate for extremely early usability testing; one such technique is called napkin testing. While talking with friends, designers can draw some rough ideas about a design and get the immediate impressions of the design (Krug, 2010). **FIGURE 5-4** illustrates a simple napkin test. Even more formal design work, such as single prototyping, parallel designs, and storyboarding, are still started on paper or using software programs to draw designs (UsabilityNet, 2006). Paper prototyping illustrates the user interface based on a set of requirements for health IT. Parallel designs illustrate more than one design based on the same set of requirements, so users can select among designs. Storyboarding shows the relationships among all screens of health

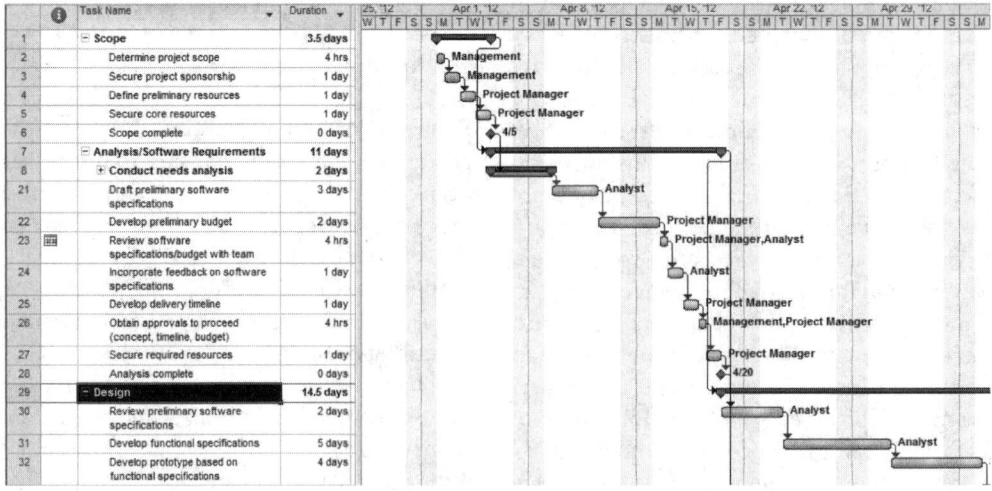

FIGURE 5-3 Example of a Gantt chart.

BOX 5-1   User-Centered Questions for the UCD Planning Phase

Who are the users of the health IT?
Why, when, and where will users access the health IT?
What are the critical needs of users for the health IT?
Which health IT features are important to users?
Which activities are core to the interaction of users with the health IT?
Which activities must be completed quickly by users of the health IT?
What is the level of satisfaction that users can expect from interacting with the health IT?
How much training on use of the health IT can end users tolerate?

Modified from U.S. Department of Health and Human Services. (n.d.). *Questions to ask at kick-off meetings.* Retrieved from http://www.usability.gov/basics/ucd/

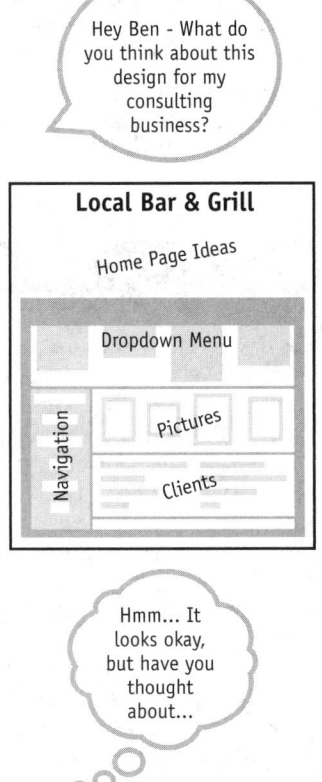

FIGURE 5-4 The napkin test.

IT. All of these methods bring user feedback to the design team and are important in the early designs to avoid the expense of rewriting code.

Testing

After the team has a working prototype, usability testing involves people outside of the design team: UX experts and actual users. Regardless of the method or the people involved in usability testing, the main point is to understand what users experience and improve health IT. Methods for the testing phase include heuristic evaluation, cognitive walkthroughs, the think-aloud method, user interviews, surveys, critical incident analysis, and satisfaction questionnaires (HHS, 2012; UsabilityNet, 2006). Frith and Anderson (2012) beta-tested nurse staffing decision-support software with five nurse managers in a community hospital. Several usability testing methods were used including cognitive walkthroughs, weekly user interviews, daily logs, and user surveys. The beta test was 3 months long, and redesign of software was batched so that users could be kept informed about changes. Users gave valuable feedback about the software. For example, the software was designed to refresh data every 4 hours, but users in the beta test wanted more frequent refresh rates (at least hourly). Usability testing also revealed other needs—nurse managers wanted graphs to trend data over time, to save and print graphs, and to annotate saved data for productivity reports. These features were not originally planned, but became priorities for redesign (Frith & Anderson, 2012).

Software programs such as Morae can record user mouse actions when users are asked to complete tasks to test the efficiency of health IT (Clearleft, 2013; TechSmith, 2013). The design team would develop structured tasks and quantify the time to complete tasks, the number of wrong mouse actions, and the completion rate for tasks by reviewing the software captures. Video cameras can add facial expressions and verbal responses to the usability testing. Specialized hardware can monitor the eye movements of users to determine if they are confused about the layout of health IT. A demo usability test recorded by Krug (2010) is freely available via YouTube, and the link to the video is found on the companion website for this text. It is worth the 25 minutes of time to watch a real usability test!

Deploying

The real test of users' experiences with health IT is when they use it in training or for the first several months. Of course, there are methods to collect data about how well health IT is performing in relation to the usability goals set for it. Usage and error logs can be collected automatically from health IT if the code for logging such activities was designed in health IT. Other manual ways to collect deployment usability data are to note problems with use during training sessions and to log calls to a support center. The usability problems noted in the deployment stage must be fixed quickly to avoid frustrating users.

▶ Examples of Usability Testing in Health Care

Health IT usability testing is appropriate for EHRs, decision-support software, medical devices, and any other health IT–supported functions.

BOX 5-2   Usability Case Study

An EBP team at a medical center wanted their sepsis protocol implemented in the electronic medical record as clinical decision support. They contacted the information technology department to work with them on the design of the clinical decision support they would call *SepCol*. The design team developed a UCD plan with three major steps that integrated different usability methods. In the first step, the evidence-based practice team translated sepsis protocol into algorithms for patient screening and treatment. Next, the EBP team developed case studies to understand how HCPs would use the algorithms in a clinical context. Meanwhile, the IT design team added SepCol to the electronic medical record software, which created prompts for HCPs to screen or treat patients for sepsis if data triggered sepsis criteria. In the second step, the IT design team asked HCPs to use a prototype of the SepCol and to think aloud while they completed several tasks. The HCPs identified confusing instructions in the decision support, so the IT design team revised the instructions to better fit the practice of nurses and physicians. In the final step of usability testing, HCPs were asked to use the SepCol with real patients. The EBP team counted the number of SepCol prompts to initiate the use of the sepsis protocol. The design team found that nurses who used the SepCol initiated significantly more treatments for sepsis as compared to the standard system used before the usability testing of the new decision support.

Check Your Understanding
1. What was the benefit of using different usability tests in the three phases of development of SepCol?
2. What other methods could have been selected to test usability?

Matrix of Usability Methods Based on Their Role in User-Centered Design

- Usability.gov: http://www.usability.gov/methods/index.html
- UsabilityNet: http://www.usabilitynet.org/tools/methods.htm
- Nielsen Norman Group: http://www.nngroup.com/articles/which-ux-research-methods/
- Nielsen Norman Group, "10 Usability Heuristics for User Interface Design": http://www. nngroup .com/articles/ten-usability-heuristics/
- Nielsen Norman Group tips for recruiting users: http://www.nngroup.com/reports/tips/recruiting
- Human Factors International: http://www.humanfactors.com/services/usabilitytestingchart.asp
- Usability Body of Knowledge: http://www.usabilitybok.org/methods

Demo Usability Test

- Steve Krug: http://www.youtube.com/watch?v5QcklzHC99Xc&feature5player_embedded

User Experience

- UX Matters: http://www.uxmatters.com/index.php
- *UX Magazine:* http://uxmag.com/

The case study presented in this chapter was reported in the literature by Anderson, Willson, Peterson, Murphy, and Kent (2010). The case study presented in this chapter illustrates the user-centered design and usability testing (see **BOX 5-2**).

If you were asked to participate in usability testing and could select only one method, which one would you select and why?

▶ Summary

Usability testing in health care is an integral part of the design of health IT. **BOX 5-3** provides helpful links to usability resources available on the Internet. Usability testing should be a regularly scheduled activity in the design plan. When usability is iterative with design, the needs of users become central to the design. The purpose of usability testing is not to prove anything; rather, it is to improve the design and function of health IT. The three dimensions of

usability testing—effectiveness, efficiency, and satisfaction—can be measured with a variety of qualitative or quantitative methods. Usability testing should improve health IT so that HCPs can give care in an efficient manner and safeguard against medical errors.

References

Anderson, J. A., Willson, P., Peterson, N. J., Murphy, C., & Kent, T. A. (2010). Prototype to practice: Developing and testing a clinical decision support system for secondary stroke prevention in a veterans health care facility. *CIN: Computers, Informatics, Nursing, 28*(6), 353–363. doi: 10.1097/NCN.0b013e3181f69c5b

Bangor, A., Kortum, P. T., & Miller, J. T. (2008). An empirical evaluation of the system usability scale. *International Journal of Human-Computer Interaction, 24*(6), 574–594. doi:10.1080/10447310802205776

Chin, J., Diehl, V., & Norman, K. (1988). *Development of an instrument measuring user satisfaction of the human-computer interface.* Paper presented at the Proceedings of ACM CHI '88 Conference on Human Factors in Computing Systems.

Cho, I., Kim, E., Choi, W. H., & Staggers, N. (2016). Comparing usability testing outcomes and functions of six electronic nursing record systems. *International Journal of Medical Informatics, 88*, 78–85. doi: 10.1016 /j.ijmedinf.2016.01.007

Clearleft. (2013). *Silverback.* Retrieved from http://silver backapp.com/

Davis, F. (1989). Perceived usefulness, perceived ease of use, and user acceptance of information technology. *MIS Quarterly, 13*(3), 319–340.

Federal Health IT Strategic Plan 2015–2020. (n.d.). Retrieved from https://www.healthit.gov/sites/default /files/FederalHealthIT_Strategic_Plan.pdf

Frith, K. H., & Anderson, E. F. (2012). Improve care delivery with integrated decision support. *Nursing Management, 43*(12), 52–54. doi: 10.1097/01.NUMA .0000422898 .37452.a4

Hornbæk, K. (2006). Current practice in measuring usability: Challenges to usability studies and research. *International Journal of Human-Computer Studies, 64*(2), 79–102. doi: http://dx.doi.org/10.1016/j.ijhcs.2005.06.002

Horsky, J., McColgan, K., Pang, J. E., Melnikas, A. J., Linder, J. A., Schnipper, J. L., & Middleton, B. (2010). Complementary methods of system usability evaluation: Surveys and observations during software design and development cycles. *Journal of Biomedical Informatics, 43*(5), 782–790. doi: http://dx.doi.org/10.1016/j.jbi.2010.05.010

Institute of Medicine (IOM). (2011). *Health IT and patient safety: Building safer systems for better care.* Washington, DC: Committee on Patient Safety and Health Information Technology, Board on Health Care Services.

International Organization for Standardization (ISO). (1998). *Ergonomic requirements for office work with visual display terminals (VDTs)—Part II: Guidance on usability.* ISO 9241-11.

Jaspers, M. W. M. (2009). A comparison of usability methods for testing interactive health technologies: Methodological aspects and empirical evidence. *International Journal of Medical Informatics, 78*(5), 340–353. doi: 10.1016 /j.ijmedinf.2008.10.002

Jones, S. S., Heaton, P. S., Rudin, R. S., & Schneider, E. C. (2012). Unraveling the IT productivity paradox—lessons for health care. *New England Journal of Medicine, 366*(24), 2243–2245.

Khajouei, R., Hasman, A., & Jaspers, M. W. M. (2011). Determination of the effectiveness of two methods for usability evaluation using a CPOE medication ordering system. *International Journal of Medical Informatics, 80*(5), 341–350. doi: 10.1016/j.ijmedinf.2011.02.005

Kjeldskov, J., Skov, M. B., & Stage, J. (2010). A longitudinal study of usability in health care: Does time heal? *International Journal of Medical Informatics, 79*(6), e135–e143. doi: 10.1016/j.ijmedinf.2008.07.008

Krug, S. (2010). *Rocket surgery made easy.* Berkeley, CA: New Riders.

Kushniruk, A. W., & Patel, V. L. (2004). Cognitive and usability engineering methods for the evaluation of clinical information systems. *Journal of Biomedical Informatics, 37*(1), 56–76. doi: 10.1016/j.jbi.2004.01.003

Lewis, J. (1993). IBM computer usability satisfaction questionnaires: Psychometric evaluation and instructions for use. *International Journal of Human-Computer Interaction, 7*(1), 57–78.

Lowry, S., Quinn, M., Ramaiah, M., Schumacher, R., Patterson, E., North, R., . . . Abbott, P. (2012). *Technical evaluation, testing, and validation of the usability of electronic health records.* Gaithersburg, MD: National Institute of Standards and Technology.

Lund, A. M. (2001). Measuring usability with the USE questionnaire. *Usability Interface Newsletter, 8*(2).

McGonigle, D., & Mastrian, K. (2012). *Nursing informatics and the foundation of knowledge.* Burlington, MA: Jones & Bartlett Learning.

Nielsen, J. (1995). *How to conduct a heuristic evaluation.* Retrieved from http://www.nngroup.com/articles /how-to-conduct-a-heuristic-evaluation/

Nielsen, J. (2000). *Why you only need to test with 5 users.* Retrieved from http://www.nngroup.com/articles /why-you-only-need-to-test-with-5-users/

Office of the National Coordinator (ONC). (n.d.). Fact sheets. HealthIT.gov. Retrieved from https://www.healthit .gov/newsroom/fact-sheets

Park, K. S., & Hwan Lim, C. (1999). A structured methodology for comparative evaluation of user interface designs using usability criteria and measures. *International Journal of Industrial Ergonomics, 23*(5–6), 379–389. doi: 10.1016 /S0169-8141(97)00059-0

Shenoy, G. (2008). *Benefits of early usability testing.* Retrieved from http://productmanagementtips.com/2008/09/15 /product-manager-usability-testing/

Shultz, S., & Hand, M. W. (2015). Usability: A concept analysis. *Journal of Theory Construction & Testing, 19*(2), 65–70.

Sinsky, C. A., Hess, J., Karsh, B. T., Keller, J. P., & Koppel, R. (2012). *Comparative user experiences of health IT products: How user experiences would be reported and used.* Retrieved from http://www.iom.edu/Global/Perspectives /2012/~/media/Files/Perspectives-Files/2012/Discussion -Papers/comparative-user-experiences.pdf

Siwicki, B. (n.d.). Nurse informaticist: We face severe usability problems. *Healthcare IT News.* Retrieved from http://www.healthcareitnews.com/news/nurse -informaticist-healthcare-it-faces-severe-problems -usability

Smallheer, B. A. (2015). Technology and monitoring patients at the bedside. *The Nursing Clinics of North America, 50*(2), 257–268. doi: 10.1016/j.cnur.2015.02.004

Sova, D., & Nielsen, J. (2003). *How to recruit participants for usability studies.* Retrieved from http://www.nngroup .com/reports/tips/recruiting

Staggers, N. (2012). Improving the user experience for EHRs: How to begin? *Online Journal of Nursing Informatics, 16*(2), 15–17.

Staggers, N., Iribarren, S., Guo, J.-W., & Weir, C. (2015). Evaluation of a BCMA's electronic medication administration record. *Western Journal of Nursing Research, 37*(7), 899–921. doi: 10.1177/0193945914566641

Staggers, N., & Sengstack, P. (2015). A call for case studies and stories about how usability impacts nurses. *Online Journal of Nursing Informatics, 19*(2), 1.

TechSmith. (2013). Morae [Software]. Retrieved from http://www.techsmith.com/morae.html

U.S. Department of Health and Human Services. (n.d.). *Questions to ask at kick-off meetings.* Retrieved from http://www.usability.gov/basics/ucd/

U.S. Department of Health and Human Services (HHS). (2012). *Usability.gov: How to & tools: Methods.* Retrieved from http://www.usability.gov/methods/test_refine/learnusa/index.html

Usability Evaluation Basics. (2013, October 8). Retrieved from http://www.usability.gov/what-and-why/usability-evaluation.html

UsabilityNet. (2006). *Methods table.* Retrieved from http://www.usabilitynet.org/tools/methods.htm

Zhang, J., & Walji, M. F. (2011). TURF: Toward a unified framework of EHR usability. *Journal of Biomedical Informatics, 44*(6), 1056–1067. doi: 10.1016/j.jbi.2011.08.005

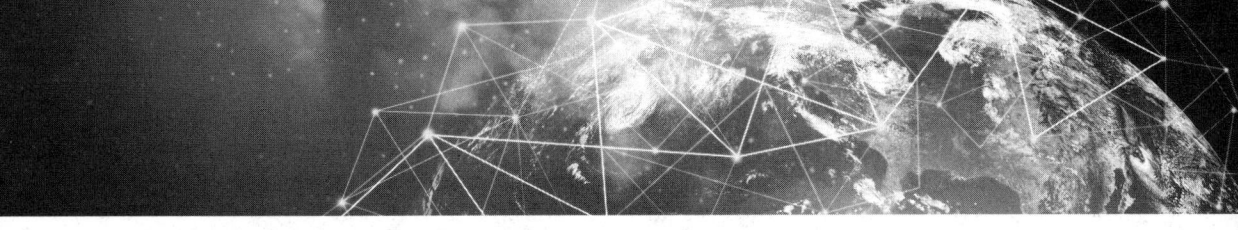

CHAPTER 6

Privacy, Security, and Confidentiality

Faye E. Anderson, DNS, RN, NEA-BC

Karen H. Frith, PhD, RN, NEA-BC

LEARNING OBJECTIVES

1. Review the requirements of laws governing protection of personal health information.
2. Describe the actions required of organizations for protecting personal health information.
3. Identify activities of nurses to protect personal health information.
4. Give examples of inappropriate uses of protected health information.
5. Analyze clinical situations for compliance with privacy and security regulations.

KEY TERMS

Biometric identifiers
Breach
Business associate
Covered entity
Ethics
Health Information Technology for Economic and Clinical Health Act (HITECH)
Health Insurance Portability and Accountability Act (HIPAA)

Law
Need to know
Notice of Privacy Practices
Patient Safety and Quality Improvement Act of 2005 (PSQIA)
Patient safety organizations (PSO)
Privacy

Protected health information (PHI)
Risk assessment
Security

▶ Chapter Overview

This chapter presents the key components of laws governing the **privacy** and **security** of patient health information, contrasting ethical and legal requirements. Components of the **Health Insurance Portability and Accountability Act (HIPAA)**, **Health Information Technology for Economic and Clinical Health Act (HITECH)**, and **Patient Safety and Quality Improvement Act of 2005 (PSQIA)** laws related to protecting health information are presented. Aspects of maintaining the security of electronic forms of health information are discussed and implications for nurses are presented.

▶ Introduction

Protecting patient information is both an ethical and a legal responsibility of nurses. Nurses are privy to very personal, intimate information about patients. The health history and physical assessment provide details of a person's life and background, and in the process of providing care, nurses gain even more information about a patient (California Nurses Association [CNA], 2011). If patients fear that health information is shared inappropriately, full disclosure may be compromised. For example, patients may not report a family history of mental illness or chronic disease if they fear the information could be used to deny a job opportunity. A history of sexually transmitted diseases, injuries resulting from violence or abuse, or drug use may be embarrassing. Thus information needed for appropriate treatment is withheld due to fear of ridicule, judgment, or misuse; such fears may even cause someone to avoid seeking care. Withholding critical information could not only impact quality of care for the individual, but could also affect public safety (Rothstein, 2012).

Maintaining patient confidentiality is a core duty of healthcare practitioners (De Bord, Burke, & Dudzinski, 2013). Patients trust that their personal information will be handled in a professional manner (CNA, 2011). Professional

healthcare associations and regulatory bodies support the ethical standards of confidentiality and privacy. The American Hospital Association (AHA, 2003) identifies protection of privacy as a patient's right. Confidentiality is a requirement in accreditation standards, such as those promalgated by The Joint Commission and the Medicare and Medicaid Conditions of Participation (Rinehart-Thompson, 2013).

The ethical duty of nurses to maintain confidentiality of patient information is set forth in the Code of Ethics for Nurses. Provision 3 of the code states, "The nurse promotes, advocates for, and protects the rights, health, and safety of the patient" (American Nurses Association [ANA], 2015, p. 9). The ethical actions of the nurse include maintaining an environment that protects both physical privacy as well as personal information. The nurse does not disclose information to individuals not involved in care of the patient or allow unauthorized access to patient information. The code does acknowledge that at times the right to confidentiality may be limited in order to protect the patient or others or by laws or regulations.

To comply with ethical and regulatory standards, healthcare organizations develop policies to ensure confidentiality of patient information. These privacy protections typically include restrictions on using patient names or likenesses without permission, disclosing private facts about a patient, providing unfavorable or false statements to the public about a patient, and causing unreasonable intrusion into a patient's affairs (CNA, 2011).

It is important to remember there is a difference between ethics and law. **Ethics**, a branch of philosophy that is concerned with the values of human behavior, can be subjective; it incorporates moral values and requires examination of the issues involved. Conversely, the **law** is an objective rule. Ethical standards are foundational and rarely change. A law may change or be overturned. A law may incorporate aspects of ethical behavior; so an ethical standard and a law may be essentially the same. Professional ethical codes of conduct are not law; but just as violation of a law can result in penalities, violations of ethical standards can also result in penalties, such as termination by an organization or disciplinary action by a state licensing board. **BOX 6-1** provides a case study to illustrate nurses' responsibilitities. **TABLE 6-1** summarizes the best practices for confidentiality with regard to health information.

BOX 6-1 Case Study

You are doing an admission assessment on an 87-year-old female patient who was admitted with pneumonia. You notice bruises on her back and arms in various stages of healing. When you question her about the bruises, she begins to cry. She states, "Please do not say anything about this. I live with my son and sometimes he gets mad at me if I don't do what he says. But he is good to me, and I have nowhere else to live. I just try to be quick when he wants something and not make him mad especially when he is drinking."

Check Your Understanding

1. What should you say to the patient?
2. What action should you take?
3. Does HIPAA cover this situation?

TABLE 6-1 Confidentiality Practices for Nurses

1. Do not discuss patient information in public places (hallways, elevators, cafeterias).

2. Keep user names and password secure. Do not share a user name or password; do not use another person's password.

3. Log off when leaving a computer; do not leave a computer open for another person to access.

4. Attend educational sessions on updates to confidentiality policies.

5. Do not take or use pictures of patients without permission.

6. Never share patient information with those without a need to know. Only provide information to caregivers involved in care of the patient or to administrative personnel authorized to receive such information.

7. Do not allow observations of care by others not involved in the care of the patient (such as a student) without the patient's permission.

8. Never post information or pictures of a patient on social media, even if the name of the patient is not used.

(continues)

TABLE 6-1 Confidentiality Practices for Nurses (*Continued*)
9.   Dispose of records containing patient information according to policy, such as shredding.
10.   Avoid unnecessary printing of protected health information (PHI).
11.   Never transfer PHI to an outside entity unless authorized to do so. Transfer according to policy.
12.   Never access records without authorization. This includes your own record or records of family members.
13.   Follow security requirements for accessing PHI remotely.
14.   Report any breaches of privacy immediately.

▶ History of Legal Protection for Privacy

Legal protection of personal health information was initially addressed in selected federal laws (Rinehart-Thompson, 2013). The Privacy Act of 1974 required federal agencies to protect personal information, but did not specifically address health information, and applied only to federal agencies. The 1970 and 1972 federal drug laws established protection of information related to diagnosis and treatment of substance abuse. The Medicare and Medicaid Conditions of Participation required agencies to maintain confidentiality of patient records, but the scope was limited. The regulation applied only to Medicare and Medicaid patients; other patients were not included (Rinehart-Thompson, 2013).

State laws provide some protection of privacy, but the regulations vary from state to state and are limited in scope (CNA, 2011; Rinehart-Thompson, 2013). States have laws that require protection of sensitive health information for conditions such as human immunodeficiency virus (HIV), acquired immunodeficiency syndrome (AIDS), or mental health disorders. State laws also require the reporting of selected health conditions for public health and safety reasons, including the reporting of communicable diseases and abuse and neglect of children, elders, and disabled persons. Reporting to maintain vital statistics, such as births, deaths, and unnatural causes of death such as homicide or suicide, is also required.

Prior to electronic communication, privacy of health information was recognized as an individual's right by federal agencies and professional organizations (Buckovich, Rippen, & Rozen, 1999). However, there was little consensus about some, but not all principles to protect health information. With the adoption of electronic health records (EHRs), new technologies brought the ability to limit access to health information; the same technologies could also make violating health information easier (Rothstein, 2012).

▶ Health Insurance Portability and Accountability Act (HIPAA)

The ethical and regulatory guidelines for confidentiality were codified into federal law in 1996 with the passage of the Health Insurance Portability and Accountability Act (HIPAA)

(McGowan, 2012). The law covered more than just privacy protections; it included sections promoting continuity of health insurance coverage for employed people, reducing Medicare fraud and abuse, simplifying health insurance administration, as well as a section (Title II) protecting the privacy and security of health information. Enactment of the legislation was significant as it established minimum national standards for protecting health information (Department of Health and Human Services [DHHS], 2005; McGowan, 2012). The privacy section received much public attention; and while it was received positively by many, it was also a cause of concern due to the costs of implementation.

Privacy and Security Regulations

The law directed the Department of Health and Human Services (DHHS) Secretary to develop both privacy and security regulations (CNA, 2011). The privacy rules focused on the rights of the patient; standards were established to protect health information communicated in any manner—verbal, paper, visual, or electronic. Security rules addressed standards for protecting health information held or transmitted electronically (DHHS, 2005). Penalties for failure to protect an individual's identifiable health information were also defined. Regulations to guide implementation of the privacy protection became effective in 2003, and security requirements became effective in 2005 (McGowan, 2012; Rinehart-Thompson, 2013).

HIPAA Omnibus Final Rule

In the years following implementation of the law, the need for additional rules and regulations was identified, with strengthening of security and enforcement incorporated into the HITECH Act of 2005. Final regulations issued in January 2013 focused on the areas of security, enforcement, and patient rights (Crandell, 2013; DHHS, 2013b; Morris, 2013; Reber, 2011). First, the mandates of the HITECH Act of 2005 were included, making business associates directly liable for compliance

with tiered penalties for violations. The penalties for civil violations were increased. Limitations on use of **protected health information (PHI)** for marketing and fund-raising were strengthened by requiring patient consent for marketing and promoting a product or treatment which the patient was not using. The rights of an individual were expanded to be able to receive an electronic copy of PHI if the **covered entity (CE)** uses an EHR and to be able to restrict disclosures for treatments paid in full out of pocket. The rules require modification and redistribution of the Notice of Privacy Practices informing patients of their rights and how information is protected. Reporting of breaches was modified to a standard based on risk rather than on harm. And finally, changes increased privacy protection for genetic information.

TABLE 6-2 lists definitions of the common terms used in the law.

Privacy

The statute applied to covered entities and to **business associates**. Covered entities are defined as: (1) providers (ranging from an individual provider to a large organization) if the provider transmits health information in an electronic form; (2) health plans that provide or pay for health care; and (3) healthcare clearinghouses. A clearinghouse processes billing transactions or processes nonstandard health information received from another entity into a standard format. A business associate is a person or organization that uses PHI to perform activities on behalf of a covered entity, but is not part of the covered entity's workforce (DHHS, 2005; Rinehart-Thompson, 2013).

To be considered PHI, three criteria must be met. First, it includes information that could reasonably identify the person such as name, address, date of birth, and social security number. Second, it includes past, current, or future information about the patient's physical or mental conditions, information about the provision of care, and information about payment for care. Finally, it must be held or transmitted electronically by the

TABLE 6-2 Selected Terms Used in HIPAA

Term	Definition
Individual	Person who is subject of protected health information
Personal representative	Person with legal authority to act on behalf of another in making healthcare decisions
Covered entity	One of three categories: healthcare provider, health plan, or healthcare clearinghouse
Business associate	Person or organization that performs activities on behalf of covered entity
Designated record set	Records used by covered entities to make decisions about an individual; includes medical records, billing records, case management records, and enrollment, payment, and claims records
Breach	Unauthorized acquisition, access, use, or disclosure of PHI

Data from U.S. Department of Health and Human Services (HHS). (2005). *Understanding patient safety confidentiality.* Retrieved from http://www.hhs .gov/ocr/privacy/psa/understanding/index.html; Rinehart-Thompson, L. A. (2013). *Introduction to health information privacy and security.* Chicago, IL: American Health Information Management Association Press.

covered entity or buisness associates (McGowan, 2012; Rinehart-Thompson, 2013).

Deidentified information does not contain data that could be used to identify an individual. It can be used or disclosed without restrictions. The law specifies two options for deidentification. One option is to use an expert to ensure statistically that any risk of identification is minimal. The other option is to remove the 18 defined identifiers of the individual, household members, or employers. The 18 elements include name; date of birth, admission, discharge, or death; addresses; email addresses; phone and fax numbers; medical record numbers; health plan beneficiary numbers; license and certification numbers; vehicle and device identifiers; **biometric identifiers** such as fingerprints and voice prints; and account numbers (DHHS, 2005; Rinehart-Thompson, 2013).

The HIPAA of 1996 and the final regulations require two privacy documents that must be used to advise patients on how PHI will be protected and obtained from other entities (DHHS, 2005; DHHS, 2013b; Muller, 2014). First, the law requires that a **Notice of Privacy Practices** be given to a patient upon the first contact with a covered entity and at other times upon request. The notice must be written in language that is easy for patients to understand, and explain how the covered entity will use the patient's protected health information. It is not necessary to provide a privacy notice upon subsequest encounters unless there are changes (Rinehart-Thompson, 2013). The second document is the authorization to share PHI. When such an authorization is required or requested by the patient, the law requires that specific components be included. It must be correct, be written in plain language, and contain all the required elements (Reinhart-Thompson, 2013). **FIGURE 6-1** shows an example form authorizing use or disclosure of protected health information.

AUTHORIZATION FOR USE OR DISCLOSURE OF PROTECTED HEALTH INFORMATION

Patient name

I , _____ , hereby give permission to disclose information from my medical record. I understand that I may revoke this authorization in writing, submitted at any time.

Sending Information	**Information to be disclosed by:**	**Receiving information**	**Provided to:**
	Name of facility		Facility or person
	Address		Address
	City, State		City, State

Reason for release of information

The disclosure is because of (check one or more):

☐ Medical care ☐ Personal use ☐ Legal advice ☐ Insurance

☐ School ☐ Disability ☐ Research ☐ Other

Part or whole of medical record to release

The information to be disclosed from my medical record:
- Only information related to: _____
- Only the events during the period of ___/___/___ to ___/___/___
- Entire record: _____

Release of sensitive information

If you would like any of the following sensitive information disclosed, check one or more below:

☐ Alcohol/drug abuse treatment/referral   ☐ Sexually transmitted diseases

☐ HIV/AIDS treatment   ☐ Psychotherapy notes only

☐ Other mental health

Signature of patient or personal representative (state relationship to patient)	Date
Signature of Witness	Date

FIGURE 6-1 Example of document for use or disclosure of protected health information.

Although PHI cannot be shared without authorization with just anyone, HIPAA was not intended to make communication among caregivers difficult. It is important to remember that the intent of the law is to protect an individual's health information. The law requires that access be given only to those with a **need to know**, and that only the minimum amount of information needed to accomplish the purpose be released. A nurse would have a greater need for access

---

BOX 6-2 Case Studies

I.   Joe Kitchens is a senior student in the local baccalaureate nursing program. He is doing a rotation in the Surgery Center and Mrs. Jones, a member of his church, comes in for the preop visit for a hysterectomy in two days. When Joe gets home that night he tells his wife that Mrs. Jones is having surgery. The next day, his wife attends a prayer meeting and puts Mrs. Jones' name on the prayer list stating when and what surgery is scheduled. Later that day, a friend calls Mrs. Jones and asks why she had not told anyone. Mrs. Jones is very upset and calls the dean of the nursing program to complain and ask that Joe be dismissed from the program for violating her rights.

Check Your Understanding

1. Did Joe violate Mrs. Jones's PHI even though he didn't share paper or electronic information?
2. What are the implications for the Surgery Center?
3. If you are the dean of the nursing program, what action would you take?

II. Ms. Adams is 75 and in good health, except for hypertension controlled by medication and an occasional cold. She still lives alone and maintains her own household and financial affairs. She tends not to discuss her private business with others. She has come to the doctor for her annual checkup and had to get a ride with a neighbor as her car was in for repairs. A new nurse is working at the doctor's office. When Ms. Adams is called to the treatment room, the neighbor follows and the nurse steps back to allow the neighbor to enter the room.

Check Your Understanding

1. Is the neighbor allowed to stay?
2. Did the nurse follow HIPAA guidelines to protect Ms. Adams' privacy?

---

to PHI than would a billing clerk. A nurse not involved in an individual's care would *not* have any need to know. Patient care, public safety, or efficient operations should not be compromised by withholding important information (DHHS, 2005; McGowan, 2012). **BOX 6-2** provides a case study illustrating the need to know concept.

The HIPAA of 1996 clearly defines situations when patient information cannot be shared without authorization, situations when information must be provided without authorization, and situations when disclosure is permitted without written authorization (DHHS, 2005; McGowan, 2012; Rinehart-Thompson, 2013). Patient authorization is not required or is permitted in situations identified in **BOX 6-3**.

No authorization is required to disclose information to the patient or to the patient's personal representative (DHHS, 2005). Patients have a right to inspect and obtain a copy of their own health records (DHHS, 2005). A fee may be charged by the covered entity for the copying or the releasing of information. The patient has the right to request an electronic copy of the record if the provider uses an electronic medical record system, and can request that the record be sent to another person (Morris, 2013).

The individual may also request that an amendment be made to PHI. Such a request is not automatically approved and may be denied under specific circumstances. For example, denial may be made if the record is already accurate or was not created or is not maintained by the covered entity. An individual may also request a list of all disclosures of PHI that were submitted electronically for the previous three years. This list includes disclosures that were authorized by the law and did not require authorization (Morris, 2013). The individual may request restrictions on uses and disclosures for administrative purposes.

BOX 6-3 Sharing of PHI Allowed by the HIPAA of 1996

- No authorization is required to disclose information to the patient or to the patient's personal representative (DHHS, 2005).
- Providing information in a directory or notification of family and friends is permitted if the patient has an opportunity to informally agree or to object.
- No authorization is needed for sharing of information for purposes of treatment, for conducting the business of the organization, or for billing.
- The HIPAA of 1996 allows for the incidental disclosure of PHI occurring as a routine aspect of doing business.
- PHI may be shared without authorization to public agencies such as the Centers for Disease Control and Prevention (CDC) for surveillance of disease outbreaks.
- No authorization is required for DHHS investigative review or enforcement activities. Rather, the information *must* be provided if requested by HHS (Reinhart-Thompson, 2013).
- Most states require reporting of PHI for vital statistics and public health purposes; HIPAA allows such reporting (CNA, 2011).
- If a state law conflicts with the federal law, the federal law has priority unless the state laws are more stringent (CNA, 2011).

Because administrative purposes are a reason for use of PHI without written authorization, these restrictions do not have to be honored; but if the covered entity agrees, the restrictions must be followed (Rinehart-Thompson, 2013). However, the individual can restrict the release of treatments that were paid for in full by the patient (Morris, 2013).

Providing information in a directory or notification of family and friends is permitted if the patient has an opportunity to informally agree or to object. According to the HIPAA, the patient can authorize that information be shared with specified individuals. Permission can be given informally, but the patient must have an opportunity to agree or object. If no objection is raised, permission is implied. This permission enables the facility to maintain a directory of patients being treated and to give the location and general condition of a patient to someone asking for the patient by name. The institution is also allowed to maintain a listing of patients with religious affiliation if no objection is raised, and clergy can be given religious affiliation information. Informal permission is often given for information to be provided to family and friends involved in the person's care. If a patient

is not capable of giving permission and is in an emergency situation, PHI can be shared if the HCPs determine it is in the best interest of the patient (Rinehart-Thompson, 2013).

In an effort to allow family, significant others, and friends to have information about the patient in the absence of the patient and without violating ethical and legal restrictions, healthcare agencies have developed processes to enable patients to indicate who can receive PHI. This information is recorded for future reference. In addition, some acute care hospitals have developed a procedure for giving patients a code word response. If a family member or other person calls to request information and gives the correct code, the information can be shared. If the code is not provided, no information is provided.

No authorization is needed for sharing of information for purposes of treatment, for conducting the business of the organization, or for billing. This includes discussions and consultations among the caregivers, quality assessment and improvement activities, care coordination, compliance programs, fraud and abuse auditing, business planning, and administration of the organization. Information should *not* be shared with HCPs not involved in the care of the patient and who are not involved with administrative functions. Casual conversations and inappropriate disposal of documents containing PHI must be avoided (DHHS, 2005).

The HIPAA of 1996 allows for the incidental disclosure of PHI occurring as a routine aspect of doing business; for example, HIPAA permits calling a patient's name in a clinic or having patient information on a whiteboard that is in a private area, which is not routinely accessible to the public. The covered entity must have implemented the minimum standards and reasonable safeguards. As long as only minimal information is given and no diagnostic information provided, disclosure is considered incidental and authorization by the patient is not required (DHHS, 2005; Rinehart-Thompson, 2013).

HCPs who are covered by HIPAA and who give care to an employer's employees can release PHI to the employer only for purposes of workplace surveillance and for evaluating an employee's work-related injury or illness, in accordance with other legal requirements (CNA, 2011). The employee must be provided with notice of the release of PHI (CNA, 2011).

Protected health information may be shared without authorization to public agencies such as the CDC for surveillance of disease outbreaks. No authorization is required for the DHHS investigative review or enforcement activities. Rather, the information *must* be provided if requested by DHHS (Rinehart-Thompson, 2013).

Most states require reporting of PHI for vital statistics and public health purposes. HIPAA allows such reporting (CNA, 2011). When authorized by state law, PHI may also be shared with individuals who may have been exposed to communicable diseases such as tuberculosis and syphilis. PHI can be shared with appropriate legal entities in cases of suspected abuse and neglect, with other facilities for the donation and transplantation of organs and tissues, with agencies to protect an individual or the public from a serious threat, in worker's compensation cases, in legal proceedings about decedents, and in research (McGowan, 2012). If a state law conflicts with the federal law, the federal law has priority, unless the state laws are more stringent.

State statutes usually require more restrictions on health information related to a diagnosis of HIV/AIDS, mental illness, or substance abuse (CNA, 2011). The case studies in **BOX 6-4** illustrate some of these HIPAA regulations about authorizations.

Security

The HIPAA security standards establish the national standards for protection of health information that is held or transferred electronically. It includes all identifiable health information that a covered entity creates, receives, maintains, or transmits in an electronic format (DHHS, 2005). It requires covered entities to protect against hazards that might affect the integrity of electronic PHI, protect against inappropriate disclosures of PHI, and ensure compliance by employees.

Karasz, Eiden, and Bogan (2013) note that whether a patient authorizes disclosure or if disclosure is allowed without authorization, transmission of electronic PHI *must* be conducted in accordance with the security rules. The law establishes safeguards to minimize the inappropriate use and disclosure as well as the incidental disclosure of PHI. Some standards are required while others are considered addressable, meaning that the organization can implement a reasonable equivalent (Rinehart-Thompson, 2013). Three types of security safeguards are required for electronic records: administrative, physical, and technical. There are requirements for organizational contracts and for policies and procedures (DHHS, 2005; Karasz, Eiden, & Bogan, 2013; Rinehart-Thompson 2013). Organizational safeguards include specific requirements for contracts with business associates and group health plans. The policy, procedure, and documentation safeguards require that policies, procedures, activities to meet standards, and responses to complaints or **breaches** be written (electronic acceptable) and be maintained for 6 years from the date of creation or date when last in effect. The policies and procedures must also be available to those who will be required to implement the policies and be reviewed and

BOX 6-4 Case Studies

I.   The surgical unit has a whiteboard in the nursing station listing the patient's last name, age, room number, diagnosis, and important activities for the day, such as scheduled X-rays, surgery, or lab tests. The unit is closed to the public, but occasionally a patient family member enters the unit looking for a specific nurse. Some of the nurses have concerns about the information on the board and question whether it is violating HIPAA regulations.

Check Your Understanding

1.   As the unit director, what action should you take?
2.   Should the board be removed?

II. The emergency department in Community Hospital has curtains separating the patients. As the new director, Carl Winslow is concerned about maintaining privacy especially as many of the patients are elderly and have hearing problems. The caregivers must talk loudly in order for the patients to understand what is said. In addition, patient information is faxed to local nursing homes when a patient is to be transferred.

Check Your Understanding

1.   Is there a potential HIPAA violation in this emergency department?
2.   What actions can be taken to ensure HIPAA privacy protections are met?

updated in response to changes that affect PHI (Rinehart-Thompson, 2013).

Administrative Safeguards

Administrative safeguards are the policies, procedures, and actions to protect the electronic PHI and manage the workforce (DHHS, 2005; Rinehart-Thompson, 2013). Components of this category are included in the following paragraphs.

Conduct a Risk Analysis

The risk analysis includes evaluation and impact of potential risks. Security measures to address the identified risks must be implemented with documentation of the measures and the rationale. The risk analysis must be continuous with regular reporting and review (DHHS, 2005; Rinehart-Thompson, 2013).

Develop a Security Management Process

A number of components are required for security management (DHHS, 2005; Rinehart-Thompson,

2013). Among requirements, two are particularly important: having a security officer and developing policies and procedures for access.

Appoint a Security Officer. The security official is responsible for developing and implementing security policies and procedures. The organization must also appoint someone to receive complaints about privacy policies, noncompliance, and violations of privacy.

Develop Policies and Procedures for Access. Policies and procedures must be developed to ensure compliance with the regulations and limit access to electronic PHI to appropriate users only. Policies must address who has access and the degree of access, how clearance for access is obtained, and how access is terminated if the employee no longer works for the organization. Policies also establish disciplinary action for employees who violate confidentiality policies, which can include termination, and procedures for security incidents must describe the actions to respond and report all security issues.

Physical safeguards are required to limit physical access to electronic health information and ensure control (DHHS, 2005; Rinehart-Thompson,

2013). Physical safeguards include facility access controls, workstation use and security, and device and media controls. Restrictions must limit unauthorized access and validate appropriate access to all areas and equipment containing electronic PHI. Access may be based on role or on the individual's identity. Use may be restricted, such as read only or read, edit, create, and print. Emergency plans must address access and restoration of data following an emergency or disaster. Any repairs or modifications of the physical areas containing PHI are to be documented and retained.

Policies and procedures must specify proper use of workstations and devices including transfer, removal, disposal, and reuse. Workstations, both in the facility and remote stations, should be in secure locations with restricted viewing by the public or those without a need for access. This can be accomplished by privacy shields, automatic log off, and returns to screensaver mode (DHHS, 2005; Rinehart-Thompson, 2013).

The organization must implement policies and procedures to inventory the receipt and removal of devices that contain electronic PHI and for disposal of the devices. These include hard drives, magnetic tapes, disks, memory cards, and flash drives. Information must be deleted from any device that is to be reused. Data backup and storage is required before equipment is moved (DHHS, 2005; Rinehart-Thompson, 2013).

Conduct Workforce Training and Management

All employees who have access to electronic PHI must have proper authorization. Training and education of security policies and procedures must be conducted.

Conduct Periodic Evaluations

An assessment must be conducted periodically to determine if the security policies and procedures continue to meet the requirements of the law.

Technical Safeguards

Required technical safeguards are access control, audit controls, integrity, entry authentication,

and transmission security (DHHS, 2005; Rinehart-Thompson, 2013). Aspects of technical safeguards are described in the following sections.

Implement Controls for Access, Audits, Integrity, and Transmission

Technical procedures must ensure access is proper, and electronic PHI is not altered or destroyed improperly. Hardware and software mechanisms that record access and alterations or destruction must be installed, and technical security measures implemented to prevent unauthorized access for PHI being transmitted electronically.

Access can be controlled through user identification, emergency access procedures, automatic log off, and encryption. Unique user identification is required in order to identify and track a user and the functions that user is performing. Emergency access enables a user to access records even if controls are in place if an emergency occurs. For example, access may be disrupted if the electrical power is disrupted or if a user needs information for which they normally do not have access. Automatic log off helps to prevent unauthorized viewing. Encryption or scrambling of data is a way to protect data from being read while in transit. Only the use of user identification and emergency access is required (DHHS, 2005; Rinehart-Thompson 2013).

Policies for disposal of PHI must be developed to ensure that both the patient and the environment are protected. The law requires that a record be maintained of the movements of the hardware and electronic media. When a piece of equipment is disposed, erasure of the PHI must be documented (Andersen, 2011).

Audit Controls

Mechanisms must be installed to examine and record activity. Audits are done after activity has occurred. There is no requirement for how often audits are conducted or what information is collected. Audits are useful in the investigation of breaches and misuse.

Integrity

Policies must address the unauthorized alteration or destruction of electronic PHI. Such actions may occur by mistake or on purpose. The policies must address all causes.

Entry Authentication

Procedures must be implemented to prevent unauthorized access to PHI. Methods include user or log-in ID, passwords, key cards, and biometric identifiers such as fingerprints, face prints, or retinal scans. Biometric markers are the most secure means to authenticate users.

Transmission Security

Electronic PHI must be protected from unauthorized access when it is transmitted via an electronic network. Firewalls, antivirus software, and encryption may be used to meet this requirement. Common organizational practices to meet the HIPAA regulations are listed in **TABLE 6-3**.

TABLE 6-3 Common Organizational Policies and Practices to Comply with HIPAA

1. Provide HIPAA training during orientation for all new employees

2. Have employees sign documents acknowledging understanding of privacy requirements

3. Conduct yearly HIPAA educational reviews and updates for all employees

4. Require that all paper documents with PHI be shredded

5. Limit access to areas holding documents with PHI (locked doors or cabinets, key cards required for access)

6. Require passwords to access computers; require passwords to be changed periodically

7. Forbid leaving patient information displayed on computers where it can be seen by others; require logging out when leaving the workstation

8. Forbid sharing of passwords

9. Install firewalls to protect servers

10. Forbid access to PHI by caregivers not involved in care

11. Monitor access to electronic medical records for inappropriate access

12. Limit information on whiteboards to the minimum necessary

13. Place general information whiteboards in designated area least accessible to those not involved in care

(continues)

TABLE 6-3 Common Organizational Policies and Practices to Comply with HIPAA (*Continued*)
14.   Install sound muffling curtains in patient areas divided by curtains
15.   Require incident reporting of all suspected policy violations or unauthorized access, disclosure, transfer, or modifications

Data from U.S. Department of Health and Human Services (HHS). (2005). *Understanding patient safety confidentiality.* Retrieved from http://www .hhs.gov/ocr/privacy/psa/understanding/index.html; California Nurses Association (CNA). (2011). HIPAA—The Health Insurance Portability and Accountability Act: What RNs need to know about privacy rules and protected electronic health information. *National Nurse, 107*(6), 20–27.

▶ Use of PHI In Marketing, Fund-Raising, and Research

The HIPAA of 1996 requires that authorization be given before PHI can be used in marketing. Marketing is defined as communications that encourage a person to purchase a product or service. Face-to-face communication or gifts of nominal value provided by the covered entity do not require authorization. However, the HITECH Act of 2009 strengthened the marketing restrictions (DHHS, 2005; Rinehart-Thompson, 2013).

Disclosure of PHI to a foundation associated with the covered entity for purposes of fund-raising is allowed. The privacy notice has to indicate that such use is possible and has to contain an option for the patient to be removed from the solicitation. The HITECH Act also strengthened the provisions related to fund-raising (DHHS, 2013a; Rinehart-Thompson, 2013).

The HIPAA regulations allow the use of patient information in research under defined conditions. The research must be reviewed by an institutional review board (IRB) and informed consents provided to the research participants. In general, care cannot be contingent upon signing an authorization for research purposes. No authorization is required if the PHI is deidentified or if the research uses a limited data set (Rinehart-Thompson, 2013).

▶ Enforcement of Privacy and Security of PHI

The focus of enforcement is on entities such as healthcare plans and clearinghouses, providers who transmit health data, and Medicare prescription drug card sponsors. Individuals can be liable for conspiracy and aiding or abetting the disclosure of PHI. The DHHS can also exclude a provider or entity from participation in Medicare and Medicaid programs for violation of standards. Authority for the enforcement of privacy standards is shared by the DHHS, Office of Civil Rights, and the Centers for Medicaid and Medicare Services (CMS) (CNA, 2011; DHHS, 2005).

The American Recovery and Reinvestment Act of 2009 imposed civil monetary penalties if violations are not corrected within 30 days, with fines ranging from $100 to $50,000 per violation, with a $1.5 million cap annually (DHSS, 2013b). In 2005, the Department of Justice clarified that criminal penalties can be brought against individuals who knowingly (has knowledge of actions that are forbidden) violate, obtain, or disclose identifiable health information. The person can be fined up to $50,000 and sentenced to 1 year in prison. If someone obtains PHI under false pretense, the fine can be increased up to $100,000, with an accompanying sentence of up to 5 years in prison. If the intent is for commercial purposes or malicious harm, the fine may reach $250,000, accompanied by a 10-year prison sentence (CNA, 2011; DHHS, 2013a).

▶ Filing Complaints

If individuals believe their rights are being denied or that PHI is not protected, they can file a complaint. The complaint can be filed with the healthcare provider or insurer or with Health and Human Services (DHHS, 2013a).

The HIPAA privacy and security provisions were comprehensive; confidentiality of health information is now mandated by federal law. However, the legal requirements did not end with the HIPAA regulations. Two more laws were enacted to enhance the protection of an individual's health information.

Patient Safety and Quality Improvement Act of 2005 (PSQIA)

The PSQIA of 2005 created a voluntary system for reporting medical errors without fear of liability. The patient safety information is considered a "patient safety work product" and can be shared by HCPs and organizations within a protected legal environment, with a common goal of improving patient safety and quality of care. The law contains provisions for the establishment of **patient safety organizations (PSOs)**. A PSO can be public or private, for profit or not for profit. Insurance companies are not eligible to be designated as a PSO. The Agency for Healthcare Research and Quality is responsible for certifying, listing, and overseeing the PSOs (CNA, 2011; DHHS, 2008).

The PSOs are to receive reports of patients' events and safety concerns from HCPs and organizations, analyze the reports, and provide the results of the analysis to the organization or HCPs who originally reported the safety event or concern. Through analysis of the data, the PSOs can identify trends and patterns and propose measures to reduce risks of adverse events (DHHS, 2005).

The act established civil penalties for knowing or reckless confidentiality violations of patient safety. Enforcement of the act is the responsibility of the DHHS Office for Civil Rights. Civil penalties up to $11,000 per violation can be imposed (DHHS, 2005).

▶ Health Information Technology for Economic and Clinical Health (HITECH) Act

The HITECH Act is a section of the American Recovery and Reinvestment Act of 2009 that was enacted to stimulate the U.S. economy (DHHS, 2013a). The health information technology (health IT) industry was identified as an area that could not only stimulate the economy but could also improve healthcare delivery (Gialanella, 2012). The act established an Office of the National Coordinator for Health Information Technology (ONC). The ONC is to oversee the development of a national health IT infrastructure that will support the use and exchange of information. The goal of this infrastructure is to improve healthcare quality, reduce costs, promote public health, reduce health disparities, facilitate health research, and secure patient health information. Increasing the availability of health information is clearly related to the stated purposes of the law. Most EHRs enhance the ability to provide care with full knowledge of previous health history. This feature of EHRs can help to minimize duplication and promote care coordination among HCP and agencies and aid in the development and comparison of performance measures. However, enhanced access to health records through such a national system also requires additional security to protect the privacy of individuals (Gialanella, 2012).

The act establishes two national committees: the Policy Committee and the Standards Committee. The Policy Committee makes recommendations on implementation of the requirements of the law. The Standards Committee is charged with establishing standards for the electronic exchange of health information. The Policy Committee must have two HCPs as members, one of whom is a physician. There is no requirement for a nurse to be a member. There are no specified membership specialties for the Standards Committee (Gialanella, 2012). The regulations of the HITECH Act cover four areas shown in **BOX 6-5**.

Under the HIPAA of 1996, business associates were regulated under the agreements with covered entities. After the HITECH Act of 2009 was passed, business associates and subcontractors to business associates are under the jurisdiction of the HIPAA law and must comply with HIPAA security rules. Patient rights were expanded to include the right to obtain an electronic copy of PHI. If not available, then the individual has a right to hard copy (Doe, 2009; Freeman, 2013).

The requirements for obtaining authorization for marketing purposes were strengthened. Under HIPAA, the sale of PHI was not specifically prohibited, so provisions in the HITECH Act imposed restrictions on the sale of PHI. If remuneration is received by the covered entity from a manufacturer for use of PHI, authorization is required from the patient. Sharing PHI for fund-raising for the covered entity is allowed, but information provided to the patient must clearly state the opt-out option. Treatment cannot be withheld if the authorization is not given or if the patient chooses to opt out (Doe, 2009; Freeman, 2013).

The law changed the requirement of a reportable breach. Following a breach, a **risk assessment** must be conducted by the covered entity. A breach is presumed unless there is a low probability that PHI has been compromised following a risk assessment. The required risk assessment includes an assessment of the PHI involved, the person who used or to whom the PHI was disclosed, whether the PHI was actually viewed, and the extent of the risk (Freeman, 2013).

Enforcement Activities

The Office for Civil Rights within the Department of Health and Human Services has responsibility for enforcement of HIPAA's civil penalties. Under the HITECH Act, state attorneys general now have authority to investigate HIPAA violations and can impose civil penalties of up to $25,000 (Gialanella, 2012; Vanderpool, 2012). Civil actions are most commonly the result of complaints from individuals (Vanderpool, 2012). Examples of civil cases are loss of patient

---

BOX 6-5 Regulations of the HITECH Act

1. Modify HIPAA regulations to make BA directly liable for compliance with HIPAA regulations, to limit the use of PHI for marketing and fund-raising purposes, and to allow individuals to receive electronic copies of PHI.
2. Establish increased, tiered civil money penalties.
3. Establish an objective breach standard.
4. Prohibit health plans from using or disclosing genetic information for underwriting purposes.

Reproduced from U.S. Department of Health and Human Services. (2013, January 25). Modifications to the HIPAA Privacy, Security, Enforcement, and Breach Notification Rules under the Health Information Technology for Economic and Clinical Health Act and the Genetic Information Nondiscrimination Act; other modifications to the HIPAA rules; final rule. *Federal Register, 78*(17).

records by an employee taking records home or a health plan failing to honor patient requests for access to their records. The criminal provisions now apply to individuals—not just to a covered entity. Criminal cases may involve accessing PHI for financial gain or for simple snooping. In a recent case, a physician and several hospital employees were individually fined and had to perform community service after inappropriately accessing records of a high-profile patient (Vanderpool, 2012).

Changes to Filing Complaints after Enactment of the HITECH Act

Complaints can be filed by anyone who thinks that a covered entity or a business associate has violated some aspect of the privacy or security rules. The complaint must be submitted to the Office of Civil Right office in writing—paper or electronically. The form and directions for use are available online and a link can be found in the companion website to this book.

▶ Unresolved Issues of Health Information

Rothstein (2012) notes that concerns about privacy continue to escalate as electronic storage, use, and transmission of health information expand. Individuals give permission to access personal records for many reasons; but individuals may have access to health information that has no relevance to a current condition or situation. For example, Rothstein questions whether an emergency physician treating a woman for a broken ankle needs to know her past sexual history. However, an insurance company would want to know her history of cervical cancer. Rothstein suggests that health records be "segmented" to grant appropriate access to a provider or an agency while protecting the privacy of the patient from inappropriate access. However, the

technical problems to implement a "segmented" approach are great and the costs are significant.

Concerns have also been identified about the penalties for violations (Sarrico & Hauenstein, 2011). Self-reporting in good faith, with actions for improvement may still result in costly fines. This can be especially devastating to individual providers such as physicians and nurse practitioners. Efforts to promote sharing of electronic health information may be hampered by strict enforcement and excessive fines. The unintended consequences of enforcement may be a reluctance to participate in health information exchanges.

Researchers have raised questions about the use of patient data for research purposes while maintaining compliance with privacy regulations (CNA, 2011). Researchers have reported drops in participation rates as a result of the implementation of HIPAA compliance consents and authorizations. Regulations from the HITECH Act have eased some of the requirements for researchers to enable patients to more easily authorize the use of PHI for research, but approaches to deidentify data that are effective and low cost are needed when authorization was not obtained or possible.

The field of telehealth is an area that poses many questions related to privacy. Hall and McGraw (2014) notes that home sensors or transmissions from an app or medical device can be a source of inappropriate transmission of personal information. Such information may be used in inappropriate ways in marketing or even criminal activity. If such events occur, public trust in telehealth would be compromised. Hall (2016) proposes that comprehensive federal regulations be developed and enforced in order to protect the public trust and enable telehealth to advance in ways that benefit the public.

The use of smartphones and social media (Facebook, Twitter, YouTube, and others) create new issues with PHI. Not only do covered entities need to have policies that employees follow, they must also consider what visitors, family members, and students might do to violate the

BOX 6-6 Case Study

Mindy Wheeler is a student nurse in her last semester of nursing school. She is working with a preceptor in a cardiothoracic intensive care unit. One day she has the opportunity to observe coronary bypass grafting from an enclosed theater. During the operation she was able to take pictures and later she posted them on Facebook. She did not provide the patient's name, but did give age, gender, and details of previous health history leading up to the need for a bypass surgery. She stated she was posting the information to encourage her friends to follow good health habits in order to avoid problems.

Check Your Understanding

1. Did Mindy violate ethical standards?
2. Did she violate HIPAA regulations? If so, in what way?
3. Is it likely there were hospital policies regarding her actions?
4. If you were the dean of the school, what would you do?

privacy of health information. Ekrem (2011) provides tips to avoid HIPAA violations using social media. The first and most important tip is to never post or tweet about patients, even in general terms. Other helpful tips include avoid mixing professional and personal lives in social media; do not complain about work online; and if the information should not be said in an elevator, it should not be posted using social media. **BOX 6-6** provides a case study about social media and PHI.

▶ Summary

Statutes and the associated regulations protecting privacy and confidentiality are detailed and include provisions beyond just the routine delivery of daily care. Organizations establish policies and technology restricting access to PHI to promote compliance with the regulations; however, details of the regulations may not always be covered completely in a policy. It is not a good idea for nurses to assume that they understand procedures for dealing with PHI; instead, questions about unique situations should be

© nednapa/Shutterstock

directed to the designated experts within the healthcare facility. Failure to adhere to ethical, legal, and policy expectations can result in severe penalties. A nurse may be terminated by the employer, the state board of nursing may take action against the nurse, and the patient may file a lawsuit against the nurse—all are possible negative effects of breaching confidentiality and privacy. The nurse is duty bound, professionally and legally, to know and adhere to confidentiality policies and procedures. Nurses must disclose information appropriately to ensure that care and continuity is promoted but should not share information with anyone who does not have a need to know. More information about law and regulations can be found in the companion website and in **TABLE 6-4**.

It is clear that protection of personal health information is complex and important. Today's laws and regulations will evolve and change as the technology changes, but the basic ethical standard for protecting privacy and confidentiality will not change. The challenge for all healthcare providers, including nurses, is to be aware of the need for privacy, to follow the policies currently in place, to keep abreast of changes, and to lead or participate in developing new approaches and guidelines for protecting privacy.

TABLE 6-4 Internet Resources to Understand Laws and Regulations About Protected Health Information

Resource	Internet Address
DHHS Health Information Privacy	http://www.hhs.gov/ocr/privacy/index.html
DHHS Guide to Privacy and Security of Health Information	http://www.healthit.gov/sites/default/files/pdf/privacy/privacy-and-security-guide.pdf
DHHS Health Information Privacy, Security, and Your EHR	http://www.healthit.gov/providers-professionals/ehr-privacy-security
Health Information Privacy Complaint	https://www.hhs.gov/hipaa/filing-a-complaint/index.html
Seven Tips to Avoid HIPAA Violations in Social Media	http://www.kevinmd.com/blog/2011/06/7-tips-avoid-hipaa-violations-social-media.html
National Council of State Boards of Nursing. *A Nurse's Guide to the Use of Social Media*	https://www.ncsbn.org/NCSBN_SocialMedia.pdf

References

American Hospital Association (AHA). (2003). *The patient care partnership: Understanding expectations, rights, and responsibilities*. American Hospital Association. Retrieved from http://www.aha.org/content/00-10/pcp_english_030730.pdf

American Nurses Association (ANA). (2015). *Code for nurses with interpretive statements*. Washington, DC: American Nurses Association Publishing. Retrieved from http://nursingworld.org/MainMenuCategories/EthicsStandards/CodeofEthicsforNurses/2110Provisions.html

Andersen, C. M. (2011). A primer for health care managers: Data sanitization, equipment disposal, and electronic waste. *Health Care Manager, 30*(3), 266–270.

Buckovich, S., Rippen, H., & Rozen, M. (1999). Driving toward guiding principles: A goal for privacy, confidentiality, and security of health information. *Journal of the American Medical Informatics Association, 6,* 122–133. doi: 10.1136/jamia.1999.0060122

California Nurses Association (CNA). (2011). HIPAA—the Health Insurance Portability and Accountability Act: What RNs need to know about privacy rules and protected electronic health information. *National Nurse, 107*(6), 20–27.

Crandell, D. (2013, May). Key provisions of the HIPAA final rule: Modifications of importance to physical therapists. *PT in Motion,* 38–41.

De Bord, J., Burke, W., & Dudzinski, D., (2013). Confidentiality, *Ethics in Medicine*, University of Washington School of Medicine.

Department of Health and Human Services (DHHS). (2005). *Understanding patient safety confidentiality*. Retrieved from http://www.hhs.gov/ocr/privacy/psa/understanding/index.html.

Department of Health and Human Services (DHHS). (2008). Patient Safety and Quality Improvement Act of 2005, *Federal Register, 73*(226). Retrieved from http://www.gpo.gov/fdsys/pkg/FR-2008-11-21/pdf/E8-27475.pdf

Department of Health and Human Services (DHHS). (2013a). *Health information privacy*. Retrieved from http://www.hhs.gov/ocr/privacy/hipaa/enforcement/examples/index.html

Department of Health and Human Services (DHHS). (2013b). Modifications to the HIPAA Privacy, Security, Enforcement, and Breach Nortification Rules under the Health Information Technology for Economic and Clinical Health Act and the Genetic Information Discrimination Act; other modificaiton to the HIPAA rules; final rule, *Federal Register, 78*(17). Retrieved from http://www.gpo.gov/fdsys/pkg/FR-2013-01-25/pdf/2013 -01073.pdf

Doe, J. (2009). HITECH meets HIPAA HITECH Act: Changes to HIPAA obligations for covered entities and business associates. *Journal of Health Information Management, 23*(4), 15–16.

Ekrem, D. (2011). 7 tips to avoid HIPAA violations in social media. Retrieved from http://www.kevinmd .com/blog/2011/06/7-tips-avoid-hipaa-violations-social -media.html

Freeman, G. (2013). Final HIPAA rule increases penalties, liability for associates. *Healthcare Risk Management, 35*(3), 25–27.

Gialanella, K. M. (2012). Legislative aspects of nursing informatics: HITECH and HIPAA. In D. McGonigle & K. G. Mastrian (Eds.), *Nursing informatics and the foundation of knowledge* (2nd ed.). Burlington, MA: Jones & Barlett Learning.

Hall, J., & McGraw, D. (2014). For telehealth to succeed, privacy and security risks must be identified and addressed. *Health Affairs, 33*(2), 216–221. Retrieved from https://elib.uah.edu/login?url=http://search.proquest .com/docview/1498231612?accountid=14476

Karasz, H. N., Eiden, A., & Bogan, S. (2013). Text messaging to communicate with public health audiences: How the HIPAA security rule affects practice. *American Journal of Public Health, 103*(4), 617–622. doi: http://dx.doi .org/10.2105/10AJPH.2012.300999

McGowan, C. (2012). Patients' confidentiality. *Critical Care Nurse, 32*(5), 61–65. doi: http://dx.doi.org/10.4037/ccn2012135

Morris, K. (2013, March/April). Sing a song of HIPAA. *Ohio Nurses Review,* 12–14. Retrieved from http:// www.ohnurses.org.

Muller, L. (2014). HIPAA compliance tips. *Professional Case Management, 19*(4),191–193. doi: 10.1097/NCM .0000000000000045

Reber, E. (2011). Five steps to achieving HIPAA compliance. *Biomedical Instrumentation & Technology, 45*(5), 360–363. doi: 10.2345/0899-8205-45.5.360

Rinehart-Thompson, L. A. (2013). *Introduction to health information privacy and security.* Chicago, IL: American Health Information Management Association Press.

Rothstein, M. A. (2012). Currents in contemporary bioethics. *Journal of Law, Medicine & Ethics, 40*(2), 394–400. doi: 10.1111/j.1748-720X.2012.00673.x

Sarrico, C., & Hauenstein, J. (2011). Can EHRs and HIEs get along with HIPAA security requirements? *Healthcare Financial Management, 65*(2), 86–90.

Vanderpool, D. (2012). Risk management: HIPAA—should I be worried? *Innovations in Clinical Neuroscience, 9*(11/12), 30–55.

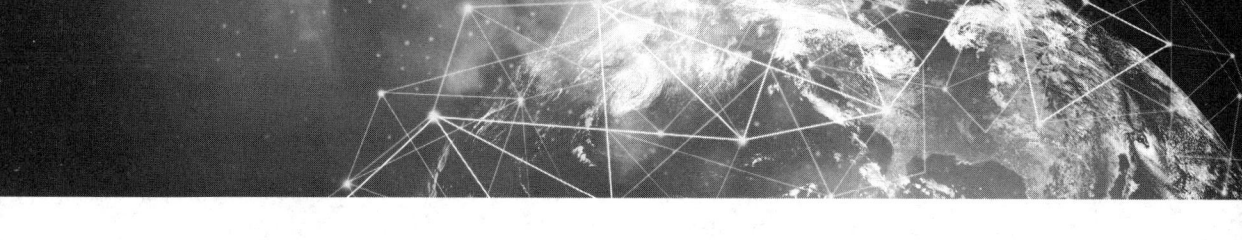

© nednapa/Shutterstock

CHAPTER 7

Database Systems for Healthcare Applications

Manil Maskey, MS
Susan Alexander, DNP, RN, ANP-BC, ADM-BC
Gennifer Baker, DNP, RN, CCNS

LEARNING OBJECTIVES

1. Comprehend concepts used to describe databases.
2. Review tools used to work with databases.
3. Describe examples of how databases can be used in healthcare settings.

KEY TERMS

Data warehouse
Database
Database management system (DBMS)
Embedded relational database
Flat database model
Form

Indexes
Integrity rules
Open source relational database
Proprietary relational database
Query

Read operation
Redundancy of data
Relational database model
Reports
Structured query language (SQL)

▶ Chapter Overview

Databases have become an essential part of everyday life, and people constantly interact with databases though they may be unaware of the interaction. Have you checked your email today? Ordered a new book from Amazon? Used Google to find the closest pizza restaurant? All of these common activities are examples of database interactions. Healthcare applications also rely heavily on databases, and the technology used to create and maintain them has made tremendous strides in the recent past. In caring for patients, nurses will have daily encounters with databases. Increased understanding about how these tools are built and used can help nurses realize the importance of these interactions in patient care. In this chapter, the basics of database systems and their components are introduced. Applications of databases in healthcare delivery systems are also reviewed.

▶ Using Databases in Healthcare Settings

Background knowledge relating to the design, implementation, and use of databases is useful for nurses in helping to understand the need for accuracy in collection and entry of content into the databases. A **database** is a term used to describe a collection of related data, ranging in size from a few entries in a Microsoft Excel spreadsheet, to the complex relational databases needed in business and retail. In healthcare communities, databases may be used by medical personnel for tasks such as the recording of patient care, patient diagnoses and treatment plans, medications, and for progress toward treatment goals. Healthcare researchers also use databases to answer complex questions, such as assessing the incidence and prevalence of disease or the efficacy of pharmacologic treatments or clinical procedures. A **database management system (DBMS)** is a set of software that enables users to create and maintain a database (**FIGURE 7-1**).

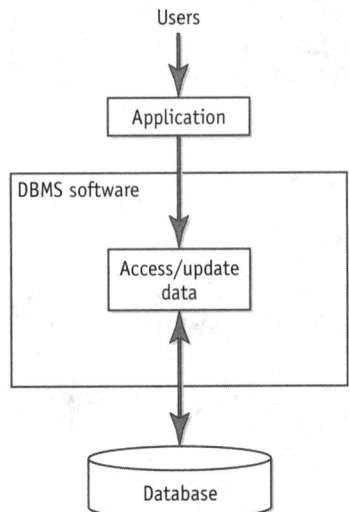

FIGURE 7-1 Elements of database design and management.

Consider a simple example of a database that might be used in a healthcare setting structured to store data about patient demographics, medical histories, and medication use (**FIGURE 7-2**).

In Figure 7-2, the database is created using columnar storage to organize three types of data: Patient, Medical History, and Medications. Precise terms are used to identify aspects of the data structure. A *table* is defined as an individual level of columnar storage. Each column in a table is a *field*. A *field* describes a particular attribute of a record (a row in a table). Records that have a relationship to each other, such as the fields in Figure 7-2, require the use of links in order to be manipulated correctly for analysis. For example, the patient records in the Patient table are related to Medical History and Medication tables. The records in the Patient table are linked to records in the Medical History table using Patient ID fields. Similarly, the records in the Medical History table are linked to records in the Medication table using Patient ID and Observation ID fields. Using the field links increases the ways in which data within the fields can be examined to answer a clinical question.

The manipulation of databases involves reading and updating the data in the tables. A specific

Patient

Name	Patient ID	DOB
Jason Smith	12	2012-12-01
Pat Hines	34	1979-02-28

Medical History

Patient ID	Observation ID	Observation Date	Diagnosis
12	3	2013-03-05	Infection
34	5	2012-12-24	Flu

Medication

Patient ID	Observation ID	Prescription
12	3	Amoxicillin
34	5	Tamiflu

FIGURE 7-2 Structure of a database used in a healthcare setting.

question is prepared as a **read operation**. An example of a read operation could be "all patients who are older than 4 years old and have been diagnosed with the flu." These kinds of questions, or read operations, can be easily and precisely constructed using **structured query language (SQL)**. SQL is the language used to communicate with databases and is considered to be the standard language used in working with relational databases. Though detailed instruction in the use of SQL, a computer language with many elements, is not within the scope of this textbook, it is helpful to understand that when an end user works with a database, virtually any task that is accomplished is done using SQL. Two common examples of SQL elements are queries and statements. Answering a clinical question about numbers of patients who were diagnosed with flu could be performed using a SQL query. End users who interact with databases, such as in entering vital signs or other details of patient information, are altering the database by using a SQL statement. Depending on the structure of the database, SQL statements can create permanent alterations.

Advantages of Using Databases

There are numerous advantages to using databases. Large amounts of data can be stored efficiently,

without taking up large amounts of disk space. Data may be easily discoverable when stored in a database, and database operations are frequently optimized to create a fast response for the user. The use of a common language such as SQL simplifies data interactions and the ease of importing/exporting and modification by other software applications. Use of SQL can also allow for simultaneous access of the database by multiple software applications.

In healthcare settings, the ubiquitous use of databases has offered a mechanism for conducting daily tasks in accounting and billing, and it has facilitated long-term storage and maintenance of patient information (histories, medications, and similar items), while enabling an efficient exchange of patient information between healthcare providers (HCPs). Databases can also be used to develop patient care applications and for research purposes.

Models of Databases Used in Healthcare Settings

Database designs can be classified into two main models: flat and relational. In a **flat database model**, only one table is used, and the attributes are defined as separate columns of the table. In a **relational database model**, a collection of tables is used and linked together by relationships between attributes within the separate tables and/or operations within the tables (see **BOX 7-1**).

While a flat database can be simple to construct, its use can be problematic if data from two (or more) databases need to be merged. When using flat databases, one may add information as necessary without affecting existing data because there is no relationship between the attributes within the flat database. This can be both an advantage and disadvantage of using flat databases.

BOX 7-1 Case Study

Mavanea has worked for the past 7 years on a medical-surgical floor. Because of her exceptional skills in initiating intravenous access (IVs), Mavanea is often called upon to assist in situations when patients have experienced multiple failed attempts by other staff members to start IVs. Mavanea's skills, and those of other nurses in the facility, have been noted by nurse leaders, and efforts to create an IV team have started. Because charting in the facility is hybrid (a mix of paper and electronic methods), documentation of the workflow surrounding IVs requires thoughtful attention to user experiences and workflow. Mavanea is appointed to participate in a team that is designated to create a new electronic IV charting pathway that will reflect desired outcomes. A flow form, or an electronic template used to chart data and clinical findings, would be used as the basis of the IV charting pathway.

Mavanea understands the need to collect and aggregate data on multiple elements per patient, such as advanced techniques used in the placement of difficult IV starts and the size and length of IV catheters used to access deeper veins. Using a proprietary relational database, an IV charting pathway is designed for efficient capture of the IV team's activities. Fields in the database have preprogrammed entries, appearing as drop-down boxes, preventing the entry of free text and minimizing error, while increasing the charting speed by the staff. For example, one field contains all possibilities of IV catheter sizes, while another contains anatomical sites for IV starts. The IV team enters data into the fields by using a form, which is often visually easier to manipulate than the data tables.

Other embedded capabilities of the relational database make the IV charting pathway useful for nurse leaders. For example, the reporting or query function can be used to generate data on specific team members, such as in validating the daily activities of the team member. Effects on outcomes are reflected in continuity of care, provider satisfaction, patient satisfaction, and financial outcomes. The electronic charting coupled with a hand-off communication report at shift change ensures the continuity of care for the patients who receive IV team services.

After reviewing data from the IV start team, it was noted that a medical/surgical unit called upon the team 35% more than any other unit in the facility. Further investigation showed that the nursing staff turnover on the medical/surgical unit had increased over the past 3 months, and that many recent hires were new graduates with little experience in initiating intravenous access. In an effort to improve education for the new graduates, the IV start team decided to create a module of basic information, covering topics including facility policies on initiation of IV access, tips on how to start an IV on patients with "difficult" veins, and proper use of vein visualization devices. The module included the content as well as posttest questions to validate understanding. The module was loaded into the facility's LMS and assigned to the new RN graduates on the medical/surgical unit with a completion deadline set at 3 weeks. After the new nurses completed the module, IV team charting data were reviewed at 4-, 8-, and 12-week intervals. A clinically significant decrease in calls to the IV team was seen across the time frame. Based on the success of the module completion and decreased numbers of calls to the IV team, nursing leadership decided to add the training to the training curriculum for new RN hires.

(continues)

BOX 7-1 Case Study (*Continued*)

Information collected in databases, which occurred with consistent use of the IV charting pathway, can be important in planning for future patient care. Data trends can be identified and proactively used to address patient needs as well as staff training needs. Reports may validate the decreased utilization of more invasive infusion catheters, which in turn can minimize the occurrence of catheter-related bloodstream infections. In the case study, important outcomes included lower overall turnover rates (and the cost savings associated with RN turnover) to the healthcare organization, increased patient satisfaction, increased employee satisfaction, and validation of the IV team's worth in its role with value-based purchasing.

Check Your Understanding
1. What pieces of data could be added to a charting database that would assist leadership in identifying opportunities for improvement in utilizing the IV start team?
2. What are examples of best practices regarding addition of data collection elements to databases to improve uniformity and retrieval?
3. In your experience, what opportunities have you observed for process improvement by initiation or revision of data collection methods that could positively influence patient care outcomes?

Relational databases are frequently the preferred solution for settings in which long-term data storage and manipulation is needed. The design of relational databases may be quite complex and require planning by multiple software engineers and other disciplines to consider the implication of various decisions within the design process. For example, **redundancy of data**, or the repetition of a field in two or more places in a database, is a phenomenon that can lead to error and eventual loss of storage space. Using a relational database can minimize redundancy of data, but care must be taken to store data in tables in such a way that the relationships between the fields are logical. Building a relational database requires overarching knowledge of how its data will be used to establish an effective design for users. The relational model describes organization of the data in terms of structure, integrity, query, manipulation, and storage. Most database design is dominated by the relational model, which has many aspects discussed later in this chapter.

▶ Working with Databases

Types of Relational Databases

There are three primary relational database systems: proprietary, open source, and embedded.

Proprietary relational databases are licensed by vendors. Frequently, proprietary relational databases provide a robust set of management tools that includes creation of a **data warehouse** (described later in this chapter). Proprietary databases are often packaged into software suites, such as Microsoft Office, which can include the Access DBMS. Other proprietary relational database systems include Oracle and Teradata. These databases allow for computation, networking, and storage simultaneously by multiple users. **Open source relational databases**, such as MySQL (http://www.mySQL.com) and PostGIS (http://postgis.net), are available for use without charge by users. Databases can also be embedded into a larger DBMS, and coded such that an end user might be able to access a specific data point while the larger database remains hidden. Known as **embedded relational databases**, this type of relational database is frequently packaged as a part of other software or hardware applications. For example, local databases used by a mobile application to store phone numbers can be considered an embedded relational database. Application vendors provide packaged databases along with the application that can manipulate the database structure.

Depending on their needs, healthcare applications may use propriety, embedded, or open source relational databases. Large healthcare enterprises tend to use proprietary relational databases owing to their needs for customization and support. Smaller healthcare facilities may prefer open source relational databases owing to their lower cost. However, more and more HCPs are also using the embedded relational databases owing to popularity of mobile applications.

Relationships Within the Database

During the design of a relational database, it is necessary to first create a conceptual model of the data and its relationships. The entity-relationship (ER) model is frequently used to visually describe the data and their relationships (**FIGURE 7-3**). The ER model describes data as entities, relationships, and attributes (**FIGURE 7-4**). An entity is the basic component in an ER model, representing an object or a thing. Properties of the entity are known as attributes. Attributes describe the entity. A patient could be considered an entity, with the patient's name and date of birth as patient attributes. In an ER model, attributes from one entity refer to attributes from another entity and are represented as relationships. Knowledge and consideration

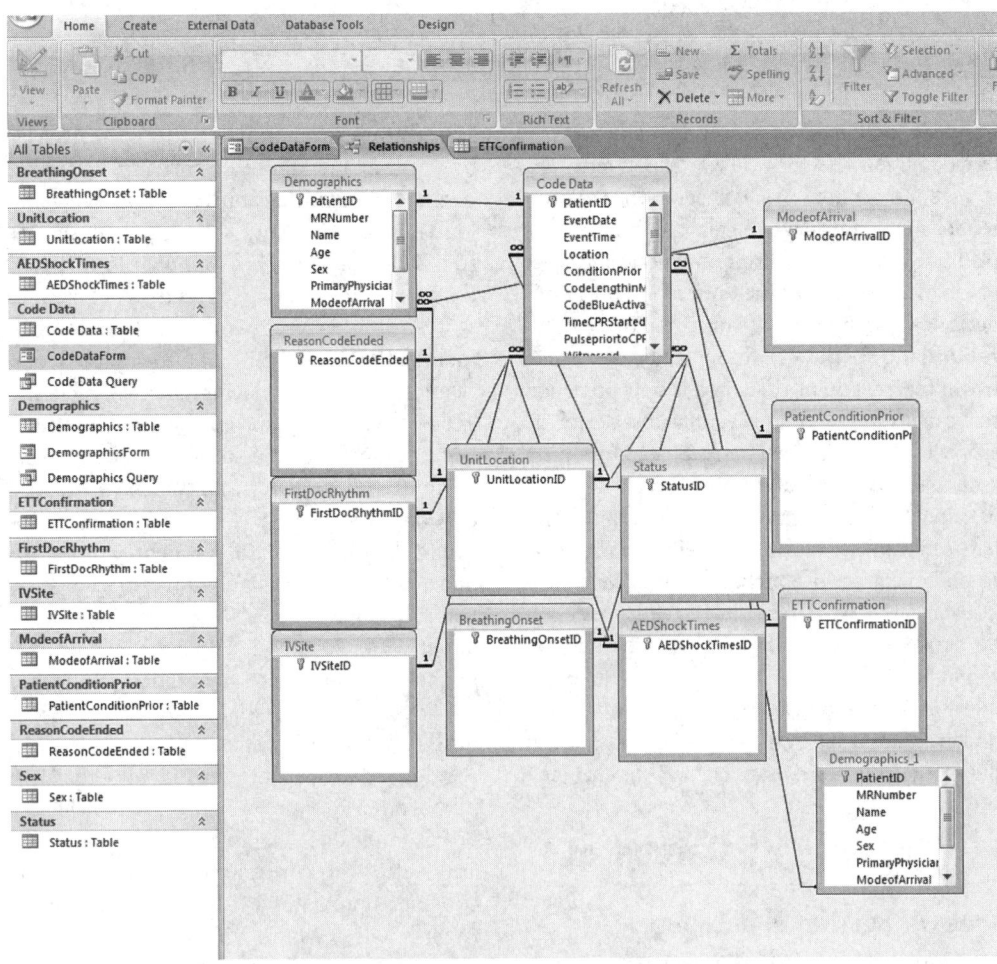

FIGURE 7-3 Illustration of relationships created in a proprietary relational database software application.

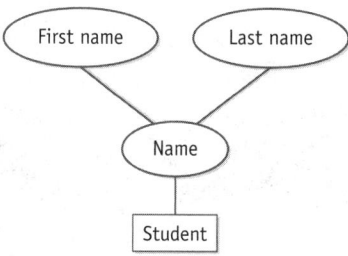

FIGURE 7-4 ER model used to describe the relationship between first name, last name, and student in a relational database.

Copyright © 2002, Dr. Angela B. Shiflet. Reprinted by permission.

of these relationships are vital to the design of successful databases and software applications.

Elements of Relational Databases

Query

A **query** is a SQL element (or operation) that is used to retrieve and update data from a database table. SQL standardizes the ways to perform such operations on various types of relational databases. Relational databases allow the user to predefine certain record fields as keys or indexes, perform an efficient search, join records, and establish integrity constraints. Queries then utilize the predefined record fields, known as the **indexes**, to perform specific operations for the user. Search queries are faster and more accurate when based on indexed values. Join queries are used to join records from multiple tables using indexed fields that are common to each table. Think of a query as a tool designed to rapidly retrieve needed data from the database. For example, a basic search query might include a list of pediatric patients who are younger than 6 years old.

Reports

Relational databases typically offer preconstructed mechanisms used for rapid retrieval and display of selected data fields, called **reports**. Compared to flat database designs, relational databases offer more robust reporting

systems that use embedded report generators to filter and display data. Applications with embedded relational databases may also offer the user the capability to build customized reporting modules. A table can be constructed and linked to data sources for multiple reports. Keeping tables up to date in relational databases makes it possible to present well-organized information in attractive formats for quick reporting. Many situations can be identified in healthcare settings in which the need for quick reports exists. For example, it would be useful in a pediatrics office to be able to generate a report illustrating a growth chart for an infant to document whether the infant is following a typical growth pattern.

Forms

The traditional interface used in databases to offer a simple visual mechanism for users to insert new data into relational databases is called a **form** (**FIGURE 7-5**). For example, at a clinic, a receptionist may need to add information on a new patient into the patient database. An advanced form can be constructed that will complete data fields based on historically filled data fields, or drop-down choices can be added. Almost all HCPs use some variation of forms to enter information into their databases.

Integrity and Security

Relational databases allow the enforcement of **integrity rules**, designed to protect the validity of the data. For example, if entity integrity is enforced, then every record will have its own specific identity and there will be no duplicated records. Referential integrity is defined using "primary" and "foreign" keys, which are fields in tables that act as links (relationships) between tables. When properly defined, these keys prevent inconsistent deletions or updates. Healthcare databases require data integrity and security. In fact, because healthcare databases store patient information, there is a need for more rigorous protection of the database. Incorrect information presented to clinicians may lead to

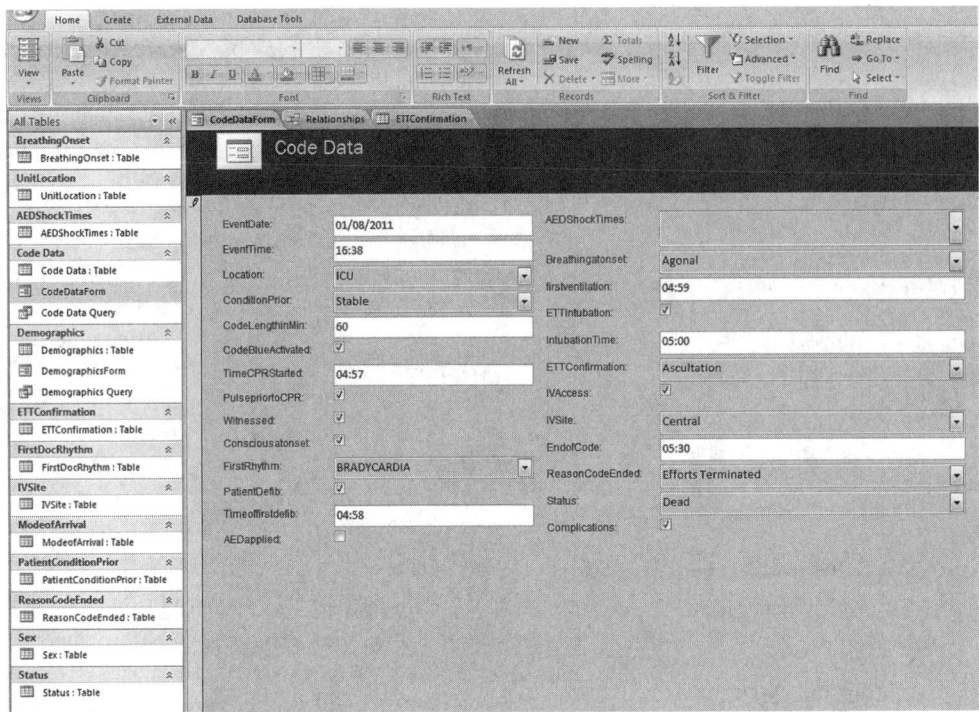

FIGURE 7-5 Example of a form that can be created using a proprietary relational database application.

misdiagnosis, incorrect treatment, and negative outcomes, including the death of patients. Many regulations govern the security of health-related patient information.

▶ Creating a Warehouse for Managing Multiple Datasets

Data Warehouses

Data warehouses are distinguished by their design and optimization with attention to specific applications (Elmasri & Navathe, 2003). A data warehouse consists of several components (**FIGURE 7-6**). The data source layer includes various databases with which users and applications interact. Implementations of the data warehouse may also contain data sources that

include data from external sources. The data that are extracted from various sources are designed to provide specific functionalities and form the structure of the data warehouse. Decision-support systems are used in the warehouse to provide specific analyses, reports, mining, and other processing that users seek from the data. In a data warehouse, queries are optimized to provide efficient access to data for analysis, reporting, and mining. Data warehouses designed to store and use data summaries and snapshots are unlike databases that store records in tables. For example, a data warehouse of a healthcare system may keep aggregated data values of all its patient records.

Often, data warehouses involve executing data analysis queries from various data sources; thus, those data analysis queries are optimized for performance and efficiency.

In a healthcare setting, each HCP may store patients' electronic health records in a

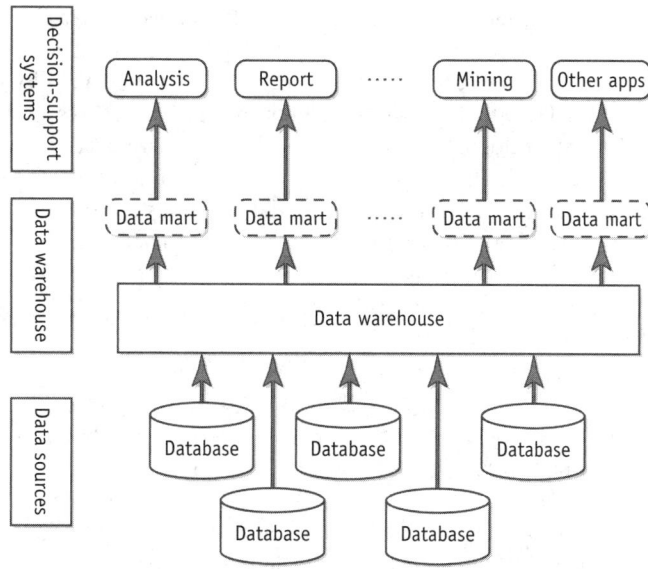

FIGURE 7-6 Elements in a typical data warehouse.

database. Such a database would be sufficient for the daily business of a small clinic. Imagine that data analysts at the Centers for Disease Control and Prevention (CDC) might want to import information relating to the treatment of influenza cases from private HCPs into a data warehouse in order to determine trends or mine for a specific event relating to influenza treatment. A data warehouse would be created, containing aggregated data from many different HCPs, in order to better understand events surrounding an outbreak of influenza. Data warehouses are increasingly finding uses in health care for tasks such as financial negotiations and comparisons, assurance of quality, achieving criteria for Meaningful Use certification, and tracking items such as electronic health record access log-ins.

Designing Data Warehouses

In general, data warehouses consist of several components but are characterized by the transmission of data to the warehouse from operational databases and other sources (Sen & Sinha, 2005, Figure 1). The design of the data

warehouse should always include the flexibility to allow for the inclusion of new databases or data marts that may be needed in the future. At the bottom of the data warehouse are operational databases, where data are updated by various sources. From the warehouse itself, specific "views" of the data warehouse are designed to provide the data needed for analyses, reports, and mining activities. Periodic summaries and reports, along with ad hoc analyses, are common functionalities that data warehouse applications provide.

Perhaps one of the great examples to date of construction of an application-driven data warehouse has been a 15-month project involving the tracking of nursing-sensitive care outcomes sponsored by the National Quality Forum (NQF, 2007). The intent of this landmark project was to describe and evaluate nurses' contributions in acute care hospitals to patient safety, healthcare quality, and professionalism in the work environment. The project used various strategies for data collection, including abstraction from electronic health records directly to the project databases, semistructured telephone interviews of project participants, and web-based surveys to gather perceptions from hospital nurses and nurse leaders on the contribution of the nursing workforce to patient safety and other outcomes. Despite the obvious importance of the nursing workforce to patient outcomes in hospitals, respondents identified barriers to adoption of NQF standards for the measurement of the quality of nursing care in hospitals, including the lack of a business case for the implementation of measurement and support by hospital administrators (NQF, 2007). Stakeholders hope that ongoing maintenance and updating of the NQF data warehouse will help to determine priorities for future research and priorities for consensus setting to promote widespread adoption of NQF standards.

As analysis of the data in the NQF warehouse continues to progress, other authors hope that this will yield specific recommendations that the nursing profession can adopt to inspire trust in the care that it provides to U.S. citizens. Kurtzman and Jennings (2008, p. 353) have proposed an agenda that includes:

- Identification of measures that quantify nurses' contributions to patient safety and quality outcomes
- Use of performance assessments derived from those measures in daily clinical management
- Regular benchmarking for hospitals' nursing quality goals
- Public reporting of nursing quality measures to key stakeholders and communities

Research in database technology is ongoing. Recent developments include the introduction of NoSQL ("Not only SQL") databases. NoSQL databases come in various flavors, each addressing a particular issue with relational databases. For example, MongoDB (http://www.mongodb.org) is a document-based database system that is very easy to use and has looser consistency in terms of relations than relational databases do. Cassandra (http://cassandra.apache.org), a database system that is designed to address performance and scalability, is another example of a new database system.

With the ever-increasing amount of healthcare data and policy changes toward mandating electronic records, scalability and performance of the relational databases will be tested. Furthermore, new and innovative devices that monitor patients' every activity will produce a different set of data relationships that may not be addressed by relational databases.

A Well-Known Example of a Data Warehouse

The Healthcare Cost and Utilization Project (HCUP), supported by the Agency for Healthcare Research and Quality (AHRQ), is a set of databases (and tools for use) comprising the largest ongoing longitudinal collection of data related to hospitalizations within the United States (AHRQ, 2017). Beginning with its initial construction and collection of data in 1988, HCUP databases combine the contributions of multiple databases describing inpatient hospital discharges, emergency department visits, hospital readmissions, and pediatric population healthcare data from 48 states across the country. HCUP partners, which may be state agencies, private healthcare data organizations, and others, transmit their state databases annually to HCUP, where analysts work to standardize data into robust tables available for use by healthcare researchers. Objectives of HCUP include the maintenance of multilevel healthcare data, including offering mechanisms for its analysis to improve decision making in health care and its delivery.

HCUP is a robust data warehouse, containing multiple tools allowing interested users to conduct queries, monitor healthcare quality measures, or use data for statistical analyses. HCUPnet is an online tool offering rapid, highly customizable queries of data about health statistics and use of inpatient and emergency department services. Users are able to find downloadable software applications and user guides using the AHRQ Quality Indicators tool that may be used in measuring their own hospital data against national quality indicators. Statistical reporting often requires the aggregation of procedures' diagnoses into meaningful elements. The Clinical Classifications Software application is freely available for downloading and can be integrated into statistical reporting applications.

▶ Applications in Healthcare Settings

While the primary job responsibility of newly graduated nurses may not be to design databases for use in healthcare facilities, it is important to recall that the chances of nurses interacting with databases in almost any variety of healthcare setting are great. The accurate entry of data into an electronic health record is arguably the most basic responsibility of any nurse and may likely represent the initial exposure of the new graduate to a database. In this section of the chapter, selected models of nurses' utilization of relational databases in aspects of patient care activities are reviewed.

Customizing Relational Databases for the Smaller Practice Setting

Relational databases can be customized to meet the needs of healthcare facilities and practices of many sizes. A small, private practice in the Southeastern United States replaced its flat database with a relational database, developed using Microsoft Access, a proprietary software package, for long-term maintenance of patient data in its outpatient diabetes self-management training program (Alexander, Frith, O'Keefe, & Hennigan, 2011). In the diabetes program, retrieval of accurate patient demographic data at 6- and 12-month intervals following initial class attendance was tied to program revenues. Variability and errors contained in the flat database had resulted in reduced revenues for the program. Implementation of the relational database required training for the practice staff, but it resulted in improved accuracy in data entry, when practice staff were surveyed (Alexander et al., 2011). Use of the relational database was reported as an economical solution to meet the long-term data storage needs of the program because costs for the purchase and installation of the software, plus staff training, were only slightly more than half of budgeted amounts.

Improving Nurse–Patient Staffing Ratios

Nurse staffing ratios, the number of nurses relative to the number of patients on a given unit, are a source of concern to patients and caregivers. In 2009 the American Nurses Association acknowledged that "the appropriate skill mix and number of registered nurses engaged in direct patient care is necessary to provide safe nursing care" (p. 4). However, such a determination can be difficult to identify, and it can change on a daily basis as nursing staff fluctuates. Retrospective analysis of data collected over months and years is often insufficient to assist a nurse manager in making real-time staffing decisions. To better characterize the relationships among nursing skill mix, the numbers of registered nurses, and patient data, researchers at an urban hospital in the Northeast United States created the Patient–Nurse Database (Radwin, Cabral, Chen, & Jennings, 2010). Using Microsoft Access, researchers created nine separate databases (five with patient data; four with nurse data) and merged them to form the Patient–Nurse Database, designed to better track patient care processes and outcomes over an 18-month period on a hematology-oncology floor. Researchers found that use of the database was effective in capturing the daily variability unique to the unit's staff and patients, also suggesting that the database and its data-capture protocol could easily be expanded to other units, such as surgical or cardiac floors, where a similar need for real-time staffing management is necessary based on census and nurse skill mix (Radwin et al., 2010).

Using Automated Systems for Nurse Competencies

Learning management systems (LMS) are relational databases that provide educational services for users, including registration, routing, and reporting (Dumpe, Kanyok, & Hill, 2007). Traditionally used in academic settings, the use of LMS has rapidly expanded to fields such as business and health care. In facility-based nursing education, where administrators struggle to maintain the competencies of nurses with variable schedules and needs, LMS can offer an economical and easily accessible solution for employers and employees. In 2003, the Cleveland Clinic Foundation partnered with the Division of Education at the Foundation in order to create an online curriculum, delivered via an LMS, that would educate all employees on the Health Insurance Portability and Accountability Act (HIPAA) and patient confidentiality. The LMS was subsequently expanded to include options such as customized assignments based on job functions, staff surveys, reporting to supervisors and human resource personnel, and automatic scoring of quizzes for tracking of progress. Use of the LMS represented cost savings for the Division of Nursing due to a reduction in overtime related to competency assessments for personnel and the use of nursing education personnel needed to complete the competency assessments (Dumpe et al., 2007).

The Virtual Dashboard

The Collaborative Alliance for Nursing Outcomes (CALNOC) is a coalition of acute care hospitals and is the largest nurse quality reporting network in the United States (Aydin, Bolton, Donaldson, Brown, & Mukerji, 2008). To date, CALNOC has 15 years of data from more than 1,700 nursing units in nine states. The CALNOC system is a secure, multi-tier, web-based system that consists of two major subsystems: a membership-management application containing demographic information for member hospitals and employees and a data-analysis application where data are stored, analyzed, and reported to CALNOC members. Member facilities submit data in spreadsheets using applications such as Microsoft Excel. Various types of reports can subsequently be generated from CALNOC data, and the reports can be drilled down to specific hospitals or units for benchmarking of performance. This reporting capacity is unique in that member hospitals can create their own virtual dashboards containing selected performance measures to meet their needs for projects such as performance initiatives, goal setting, or root cause analysis (Aydin et al., 2008).

Nursing Quality Benchmarks as Clinical Dashboards

The power of databases can truly be demonstrated when used to improve care for patients. Pressure ulcers and patient falls are two conditions that have been identified as key indicators of nursing care quality in hospitals by the NQF. In further study of the potential utility of the CALNOC databases, Donaldson, Brown, Aydin, Bolton, and Rutledge (2005) reported on a project designed to transform data analysis into useful information. Pressure ulcers and patient falls are examples of nurse-sensitive quality measures; NQF has recommended that all hospitals collect data on these measures (NQF, 2007). One CALNOC site decided to transform its own data on patient falls and pressure ulcers into an internal performance improvement project by adding these clinical benchmarks to its virtual dashboard. The addition of data on these indicators aided the facility in quickly evaluating baseline performance measurement across its specific units. In subsequent data analysis, Donaldson and colleagues (2005) found that half of the patients who developed pressure ulcers during inpatient stays at the facility were found to be "at risk" upon admission. The authors further noted that a quarter of the patient falls in the facilities occurred in critical care/step-down units, which are areas traditionally associated with closer patient monitoring and reduced fall risk. The facility was able to implement highly specific performance-improvement activities and use the clinical dashboards in ongoing follow up of the activities.

▶ Summary

Nurses, as part of the larger healthcare community, can benefit from knowledge about the uses of databases in healthcare settings. Though there is a learning curve in designing and integrating customized relational databases into practice; many common software applications that use relational databases hide complicated steps and make it easier for HCPs to use these types of databases. Although relational databases and data warehouses seem to be the ideal solution for healthcare applications, the increasing volume of healthcare data that are collected will influence the needs for new types of applications and analyses of such data. To support these new applications and analyses, systems that complement relational databases will need to be developed.

References

Agency for Healthcare Research and Quality. (2017). Overview of HCUP. Retrieved from https://www.hcup-us.ahrq.gov/overview.jsp

Alexander, S., Frith, K. H., O'Keefe, L., & Hennigan, M. A. (2011). Implementation of customized health information technology in diabetes self-management programs. *Clinical Nurse Specialist, 25*(2), 63–70. doi: 10.1097/NUR.0b013e31820aefd600002800-201103000-00005

American Nurses Association. (2009). Position statement: Rights of registered nurses when considering a patient assignment. Retrieved from http://nursingworld.org/rnrightsps

Aydin, C., Bolton, L., Donaldson, N., Brown, D., & Mukerji, A. (2008). Beyond nursing quality measurement: The nation's first regional nursing virtual dashboard. In R. Hughes (Ed.), *Patient safety and quality: An evidence-based handbook for nurses.* Rockville, MD: Agency for Healthcare Research and Quality. Retrieved from http://www.ahrq.gov/qual/nurseshdbk/

Donaldson, N., Brown, D., Aydin, C., Bolton, M., & Rutledge, D. (2005). Leveraging nurse-related dashboard benchmarks to expedite performance improvement and document excellence. *Journal of Nursing Administration, 35*(4), 163–172.

Dumpe, M. L., Kanyok, N., & Hill, K. (2007). Use of an automated learning management system to validate nursing competencies. *Journal for Nurses in Staff Development, 23*(4), 183–185. doi: 10.1097/01.NND.0000281418.50472.2e

Elmasri, R., & Navathe, S. (2003). *Fundamentals of database systems* (4th ed.). Boston, MA: Addison-Wesley Longman.

Kurtzman, E., & Jennings, B. M. (2008). Trends in transparency: Nursing performance measurement and reporting. *Journal of Nursing Administration, 38*(7/8), 349–354.

National Quality Forum. (2007). *Tracking NQF-endorsed consensus standards for nursing-sensitive care: A 15-month study.* Retrieved from http://www.qualityforum.org/pdf/reports/Nursing70907.pdf

Radwin, L. E., Cabral, H. J., Chen, L., & Jennings, B. M. (2010). A protocol for capturing daily variability in nursing care. *Nursing Economics, 28*(2), 95–105.

Sen, A., & Sinha, A. (2005). A comparison of data warehousing methodologies. *Communications of the ACM, 48*(3), 79–84.

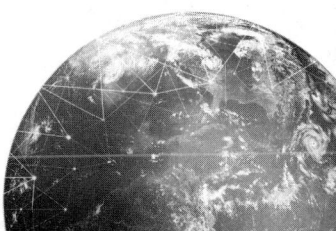

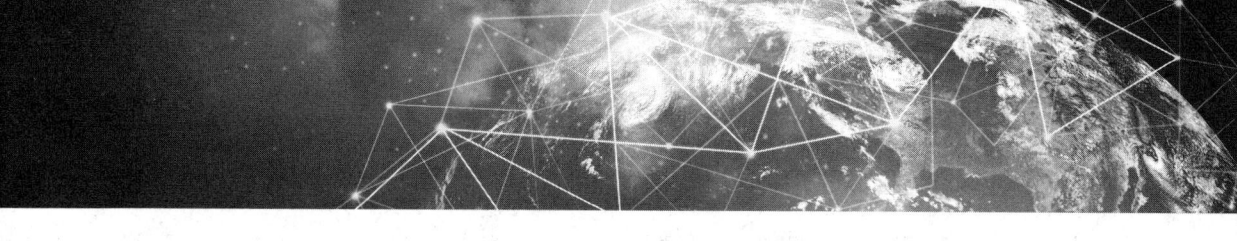

CHAPTER 8

Using Big Data Analytics to Answer Questions in Health Care

Susan Alexander, DNP, ANP-BC, ADM-BC
Rahul Ramachandran, PhD
Diana Hankey-Underwood, MS, WHNP-BC

LEARNING OBJECTIVES

1. Describe basic principles of analytics for answering healthcare questions.
2. Review use scenarios for which data analytics can answer.
3. Discuss how algorithms are created using healthcare data to address clinical questions.

KEY TERMS

Algorithms
Artificial neural network
Association rules
Bayesian modeling
Business intelligence
Clustering rules
Conditional dependence

Data analytics
Data mining
Decision tree
Descriptive algorithm
Index patient
Information gain
Instance-based learning classifiers

K-means
Modeling
Predictive algorithm
Simulation
Support vector machine
  modeling

▶ Chapter Overview

Health care is famous for its history of storing data; those who have visited medical records departments in hospitals likely can recall numerous shelves of patient records. The practice of storing healthcare data in the 21st century has largely transitioned to digital methods, offering new opportunities for healthcare professionals, administrators, and researchers to use the data in answering clinical questions. To do so, health care is increasingly adapting tools used from other fields, such as business, learning the techniques of data analysis to understand why buyers make decisions, and to identify key processes that can make a business financially successful. Known as **business intelligence**, these techniques of data analytics are being adapted for the healthcare environment for tasks such as the description of trends, prediction of future needs, and support of decisions designed to improve performance and safety in healthcare organizations.

Using data to predict future needs is often done with techniques such as **modeling** and **simulation**. Modeling can be used in many fields of science, employed in diverse tasks, such as forecasting the track of a hurricane, to predicting sports championship winners. While modeling may sound complicated, in concept, it is the application of a set of mathematical terms used in creating a computer application to predict a response in a selected situation. In simulation, one example of modeling, reality is imitated for purposes such as training or entertainment. In some cases, artificial environments are used to mimic real-world experiences. For example, a Wii game entitled Hysteria Hospital Emergency Ward is now available, in which players attempt to manage the constant flow of people into an emergency department. The game is structured so that no matter how good the "nurse" player becomes at carrying out the order of nursing tasks, the patients will come faster and some will turn green for lack of care. While the scenarios are carried out in a comical manner, for the sake of entertainment, the game is an effective example of the possibilities of both modeling and simulation in health care. This chapter reviews basic concepts and applications of data analytics, adapted from business intelligence, which are also used in the healthcare environment.

▶ Basic Principles of Big Data Analytics

Healthcare data is being amassed at an astonishing speed. At its present rate of growth, data accumulation in the healthcare environment is expected to be measured in zetabytes (10^{21} gigabytes) and eventually yottabytes (10^{24} gigabytes) (Institute for Health Technology Transformation [IHTT], 2013). Using vast amounts of data, often termed, Big Data, in meaningful ways is an ongoing challenge. While the definition of Big Data continues to evolve, it is generally agreed to be characterized by the three Vs: volume, velocity, and variety (Zikopoulos, Eaton, deRoos, Deutsch, & Lapis, 2011). Data mining and data analytics are terms that are often used interchangeably to describe the process of knowledge discovery using large databases, yet there are slight and important differences between the terms (Fayyad, Piatetsky-Shapiro, & Smyth, 1996). Fayyad, an accomplished researcher in the field, defined **data mining** as the process of identifying valid, and likely useful, patterns in data. **Data analytics** is a more focused process, concentrating on the customization of data mining in response to the specific needs of end users or those who seek to gain knowledge from manipulation of the data or application (Kohavi, Rothleder, & Simoudis, 2002). Such customization should enable an end user, irrespective of the data source and field of study, to use the results of an analysis in a way that is meaningful, or that produces a positive impact.

Business has long used data analytics principles to gain competitive advantages. For example, Amazon became the largest Internet retailer by using big data on customer preferences and purchasing history to make relevant recommendations to its shoppers. The customer experiences increased shopping satisfaction while Amazon makes record-setting sales. Other business analytics are used to examine questions ranging from personnel performance to business processes for improving efficiencies, lowering costs, and improving hiring strategies to retain new employees (Walker, 2012). In many instances, data are used as the basis for the quantitative evaluation of decisions, on both small and grand scales, that affect the performance of the organization. Since the early 2000s, federally funded large-scale projects involving the application of data analytics from healthcare sources have been conducted. Results from these projects, which are discussed later in this chapter, have strongly influenced the delivery of health care across the nation.

Using Algorithms in Data Analytics

Data analytics components consist of descriptive and predictive models for analyzing data. Data-mining algorithms are sets of mathematical rules and are often used in combinations for building predictive and descriptive models. Algorithms are used everywhere in the digital and temporal worlds. An **algorithm** is nothing more than a set of instructions used to accomplish a task. Think back to the last time you worked in your kitchen. Did you use a recipe? If your answer is yes, then you used an algorithm. Varying in complexity, algorithms are the basis of many common digital activities used in health care (and everyday life), such as downloading files from the Internet, encrypting data, and creating scoring systems that can help in monitoring and predicting patient prognoses (Utah Center for Health Sciences, n.d.) An example of a simple algorithm could measure patient movements, such as the timing of rising from a chair and ambulating a short distance, which can give clues about an older adult patient's risk for falling. The algorithm would guide an application to record the times to accomplish the specific activity for older adult patients with a history of falls and to compare the time records to those of older adult patients without a history of falls. The algorithm would be a mathematical calculation yielding a ratio describing the patient's risk of falls. In this situation, the algorithm would provide a clinician with additional information on whether an individual patient might reduce his or her risk of falls by using an assistive device for ambulation.

This example is deceptively simple, as many data points would actually be needed, such as age, gender, past medical history, medication use, and others to optimize the predictive value of the clinical algorithm. Although humans can intuitively understand the need for collection of multiple data points to illustrate differences, mathematical models using algorithms offer more insight into the appropriate numbers of variables to use in specific types of equations. In the example of evaluating rising from a chair and ambulating, a larger number of data points and sample patients used in each group would help create a better "model" of risk for falls, therefore providing a warning if a particular patient is far from the "normal" range. In the next section, an overview of the analytics process and discussion of data-mining algorithm concepts that are used in analytics are presented.

Using Data Analytics in Health Care

Before describing the data analytics process, definitions for basic terms are needed. Specific uses of terms have been updated to address the emerging paradigms of data-intensive science and big data (Bell, Hey, & Szalay, 2009) (**BOX 8-1**). Recall that data are used to derive information needed to support or negate a hypothesis. Data cannot formulate a hypothesis; new patterns discovered in data combined with knowledge about a particular domain of interest are used to formulate new hypotheses. Data analytics is the toolbox that allows for management of data to discover new knowledge in a specific setting, such as a healthcare organization. The process of using data analytics tools for answering clinical questions is composed of multiple steps, with contributions from multiple stakeholders in health care as the question is refined and strategies are selected.

Data mining is an important component within the process of analytics, in which a particular mining algorithm is used to extract patterns from the dataset. The first step requires the user to closely define the objective of analysis

BOX 8-1 Types of Data

Data are observable and therefore measurable and factual. It is sometimes a significant challenge to convert subjective information into objective data.

Knowledge is a statement about a hypothesis, and science is organized knowledge, that is, a collection of one or more hypotheses in some logical order. Consider the statement, "A nurse, Susan, knows that women experience pain 24 hours after a C-section." Susan has experience with previous patients, so she has confidence in her prediction of future patients reacting in the same way. Because we do not have data on the future, Susan is predicting based on previous data, which in science is termed a *hypothesis.* Nursing knowledge is gained by testing a hypothesis based on suitably organized data.

Information is a measure of uncertainty about a hypothesis; the role of data is to change the amount of information.

Knowledge management and discovery are the systematic use of data to test a hypothesis and/or help formulate new hypotheses.

Analytics dashboards, or simply "dashboards," are used as visualization components to effectively communicate and display analysis results, usually to end users. Much like the dashboard of a car provides information on the operating condition of the car and the driver's speed, analytics dashboards provide information in usable picture-like illustrations so that adjustments can be made as appropriate.

and select the correct dataset. The second step consists of data preparation, which involves cleaning and preprocessing of the target data. Very often, data preparation represents the most time-consuming step of the process. The final step is manipulation and analysis of the dataset to identify patterns, which may be used for descriptive and predictive purposes.

Consider the extraction of data from an electronic health record (EHR). The removal of personal identification information from the EHR should be fairly simple if the dataset is limited to a single provider or small office, but the process can be far more complex if the record contains information generated by multiple healthcare providers (HCPs). If the data abstraction requires the retrieval of data from multiple EHR systems, considerable preprocessing effort would be required to generate a usable dataset.

When multiple datasets are combined, the discovery of relevant patterns from the data often requires the use of term definitions that are consistent across the datasets. One of the best examples of the application of term definitions used in health care would be in the use of the *International Classification of Diseases, 10th Revision, Clinical Modification* (ICD-10-CM).

ICD-10-CM codes are lists of terms used to represent diagnoses in patients and have many uses across the healthcare environment. Widespread use of ICD-10-CM codes makes these data retrievable for many patient visits, even though use of a particular ICD-10-DM code may not contain all of the information needed for accurate data processing. For instance, there are many ICD-10-CM codes that could be applied to a patient who has a diagnosis of back pain (**BOX 8-2**). If a program were designed to identify patients who visited an HCP with a complaint of back pain, could those visits be isolated by using only one ICD-10-CM code, or term, to describe back pain? The answer is no—many term definitions would be needed to accurately capture all patients with the similar complaint.

▶ Overview of Algorithms Generated by Data-Mining Methods

Nurses' skill sets constantly evolve to meet the needs of patients and the healthcare environment

BOX 8-2 ICD-10-CM Codes That Can Be Used to Describe the Diagnosis of Back Pain

Lumbosacral spondylosis without myelopathy

- M47.26–M47.28
- M47.816–M47.818
- M47.896–M47.898

Spondylosis of unspecified site without mention of myelopathy

- M47.20
- M47.819
- M47.899–M47.9

Displacement of lumbar intervertebral disc without myelopathy

- M51.26
- M51.27

Degeneration of lumbar or lumbosacral intervertebral disc

- M51.36–M51.37

Degeneration of intervertebral disc, site unspecified

- M51.34–M51.37
- M51.9

Other unspecified disc disorder of lumbar region

- M46.46–M46.47
- M51.86–M51.87

Spinal stenosis of lumbar region

- M48.06–M48.07
- M99.23, M99.33
- M99.43, M99.53
- M99.63
- M99.73

Lumbago

- M54.5

Sciatica

- M54.30–M54.42

in providing efficient, high-quality care. In 1990, it was likely that the skill set of an experienced and educated nurse did not include the ability to create a presentation using Microsoft PowerPoint. However, within only a few years' time, familiarity with the use of Microsoft Office programs, including PowerPoint, became a standard skill for many nurses. Nurses are becoming more involved in using advanced techniques in data management to address important clinical questions. Understanding more about the construction and utilization of

algorithms can help to capture and inform the intricacies of clinical judgment nurses develop in working with patients.

Algorithms can be categorized based on their purpose of mining datasets: to describe or predict phenomena (Dunham, 2003). **Descriptive algorithms** are generally used to explore data and identify patterns or relationships within them. Examples of descriptive algorithms include clustering, summarization, and association rules. **Predictive algorithms** make predictions about values of data using a set of known results.

Though the baccalaureate-prepared nurse may not be expected to design and implement such algorithms, a familiarity with these concepts will likely prove useful as data analytics tools continue to permeate healthcare delivery systems. The following sections present a brief overview and examples of algorithms that are commonly used in health care.

Examples of Predictive Algorithms

Decision Trees

Represented as a tree-shaped diagram, **decision trees** are often used for patient protocols as an aid to decision making, and they are used in analytical research. In decision tree diagrams, each branch may be used to represent a possible decision or occurrence, and the structure of the branches can illustrate how one decision may lead to another. Because the branches are separate, each choice can be seen as a stand-alone decision. Using decision trees allows clinicians to examine all the possibilities of outcomes, their likelihood of occurring, and results of each outcome. They are particularly useful in situations when there is sufficient time to review all decision-making possibilities, such as in cost-effectiveness research in health care.

Envision the trunk of the decision tree as including all patients having avian flu at Hospital X **(FIGURE 8-1)**. On the trunk are three branches designating patients who were born in 1900–1960 (65 patients), 1960–2000 (7 patients), and 2001–2014 (38 patients). Under each of the branches are three leaves that separately designate patients who received immediate antiviral medications (costing $150), patients who received antiviral medications by day 3 of symptom onset, and patients who did not receive antiviral medications until a postlaboratory confirmation of diagnosis. Below each of the leaves are designations for patients whose lengths of hospital stay were 1–14 days, 14–45 days, and those patients who died during their hospital stays. Hospital reimbursement is assigned to each leaf as a total of the patients within that leaf. Analysis reveals that patients who received antiviral medications

had a length of stay that was one-third less than those who did not receive antiviral medications. Their hospital bills were less than half of those patients who did not receive antiviral medications, regardless of the age range. Does this mean that all patients should receive antiviral medications immediately? Would the answer change if only one patient died and the patient was in the group that received antiviral medications immediately? What other leaves should be on the decision tree to help decide for whom antiviral medications are the best choice? Would analysis of a larger data pool help? Would dividing the groups into male and female patients make a difference? Use of an algorithm such as the decision tree can help to inform HCPs of the important leaves and enable more effective decisions.

Another important concept used in the evaluation process is a statistical property known as **information gain**. Information gain is a measure of how well a given attribute separates a subset of the whole dataset (also known as training sample data) to achieve the target classification. The best attribute is selected and is used as the root node of the tree. Descendant nodes are created for all possible values of the root node. The entire process is repeated with more data to create the tree using the training samples. This program might inform us that patients are likely to benefit most from the antiviral based on month of admission, weight of 50 pounds or more or a BMI of over 24, and a cough when entering the hospital. It might inform us that patient sex and smoking status are irrelevant—in other words those data were found to be a poor fit to the model of the tree that it created. Based on the decision tree formulated, the best time to use the antiviral would be in January and February, making sure to dose larger patients and all of those with a cough of any kind upon entering the hospital to achieve the target classification of a shorter hospital stay.

Artificial Neural Networks

An **artificial neural network** is an information-processing system that is based on biological

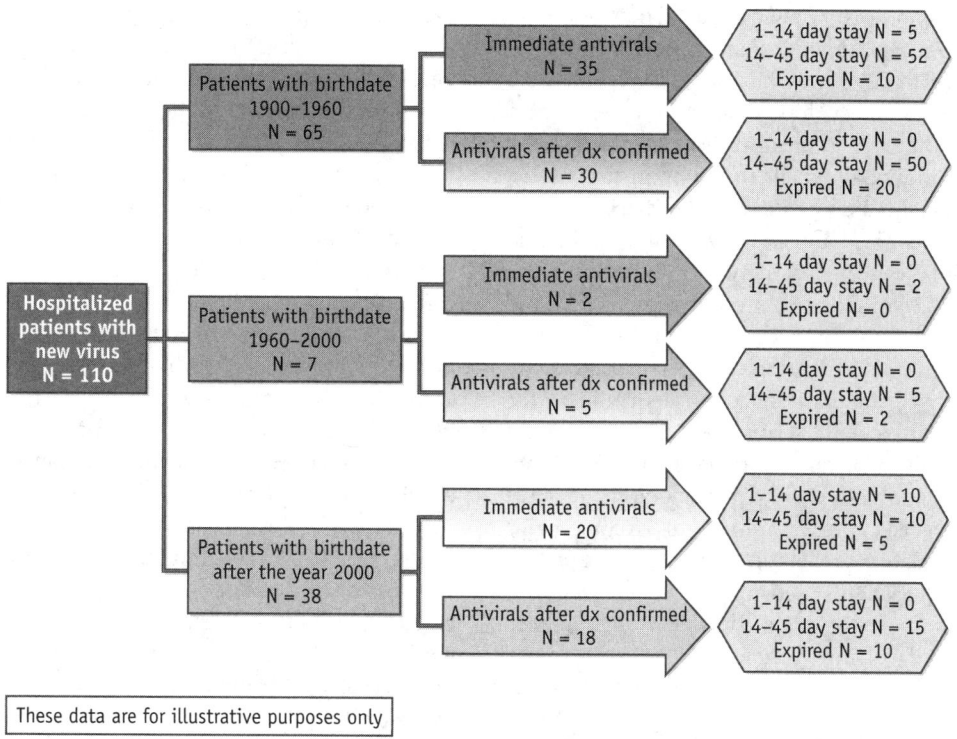

FIGURE 8-1 Decision tree applied to the treatment of avian influenza.

neural networks such as those present in the human nervous system. These networks have been developed as mathematical models of human cognition. Artificial neural networks are most useful when pattern recognition or prediction is necessary or when it is not possible to create a conventional, straightforward algorithm that could be used to describe a problem. An artificial neural network is constructed upon the assumptions that information processing involves many simple elements, called neurons, and that signals are passed between these neurons over connection links (Fausett, 1994). These connection links have associated weights that influence how quickly the signal is transmitted, similar to the transmission of signals along axons in the human nervous system. Artificial neural networks can also be classified according to the direction in which the signal is transmitted across the connection links, as either forward or

backward. The back propagation neural network (BPNN) is a commonly used artificial neural network algorithm in data mining.

In health care, artificial neural networks are used in clinical diagnosis, image and signal analysis, and drug development. They are useful when multiple relationships between data are not necessarily linear. Using an artificial neural network, Jiang and colleagues (2013) identified a group of five serum protein markers that could be used to detect early stage ovarian cancer, a disease for which there is presently no screening protocol and which is commonly undiagnosed until it reaches an advanced stage. Artificial neural networks have also been used to study the phenomenon of burnout in nurses, finding that variables such as age, work status, experience of conflictual interactions, and others, predicted the sensation of burnout in nurses in highly complex and interactive ways (Ladstatter, Garrosa, Badea, &

Moreno, 2010). Artificial neural networks have also studied functional magnetic resonance images (fMRI) of the brains of adult patients with attention deficit disorder, supporting researchers' hypothesis that the disorder is associated with maturational deficits in the brain that persist throughout life (Sato, Hoexter, Castellanos, & Rohde, 2012). Image analysis can be enhanced with the use of these networks. Borujeny, Yazdi, Keshavarz-Haddad, and Borujeny (2013) used wireless sensors attached to the arms and thighs of epileptic patients to collect data used in creating an automatic detection algorithm for the onset of epileptic seizures. Results of the project yielded important information for the patients' HCPs on the nuances of behavioral changes that preceded the onset of seizures and for improving the safety of patients in the post-seizure period. Artificial neural networks have even been used to improve the quality of tablet design in drug manufacturing (Aksu et al., 2012).

Other Types of Predictive Algorithms

Instance-based learning classifiers store labeled training data. As a new sample is presented to these classifiers, it is matched against a set of similar stored instances in order to assign a classification label. This is similar to a computerized scholastic test with which many students may be familiar. The answers are given to the program, and when a new "sample" is presented, the program can correctly detect and classify "fail" and "pass." If a test contained only 25 items, it is likely that a human could do the work almost as fast, but comparing various complex genetic codes to ascertain "easily transmissible" or "poorly transmissible" traits, for example, can be done only by using computer analysis. This type of descriptive algorithm has also been used in creating medical diagnostic applications.

Classifiers use many different methods. **Support vector machine modeling** informs the program to learn from the data. Support vector analysis has been used recently in analyses of healthcare coverage in large populations of people. In addition, this modeling technique

has been used to identify those people who are without health insurance in the populations that were studied and to offer explanations for the lack of healthcare coverage in the groups (Delen & Fuller, 2013).

Bayes' theorem is the underpinning of the **Bayesian modeling** classifier. Bayes' theorem is used to estimate the conditional probability of a given data point belonging to a particular class. Bayesian classifiers use a probabilistic approach for data classification and are based on the assumption that attributes in the training examples are governed by probability distributions. Classification decisions can be made by using these collective probabilities. Bayesian classifiers allow prior knowledge, also known as initial probability, to be combined with observed data to determine conditional probability. When predicting disease outbreaks, the aspect of numbers, such as the sheer amount of contagious people present in the population, is important. The probability of an individual becoming ill after exposure, however, is gained from the analysis of past epidemics. This information can also be used in predicting pandemics, though the numbers may not always be accurate.

When initial probabilities are unavailable, assumptions have to be made regarding the underlying distribution. Sometimes assumptions are made that the attribute values are conditionally independent. When three cases of a new gastrointestinal ailment arrive and two of the three people die within days or weeks, there can be no way to know immediately if these cases have any relationship, but there will be intense scrutiny to determine ways that the cases may be related, which is also known as **conditional dependence**. For example, perhaps the patients all became ill after sharing a pizza at the same restaurant. To find out more about the potential need to prepare for extensive outbreaks of illness in a community, it is important to discover if a common source of infection is present. Even if the cases appear at first glance to be conditionally independent, meaning that they do not share obvious history, characteristics, or other connecting conditions, detailed assessments are often helpful. Bayesian computer modeling can use known data to "fill in the blanks" and to provide models with "created" missing data. As data on new cases are loaded into the application, the models and projections continuously change, which can be helpful in a situation where some or many of the "knowns" are not known.

▶ Descriptive Algorithms

Descriptive algorithms can be broadly divided into rules of clustering and association. The detection and tracking of an influenza outbreak can be used to offer examples of applications of various descriptive algorithms.

Clustering Rules

Descriptive algorithms can be broadly divided into rules of clustering and association. Examples of **clustering rules** used in descriptive algorithms include single-link clustering, density-based spatial clustering of application with noise, and K-means clustering. The clustering algorithm discovers the groupings in the data based on similarities in the attributes of the data. These types of algorithms are often useful as exploratory tools, where the general behavior of the data can be observed by the cluster results and can also be used to summarize the data.

When outbreaks of disease occur, epidemiologists gather large amounts of data on many aspects related to the first known case of the disease, known as the **index patient**, and subsequent cases in an attempt to identify the origin of the disease and its associated exposure risks. In the Guangdong province of China, a rural area bordering Hong Kong and eastern China, health officials noted an outbreak of serious avian influenza A(H7N9) infections in March through April 2013 (Cowling et al., 2013). Officials further noted that the first cases occurred in older men, many of whom had been in close contact with unvaccinated sick or dead poultry found in small, backyard farms. Viral samples from the index patients were analyzed, with

results suggesting that the virus likely emerged from "reassortment," a process in which two or more influenza viruses coinfect a single host and exchange genes (Cowling et al., 2013). Descriptive algorithms were used to help in identifying the genetic changes found in the H7N9 virus causing infection in the index cases. These algorithms are helpful, because they can also identify outlier data points that vary substantially from the rest of the data. If all the patients have a virus that is genetically identical, it suggests a simultaneous exposure, but as the virus proceeds through patients, it acquires subtle changes, which can be identified with descriptive algorithms. These changes provide clues about the age and source of the new viral illness.

Association Rules

Association rules are designed to capture information about items that are frequently associated with each other. Association rules have been used in business applications such as market-basket analysis to find relationships present among attributes in large datasets. Companies may review credit card receipts, for instance, and find that if someone buys peanut butter, they are more likely to buy jelly. Analyzing the increase in sales of over-the-counter medications for influenza or cold symptoms and related products can use association rules and clustering to visualize movement of an influenza epidemic across the nation.

K-means is an example of a partitional clustering algorithm where the desired number of clusters to partition the data is specified. Initial cluster means are randomly selected and patterns are assigned to these closest cluster means. New cluster means, referred to as K, are then calculated. K-means is one of the most widely used clustering algorithms. Sometimes the assigned K will be given colors so that data can be visually separated. Using the K-means algorithm, investigators can assign case numbers and ages of patients affected with influenza-like illnesses across a specified region, such as a state, so that flu activity surveillance can be quickly visualized.

While the examples described in the previous paragraphs may seem complex, it is common for analytics projects to compare several factors simultaneously. For instance, much information is needed to reliably forecast the spread of influenza. The migratory pathways of birds (because droppings are contaminated with influenza viruses), human traffic patterns, the temporal distribution of influenza cases in patients, data on the rapidity of human-to-human transmission, and even weather patterns are all needed to improve predictions of influenza outbreaks and to target efforts to control those outbreaks. These data can be used to improve planning and surveillance efforts, such as the purchase of adequate amounts of protective equipment and vaccinations. Modeling can even be used to calculate what occurs when the population is vaccinated at different rates and to predict the method of social distancing (quarantine) that will work best in epidemics.

▶ Using Data Analytics in Health Care

There are great possibilities for the adoption of data analytics to work with big data in health care. Reductions in fraud and waste, earlier detection of disease, and improvements in healthcare efficiency and quality have been associated with use of data analytics tools adapted for healthcare organizations (IHTT, 2013). Finding new ways to use static and real-time data in health care to construct evidence-based architecture for analytics tools has created an emerging discipline in healthcare data management and analysis.

Computer scientists and statisticians can analyze real and projected data to visibly demonstrate consequences of various business decisions. Yet, it is the responsibility of the current generation of nurses and other HCPs to help ensure that quality data exist, to use creativity in devising methods to apply data, and to use the information that is produced with data analytics tools in a constructive manner. The idea that

tracking and monitoring can be conducted may be uncomfortable, and some nurses object to a perceived intrusion upon privacy (AbdelMalik, Boulos, & Jones, 2008). Nurses can feel that data collection is burdensome, even with the knowledge that the data could have some importance to someone else or have significance in the future. These discomforts are important because nurses need to be sensitive to the great potential for use and the great potential for abuse that come with almost all great inventions. Just as narcotics can make lengthy surgeries possible and thereby save millions of lives, they can also be abused and have destroyed many peoples' lives. Understanding the dichotomy can aid nurses in protecting patients while gaining huge advantages. Many articles have been written about the potential abuses of large datasets in the media, but few nurses have acquaintance with the ways large datasets are created, used, or provide the amazing possibilities for the improvement of health care for mankind or for their individual patients and even for their own safety. With this in mind, a review of the ways in which large datasets might have an impact on nursing safety, community planning, and hospital management in the near future is needed. **BOX 8-3** provides a clear example of responsible use of data and data analytics.

Improving Patient Care and Efficiency

By using data from radio frequency identification (RFID) device tags, researchers tracked the movements of nurses throughout a unit, documenting the time spent with patients and performing other tasks within the unit. Hendrich, Chow, Skierczynski, and Lu (2008) combined the data gathered from the use of the RFID tags with modeling and simulation techniques to better describe the movements of nurses over architectural and unit layout schematics. Techniques such as these can improve the design of units, or even entire hospitals, and maximize efficiency.

Project Artemis, named for the Greek goddess charged with the protection of infants and children and developed by researchers at

BOX 8-3 Case Study

Teri, the new nursing informatics officer of a large urban hospital, is asked to help prepare for the chief executive officer's meeting with several division directors, including the pharmacy director. Preparation for the meeting necessitated the analysis of large datasets containing details on the types and amounts of medications purchased by the hospital over past years. After the analysis was complete, Teri discovered that the purchase of opiate medications increased by 25% last year. The nursing counts for opiate medication use on each floor were consistent with the main pharmacy counts, with zero discrepancies, yet the pharmacy count revealed a decrease of 3,000 doses of oxycodone from the total purchased this year. Costs per pill rose 29.3%.

Teri needs to know which nursing unit had significantly higher rates of oxycodone use when compared to the unit's past use and to use in other units. Should Teri be concerned about possible misuses of the oxycodone medication? Could employees in the pharmacy be involved?

Teri understands that data can be misused, and interpretation of analysis of large datasets can be skewed. In this case, fortunately for the pharmacy director, Teri was wise enough to look at additional data before speaking to anyone about this. The new orthopedic center, which opened 10 months ago, increased revenue by $6 million, and the cost of extra pain medications as part of the increased operating costs was $500,000. All other units are within 5% of the trends from previous years. When Teri's hospital bought out the nearby smaller hospital in an adjacent county, they asked to "borrow" several sets of medications that were in short supply nationally. Teri went into the meeting and congratulated the pharmacy director on his amazing competence at overseeing his pharmacy and the merger with all the extra work that entailed. Arrangements were made to complete the return of medications to normalized counts and also to work on surge management in case of community disasters or pandemics. Data can harm others even when there is no malicious intent. Nurses must be prepared to research carefully and fully before assuming or repeating any harmful conclusions based on data analysis.

the University of Ontario, uses patients' physiological live data streams to conduct real-time analytics (2010). Developed in a partnership with data scientists and clinicians, the Project Artemis platform enables clinicians to make better, faster decisions using streaming data from the patient's bedside. The platform is presently being tested at SickKids Hospital in Toronto, Ontario, where is it being used to identify the development of nosocomial infections in premature infants, identifying barely perceptible changes in the heart rates of infants that are demonstrated 12–24 hours before other signs of infection arise (IBM, 2010).

Monitoring of Adverse Drug Events

Over the course of a nurse's career, it is likely that he or she will administer thousands of medications to patients, representing classes of drugs used to treat everything from the pain

of a myocardial infarction to infection in a wound. While it is likely that many patients will be given medications with no ill effects, some will experience severe adverse reactions that should be reported. Healthcare professionals and consumers (or their family members) can voluntarily report adverse occurrences to pharmaceutical manufacturers or directly to the U.S. Food and Drug Administration (FDA). If a pharmaceutical manufacturer receives a report of an adverse drug event, it is required to then forward this information to the FDA. Reports of adverse drug events are maintained in a database known as the FDA Adverse Event Reporting System (FAERS). Because it contains data contributed by pharmaceutical manufacturers, healthcare professionals, and consumers, the FAERS database is considered to be quite robust. FAERS data are available to the public for retrieval in the form of statistics, files of raw data, or case study reports (FDA, 2012).

The FAERS database is an excellent resource for research in pharmacoepidemiology, the study of the effects of drugs in populations. Pharmacovigilance, which is defined as the use of scientific methods to study and maintain the quality of medications (Partnership for Safe Medicines, 2002–2011), is a process that requires early detection of adverse drug events. Despite the wealth of information contained in the FAERS database, there are deficiencies that make the rapid recognition of adverse drug events difficult. The lag between the time data are reported to FAERS and released to the public, file types in which data are released, and duplication of data in files or reports have been cited as examples of difficulties in manipulating the FAERS database to yield relevant clinical information (Bate & Evans, 2009; Böhm, Höcker, Cascorbi, & Herdegen, 2012; Making a Difference, 2009; Pratt & Danese, 2009). To examine the utility of the FAERS database in detecting adverse drug events, Sakaeda, Tamon, Kadoyama, and Okuno (2013) created four data-mining algorithms designed to analyze reports of hemorrhage, hematemesis, melena, and hematochezia associated with use of common anticoagulants (aspirin, warfarin, and clopidogrel). In the analysis, higher numbers of adverse events were detected as "signals." Statistically significant associations, meaning that the adverse events were detected as signals, were found between the use of warfarin and hematemesis, consistent with reports elsewhere in published literature of adverse reactions associated with the drugs (Sakaeda et al., 2013).

Sakaeda and colleagues (2013) acknowledge that there are advantages and limitations related to data mining of the FAERS database. The existence of the database is not well publicized, which leads to underreporting of adverse events by healthcare professionals and consumers, and the numbers of adverse events may be increasingly reported on two separate occasions: in the first 2 years after a drug is launched and immediately after an adverse event receives wide publicity (Hauben, Reich, & Gerrits, 2006; Pariente, Gregoire, Fourrier-Reglat, Haramburu, & Moore, 2007; Raschi, Piccinni,

Poluzzi, Marschesini, & De Ponti, 2013; Sakaeda et al., 2013). Yet, potential advantages related to data mining of the FAERS database remain. While the preferable method to determine the risks of adverse reactions associated with a drug is with a randomized, controlled trial, this method is not always feasible due to financial and temporal constraints, particularly when the event is rare. Regular mining of the database could offer insight into important associations between the uses of drugs and adverse events, and mining can serve as a mechanism of directing further clinical investigation of those relationships (Sakaeda et al., 2013).

▶ Challenges in Using Data Analytics Tools in Health Care

Creating meaningful information for patients, organizations, clinicians, and payers poses a multidimensional challenge in adapting data analytics tools from the world of business to health care's Big Data. The lag between data collection and processing, integrity and quality of data collected, and data confidentiality and privacy are issues that must be addressed throughout the industry so that improvements can be realized.

A recent example of the use of social media queries to estimate disease outbreaks demonstrates the inherent challenges of rapidly collecting, processing, and interpreting data in real-life situations. Google Flu Trends, a web service operated by Google, provided predictions about trends in influenza outbreaks for more than 25 countries by aggregating Google search queries. Launched in 2008, the service was discontinued in 2014 after concerns regarding accuracy of the predictions emerged, illustrating an important concept relating to collection of data used in analytics tools. The search queries used as data points to construct the underlying algorithms of Google Flu Trends were generated by individuals

BOX 8-4

"Pray, Mr. Babbage, if you put into the machine wrong figures, will the right answers come out?"

Reproduced from Babbage, C. (1864). *Passages from the life of a philosopher*. London: Longman and Co., p. 67.

who entered terms that could easily be associated with diseases other than influenza. Practically speaking, not everyone who used *fever* as a search term was diagnosed with the flu—leading to an overestimation of occurrence rates in years 2011–2013 (Wheatley, 2014). Use of inaccurate data cannot yield accurate results (**BOX 8-4**).

▶ Summary

While the nurse's responsibility in creating algorithms underlying data analytics tools may be limited, nurses can play essential roles in other aspects of analytics design and application. Of key importance is the collection of the most accurate data possible to maintain patient safety. Patient privacy and data security are sensitive and critical components of good nursing care. A team approach is needed to design healthcare delivery systems that can reduce danger to patients, families, communities, and even nations. An understanding of the concepts of advanced data analytics techniques, including the algorithms used to generate various models used in health care, can assist the generalist nurse who may work in tandem with informatics specialists or computer analysts. Nurses can assist in designing ways to eliminate time wasters and work in teams to discover which treatments work best for patients based on genetic composition, age, gender, and weight. These methods may benefit every member of the healthcare team.

References

AbdelMalik, P., Boulos, M. N. K., & Jones, R. (2008). The perceived impact of location privacy: A web-based survey of public health perspectives and requirements in the UK and Canada. *BMC Public Health, 8,* 156. doi: 10.1186/1471-2458-8-156

Aksu, B., Paradkar, A., de Matas, M., Ozer, O., Guneri, T., & York, P. (2012). Quality by design approach: Application of artificial intelligence techniques of tablets manufactured by direct compression. *AAPS PharmSciTech, 13*(4), 1138–1146. doi: 10.1208/s12249-012-9836-x

Bate, A., & Evans, S. J. (2009). Quantitative signal detection using spontaneous ADR reporting. *Pharmacoepidemiology and Drug Safety, 18,* 427–436.

Bell, G., Hey, T., & Szalay, A. (2009). Beyond the data deluge. *Science, 323.*

Böhm, R., Höcker, J., Cascorbi, I., & Herdegen, T. (2012). OpenVigil—free eyeballs on AERS pharmacovigilance data. *Nature Biotechnology, 30,* 137–138.

Borujeny, G. T., Yazdi, M., Keshavarz-Haddad, A., & Borujeny, A. R. (2013). Detection of epileptic seizure using wireless sensor networks. *Journal of Medical Signals and Sensors, 3*(2), 63–68.

Brimmer, K. (2013, February 28). 5 ways hospitals can use data analytics. *HealthcareIT News.* Retrieved from http://www.healthcareitnews.com/news/5-ways -hospitals-can-use-data-analytics

Centers for Disease Control and Prevention. (2013). Emergence of avian influenza A(H7N9) virus causing severe human illness—China, February–April 2013. *Morbidity and Mortality Weekly Reports, 62*(18), 366–371. Retrieved from http://www.cdc.gov/mmwr/preview/mmwrhtml /mm6218a6.htm?s_cid=mm6218a6_w

Cowling, B. J., Freeman, G., Wong, J. Y, Wu, P., Liao, Q., Lau, E. H., . . . Leung, M. (2013). Preliminary inferences on the age-specific seriousness of human disease caused by avian influenza A(H7N9) infections in China, March to April 2013. *EuroSurveillance, 18*(19), 1–6. Retrieved from http://www.eurosurveillance.org/ViewArticle. aspx?ArticleId=20475

Delen, D., & Fuller, C. (2013). An analytic approach to understanding and predicting healthcare coverage. *Studies in Health Technology and Informatics, 190,* 198–200.

Dunham, M. H. (2003). *Data mining: Introduction and advanced topics.* Boston, MA: Pearson Education.

Fausett, L. (1994). *Fundamentals of neural networks.* Englewood Cliffs, NJ: Prentice Hall.

Fayyad, U. M., Piatetsky-Shapiro, G., & Smyth, P. (1996). From data mining to knowledge discovery: An overview. In U. M. Fayyad, G. Piatetsky-Shapiro, &

P. Smyth (Eds.), *Advances in knowledge discovery and data mining.* Cambridge, MA: MIT Press.

Hauben, M., Reich, L., & Gerrits, C. M. (2006). Reports of hyperkalemia after publication of RALES—a pharmacovigilance study. *Pharmacoepidemiology and Drug Safety, 15,* 775–783.

Hendrich, A., Chow, M. P., Skierczynski, B. A., & Lu, Z. (2008). A 36-hospital time and motion study: How do medical-surgical nurses spend their time? *The Permanente Journal, 12*(3), 25–34.

IBM. (2010). University of Ontario Institute of Technology: Leveraging key data to provide proactive patient care. Retrieved from http://www.ibmbigdatahub.com/sites/default/files/document/ODC03157USEN.PDF

Institute for Health Technology Transformation. (2013). *Transforming health care through Big Data strategies for leveraging big data in the health care industry.* Retrieved from http://c4fd63cb482ce6861463-bc6183f1c18e748a49b87a25911a0555.r93.cf2.rackcdn.com/iHT2_BigData_2013.pdf

Jiang, W., Huang, R., Duan, C., Fu, L., Xi, Y., Yang, Y., ... Huang, R.-P. (2013). Identification of five serum protein markers for detection of ovarian cancer by antibody arrays. *PLoS One, 8*(10), e76795. doi: 10.1371/journal.pone.0076795

Kohavi, R., Rothleder, N. J., & Simoudis, E. (2002). Emerging trends in business analytics. *Communications of the ACM, 45*(8), 45–48.

Ladstatter, F., Garrosa, E., Badea, C., & Moreno, B., (2010). Application of artificial neural networks to a study of nursing burnout. *Ergonomics, 53*(9), 1085–1096.

Making a difference. (2009). [Editorial]. *Nature Biotechnology, 27,* 297.

Pariente, A., Gregoire, F., Fourrier-Reglat, A., Haramburu, F., & Moore, N. (2007). Impact of safety alerts on measures of disproportionality in spontaneous reporting databases: The notoriety bias. *Drug Safety, 30,* 891–898.

Partnership for Safe Medicines. (2002–2011). What is pharmacovigilance? Retrieved from http://www.safemedicines.org/what-is-pharmacovigilance.html

Pratt, L. A., & Danese, P. N. (2009). More eyeballs on AERS. *Nature Biotechnology, 27,* 601–602.

Raschi, E., Piccinni, C., Poluzzi, E., Marschesini, G., & De Ponti, F. (2013). The association of pancreatitis with antidiabetic drug use: Gaining insight through the FDA pharmacovigilance database. *Acta Diabetologica, 50*(4), 569–577. doi: 10.1007/s00592-011-0340-7

Sakaeda, T., Tamon, A., Kadoyama, K., & Okuno, Y. (2013). Data mining of the public version of the FDA adverse event reporting system. *International Journal of Medical Sciences, 10*(7), 796–803. doi: 10.7150/ijms.6048

Sato, J. R., Hoexter, M. Q., Castellanos, X. F., & Rohde, L. A. (2012). Abnormal brain connectivity patterns in adults with ADHD: A coherence study. *PLoS ONE, 7*(9), e45671. doi: 10.1371/journal.pone.0045671

U.S. Food and Drug Administration. (2012). Protecting and monitoring your health. Retrieved from http://www.fda.gov/Drugs/GuidanceComplianceRegulatoryInformation/Surveillance/AdverseDrugEffects/default.htm

Utah Center for Health Sciences. (n.d.). 10 Algorithms that are changing health care. Retrieved from http://healthsciences.utah.edu/innovation/tenalgorithms/

Walker, J. (2012). Meet the new boss: Big data. *Wall Street Journal.* Retrieved from http://online.wsj.com/news/articles/SB10000872396390443890304578006252019616768

Wheatley, M. (24 March 2014). Google Flu Trends: a case of big data gone bad? Retrieved from https://siliconangle.com/blog/2014/03/24/google-flu-trends-a-case-of-big-data-gone-bad./

Wong, D. L., Hackenberry-Eato, M., Wilson, D., Winkelstein, M. L., & Schwartz, P. (2008). Wong-Baker FACES Rating Scale. In *Wong's essentials of pediatric nursing* (6th ed.). St. Louis, MI: Mosby.

Zikopoulos P., Eaton C., deRoos D., Deutsch T., & Lapis, G. (2011). *Understanding Big Data: Analytics for enterprise class Hadoop and streaming data.* New York: McGraw-Hill Osborne Media.

CHAPTER 9

Workflow Support

Karen H. Frith, PhD, RN, NEA-BC

LEARNING OBJECTIVES

1. Define workflow in a healthcare delivery system.
2. Identify appropriate methods for workflow analysis.
3. Select charts, tables, or other tools to display workflow data.
4. Describe the rationale for workflow redesign after implementation of health IT.
5. Identify technology that automates workflow.

KEY TERMS

Clinical decision-support
  systems (CDSS)
Data display
Defects
Effectiveness
Efficiency
Flowchart

Gap analysis
Inefficiency
Logistics
Patient throughput
Process mapping
Productivity
Satisfaction

Supply chain management
Systems thinking
Task analysis
Workarounds
Workflow
Workflow analysis
Workflow redesign

▶ Chapter Overview

Healthcare providers (HCPs) need to be involved in the planning and implementation of health information technologies (health IT) so that clinical processes (**workflow**) can be supported instead of hampered by health IT. This chapter outlines **workflow analysis** in a health IT planning framework as a method to avoid the consequences of poorly designed health IT and its impact on workflow. Nurse informaticists need to examine workflow prior to implementation of health IT, measure **productivity** after health IT implementation, and redesign workflow when needed. The chapter concludes with a discussion of using health IT to automate the workflow for clinical and business processes.

▶ Need for Workflow Support in Single Hospitals and Networked Hospital Systems

A primary innovation in health care during the early part of the 21st century has been the rapid implementation of health IT. Proponents of health IT believe its use can transform health care from a fragmented, error-prone system to an integrated system capable of consistently delivering high-quality, low-cost care (Bowens & Jones, 2010). However, early research shows mixed results about time and cost savings, patient safety, and consumer satisfaction (Jones, Heaton, Rudin, & Schneider, 2012).

Because the nature of health IT is radically different from the paper systems it replaces, implementation of health IT causes big changes in the way things get done. In other words, health IT affects workflow—the sequence of tasks, communications, and interactions needed to accomplish desired work (McGonigle & Mastrian, 2012). Depending on how well the health IT is implemented, changes in workflow ripple or rip through every part of a healthcare organization and can cause substantial problems for continuity of care.

As hospitals have adopted more health IT or joined networked health systems, their information management needs have risen sharply. For example, over the last 10 years, a large public hospital in Alabama has set up physician practices and purchased hospitals to create the eighth largest public healthcare network in the United States. At the time of purchase, none of the hospitals or practices had the same

electronic health records (EHRs), making the exchange of information between providers and hospitals impossible. The networked health system has had to face the complexity of making information accessible to any provider, at any location, at any time in the health system. This challenge calls for attention to workflow, interoperability, and provider satisfaction with health IT. If this example were an isolated case, then these issues would not rise to the level of national attention (Thune, Alexander, Roberts, & Enzi, 2015).

▶ The Promise of Health IT

Throughout the beginning of the 21st century, reports about patient safety and escalating costs of medical care in the United States have resulted in a call for more efficiency in health care (Institute of Medicine [IOM], 1999, 2011; Page, 2004). Believing that health IT can bring about the needed changes, the federal government used its power to induce hospitals and HCPs to adopt health IT. Under the Health Information Technology for Economic and Clinical Health (HITECH) Act of 2009, the federal government invested $35 billion in health IT by providing incentive payments to hospitals and providers for adopting health IT and meeting meaningful use criteria (Thune, Alexander, Roberts, & Enzi, 2015). This large investment provided the needed incentive for widespread adoption of health IT in the U.S. healthcare system.

Health IT plays an integral part of any healthcare system because it is used to store, process, and aggregate healthcare data. Widespread use of health IT is believed to improve communication between healthcare organizations, leading to more integration and reducing fragmentation of care for patients (IOM, 2011). Improved communication among providers in a healthcare organization is also possible with health IT when documentation from one provider is accessible and can be reused by others in their clinical processes. When designed properly, health IT can shorten time for delivery of medications, supplies, and equipment using supply chain management and make patient movement through the system more efficient, particularly in areas such as surgery, imaging, and procedures. These processes are termed *workflow,* and are the focus of this chapter (IOM, 2011).

Negative Consequences of Health IT

Although the promise of health IT is positive, its delivery on that promise is not guaranteed. Three major factors influence the outcomes: the usability of the health IT, interoperability of systems, and the plan for implementation, also called the system development life cycle.

Problems with usability affect every part of human interaction with health IT, from training sessions to long-term use in a healthcare facility (Boone, 2010). In order to achieve maximum **effectiveness**, **efficiency**, and provider **satisfaction** with health IT, the user interface should be designed with a simple and consistent appearance so that the provider does not have to remember a series of steps to complete a task or to search the interface for needed information (Boone, 2010). The health IT needs to allow for efficient interactions, allow for corrections, provide immediate cues if information entered by providers is outside normal ranges, and use language that is understood by providers (Boone, 2010). For example, health IT that requires a provider to enter medication information on six different screens is not as usable as one that requires the same input on one screen. Health IT that fails to automatically fill data-entry fields with information collected from other providers requires duplicate documentation and can lead to errors.

Interoperability is a term used to describe the "extent to which systems and devices can exchange data and interpret that shared data. For two systems to be interoperable, they must be able to exchange data and subsequently present that data such that it can be understood by a user" (Healthcare Information and Management Systems Society [HIMSS], 2005). Interoperability of systems is critical to health IT's ability to increase efficiency and promote quality. Systems that fail to pass understandable information back and forth reinforce the fragmented care processes that currently plague the healthcare system in the United States (Thune, Alexander, Roberts, & Enzi, 2015)

Failures in health IT design and implementation to support workflow and practice patterns of providers will decrease the efficiency of HCPs and increase costs associated with clinical processes. For example, the number of nonproductive hours paid for providers to learn new health IT will be higher with a system that is poorly matched to provider roles and responsibilities (Lee & McElmurry, 2010). When unexpected workflow issues surface during the initial "go live" period, additional providers may be necessary to continue giving care during the initial months of health IT implementation. An even more severe problem occurs when there is a failure to understand provider workflow and a failure to bridge the gap to the desired future state of workflow with health IT (Kohle-Ersher, Chatterjee, Osmanbeyoglu, Hochheiser, & Bartos, 2012; Unertl, Johnson, & Lorenzi, 2012). Poor design for the workflow and practice patterns cannot be reconciled to a new health IT with more practice (Kjeldskov, Skov, & Stage, 2010), and lost productivity of providers becomes integrated into the healthcare delivery system. Health IT that is poorly matched to workflow can even introduce new errors into care processes (Helmons, Wargel, & Daniels, 2009).

▶ Planning for Health IT

The adoption of health IT can be planned to avoid many problems, but understanding workflow must be a primary driver of system selection and implementation. A successful planning process requires nurses and other stakeholders to adopt **systems thinking**. Systems thinking is the "dynamic interaction, synchronization, and integration of people, processes, and technology" (Trbovich, 2014). A nurse and other members of the healthcare organization who have the ability to use systems thinking can recognize how to understand the current system and plan for a better system with the help of health IT. The systems approach calls for the identification of the inputs (elements of a system), task dependencies, work sequencing and work coordination to maximize the effects on the organizational outcomes. Systems thinking has to be cultivated and embraced by an organization so that care processes are not viewed as isolated parts, but rather as a whole system with dependent microsystems.

When system thinking is truly an established culture in a healthcare organization, planning for health IT can be approached in a methodical way. One method is to use a workflow analysis. A workflow-oriented framework illustrates the importance of workflow analysis (see **FIGURE 9-1**). The framework shows that workflow analysis precedes health IT configuration. An adaptation process follows where members of the health IT implementation team test the system with a small group of providers to decide if it performs as expected. If it does not, then adaptation continues. If the system is satisfactory, then full implementation occurs. The health IT system continues to be adjusted as more providers use the system. If the system meets providers' needs, then it is maintained by an IT department. If the system is not satisfactory to providers, adjustments to the system continue until providers can use the system without sacrificing satisfaction, productivity, and patient safety.

Role of Nurse Informaticist

One of the responsibilities of nurse informaticists is workflow analysis and process redesign for health IT implementation. Nurse informaticists are members of process redesign teams and have the requisite clinical and analytical knowledge to map workflow successfully. Other skills of nurse informaticists are the ability to lead or moderate groups, organize concepts, manage details, and generate solutions in consultation with HCPs.

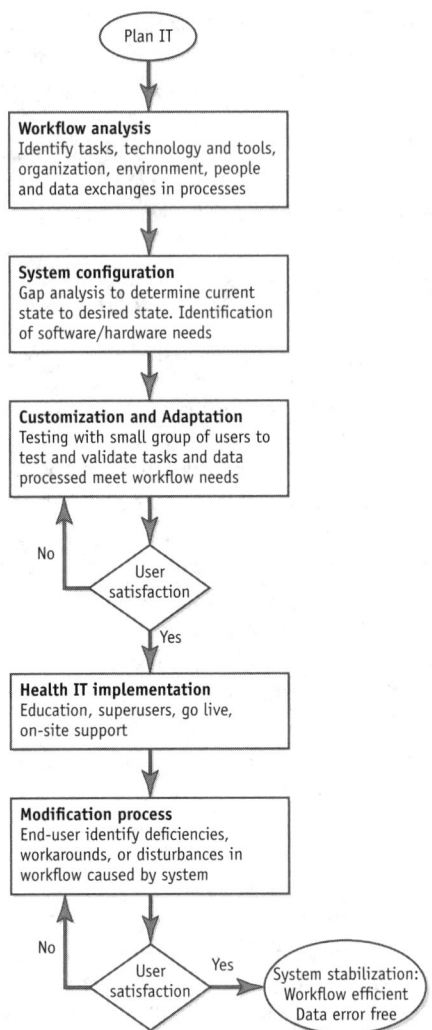

FIGURE 9-1 Workflow-oriented framework of health IT implementation.

Data from Choi, J., & Kim, H. (2012). A workflow-oriented framework-driven implementation and local adaptation of clinical information systems: A case study of nursing documentation system implementation at a tertiary rehabilitation hospital. *Computers, Informatics, Nursing, 30*(8), 409–414.

▶ Workflow Analysis

Definition of Workflow

Workflow is any process that occurs in a healthcare system. Workflow is not a linear process (although it is often depicted as such); rather, it is dynamic, moving between different levels of the organization. Workflow is defined as:

> The flow of people, equipment (including machines and tools), information, and physical and mental tasks, in different places, at different levels, at different timescales continuously and discontinuously, that are used or required to support the goals of the clinical work domain. Workflow also includes communication, coordination, searching for information, interacting with information, problem solving, and planning. (Carayon, 2012, pp. 509–510)

Workflow analysis is the assessment of workflow using specific tools for health IT planning, implementation, and continuous improvement. The analysis should be led by a health IT core team (including a nurse informaticist) with representatives from clinical disciplines in the healthcare system.

Nature of Healthcare Provider Workflow

Workflow of HCPs varies widely based on the discipline (nursing, medicine, physical therapy, etc.) and setting (inpatient or outpatient). The most chaotic workflow is experienced by nurses in inpatient hospitals (Buchini & Quattrin, 2012; Cornell, Riordan, Townsend-Gervis, & Mobley, 2011; Holden et al., 2011; Varpio, Kuziemsky, MacDonald, & King, 2012). The workflow is characterized as having a rapid pace with abrupt switching between tasks (Cornell et al., 2010). For example, Cornell and colleagues (2010) reported that 40% of observations of nursing tasks lasted only 10 seconds, and the majority of tasks were interrupted by a switch.

Interruptions are a type of switch that is not initiated by the HCP. Interruptions are reported in the literature describing medication errors because an interruption during medication calculation or other cognitive processes of a nurse is particularly risky (Buchini & Quattrin,

2012; Elganzouri, Standish, & Androwich, 2009). Interruptions during medication administration in a rehabilitation unit were studied to count the number of interruptions. Observers watched 29 nurses as they administered medications to 250 patients. During 3,000 hours of observation, there were 1,170 documented interruptions, representing one interruption every 3 minutes. Another study found that nurses were interrupted on average 1.2 times per medication pass (Elganzouri et al., 2009).

Another unique aspect of HCP workflow is the amount of walking involved in patient care. Researchers have reported that nurses who work in hospitals routinely walk 5 miles in a 12-hour shift due to supplies and equipment being stored away from patient rooms (Elganzouri et al., 2009). In another study, observers recorded activities of nurses and found that walking represented 20% of the activities. Walking was common to administer medications, seek supplies and equipment, and respond to calls from patients (Cornell et al., 2010).

Interruptions, switching, and walking are just a few human factors to be considered in workflow. A nurse informaticist with education about human factors will understand that the HCP's knowledge, skills, experience, attention, stress, and physical capabilities influence the workflow (Carayon, 2012). Other relevant factors in workflow include the HCP's tasks, the physical environment (lighting, noise, and physical layout), and the organizational characteristics (teamwork, scheduling, culture of safety, and management style). The factors of person, task, technology, physical environment, and organization interact and influence the clinical workflow (Carayon, 2012). A thorough workflow analysis will include as many of these factors as possible so that the proposed health IT is suited to conditions in which it will be used.

Methods of Workflow Analysis

Workflow analysis is the examination of tasks, interactions among providers and between providers and patients, and the exchange of information using quantitative and qualitative methods (National Institute for Health Care Management Foundation, 2005). Workflow analysis should start before discussions with vendors commence because healthcare organizations and their providers first need to understand their own care processes and then design ways that health IT can bridge the gap between the current and desired workflow. The analysis should include representatives from all stakeholders who share the responsibility for setting goals for the health IT implementation process and outcome. Products of workflow analysis should include written requirements for the proposed health IT, including all tasks that the health IT must support or achieve (that is, the cognitive processes, communication exchanges, and procedures or actions). Each requirement should be analyzed for its utility in achieving the overall goal. Any redundant and unnecessary tasks should not be included in requirements. All requirements that are retained should have time and cost estimates associated with them. After completing an extensive workflow analysis, nurses and other decision makers can make more informed choices about selecting the health IT. As described previously, workflow analysis is appropriate when planning for health IT, but it is also useful after health IT has been implemented. Workflow analysis methods include observing providers as they work, interviewing providers, and collecting structured data with questionnaires. The Agency for Healthcare Quality and Research (AHRQ) and the Health Resources and Services Administration provide free guides, toolkits, and other resources to support workflow analysis.

A study conducted by Watkins and colleagues (2012) illustrates the use of mixed methods in workflow analysis. The researchers examined the physical layout of nursing units and nurse workflow patterns in three phases before the implementation of new health IT (Watkins et al., 2012). In Phase 1 the researchers gave questionnaires to nurse–patient pairs to examine perceptions of workflow and patient-centered care. In Phase 2, each nurse was given a personal digital assistant (PDA) that automatically queried nurses about their activity 30 times in a 12-hour shift. Nurses also wore pedometers to measure the number of steps in a 12-hour shift. In this way, the researchers gathered data that were representative of nurses' activities during their shifts. This method is called work sampling. In the final phase of the research, nurses participated in focus groups to discuss the results of the first two phases and to provide feedback on their perceptions of the "best" fit of the health IT with their current unit layout and workflow. Nurses suggested several changes in the physical environment, including decentralization of medications, supplies, equipment, and computer access to reduce inefficiencies, reduce walking distances, and keep nurses closer to their patients.

Tools for workflow analysis are classified into 11 categories that can be used in specific phases of health IT from planning through continuous improvement (Carayon, 2012). The tool categories are **task analysis**, **process mapping**, **data display**, data collection, idea creation, problem solving, project planning, risk assessment, statistical analysis, and usability. For the purposes of this chapter, three categories of workflow analysis tools will be discussed: task analysis, process mapping, and data display.

Task Analysis

Task analysis is a qualitative and quantitative method for understanding the activities associated with a particular patient care goal. A common method to conduct a task analysis is to start with a detailed list of activities and then observe providers as they perform the tasks to measure time to completion and incidence of interruptions. In a study by Dasgupta and colleagues (2011), task analysis was conducted on medication administration with barcode technology to understand its effects on quality of care and time spent in direct patient care. The data collector observed eight nurses as they treated 29 patients on the day shift for a total of 20 hours. The data collector used a stopwatch to measure time associated with each part of medication administration.

The analysis revealed the most frequently occurring tasks were medication preparation, giving medications, and documenting medications. Of the three, documenting medications took the longest time. There were few interruptions, but telephone calls and delivery of meals to patients were the causes of the interruptions.

Work can be cognitive in nature, making it difficult to analyze using customary task analysis methods. In this case, interviews are an effective method to understand the thinking processes required by providers (Effken, Brewer, Logue, Gephart, & Verran, 2011). Effken and colleagues interviewed nurse managers, directors of nursing, IT managers, and quality managers in three acute care hospitals. These managers revealed an overall cognitive goal of "efficient, safe, high-quality patient care in context of nursing shortage, organizational culture, census variation, public opinion, regulations, and budget limits" (p. 702). Based on the goal, the managers had values and priorities, purpose-related functions (e.g., communication and quality improvement), and object-related processes (information management and care coordination). Using a cognitive work analysis, the researchers were better able to understand managers' needs for decision support tools.

Process Mapping

Workflow is often mapped using **flowchart** tools to show documents, tasks, decisions, and interactions associated with care delivery. A flowchart that shows work across time and roles is called a swimlane chart. Such a flowchart is helpful for illustrating the relationship of tasks among providers (see **FIGURE 9-2**).

Diagraming workflow with a flowchart follows a certain convention: Movement forward in time can either be diagramed from left to right or top to bottom. Symbols on flowcharts have specific meanings to improve understanding of workflow. The symbols are not interchangeable.

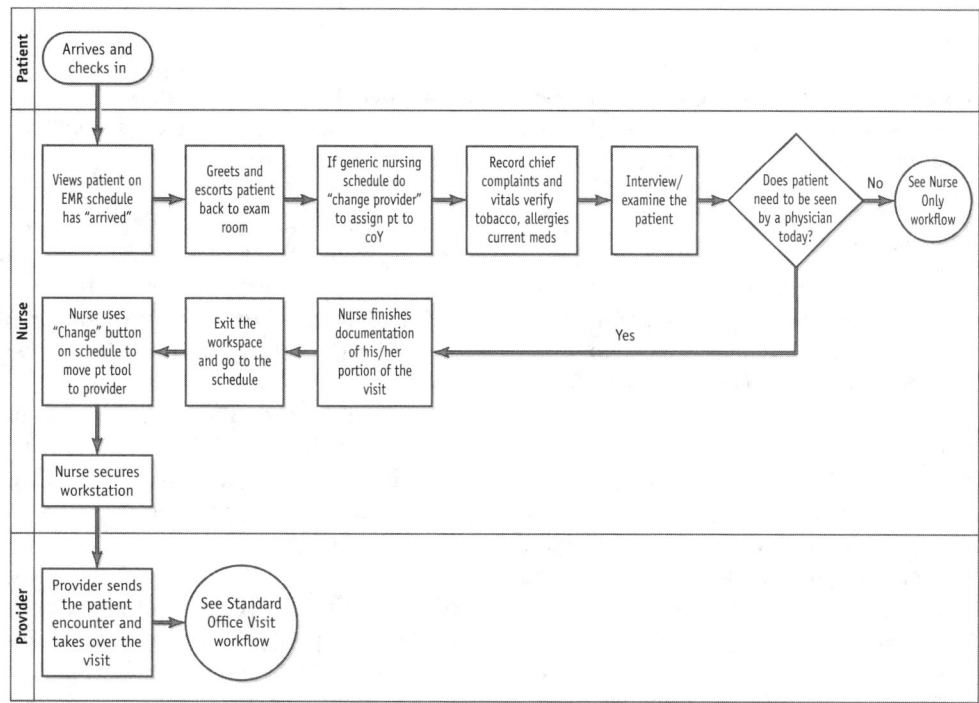

FIGURE 9-2 Simple swimlane flowchart.

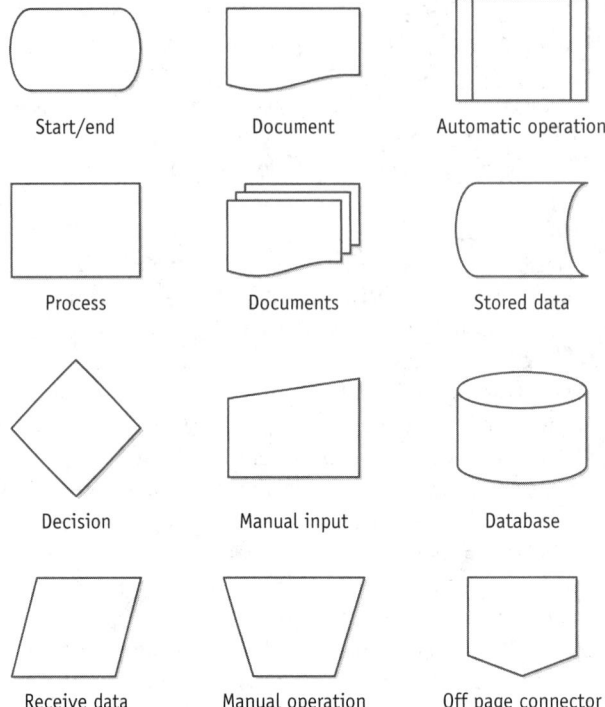

FIGURE 9-3 Common symbols used in flowcharts.

Data Display

For example, a diamond shape is always used to document a decision point. **FIGURE 9-3** shows the customary symbols to document workflow.

Data collected from observations of workflow and from interviews with providers need to be presented in an understandable manner. Common methods include flowcharts (previously discussed), Pareto charts, Gantt charts, run charts, control charts, scatterplots, force field analysis, and fishbone charts. Each of the presentation methods has a particular purpose.

A Pareto chart is useful for displaying the most important areas for **workflow redesign** or safety improvement activities. The principle behind a Pareto chart is that improvement activities should focus on 80% of problem areas, not the less frequently occurring problems. **FIGURE 9-4** shows a Pareto chart with medication errors. Based on the results illustrated in the Pareto chart, safety improvement should focus on administering and transcribing medications.

Gantt charts are used primarily for project management. For example, workflow analysis before implementation of health IT requires a review of all other technologies and processes in a health system before the introduction of a new information system. **FIGURE 9-5** shows a Gantt chart illustrating tasks, duration of tasks, start and end dates of tasks, persons responsible for tasks, and a graphical display of duration of tasks. The Gantt chart keeps the health IT implementation team informed about the progress toward task completion.

Run charts and control charts display change in data over time. These charts are important to use when monitoring a process for quality improvement. For example, if a nursing unit were trying to reduce the time from request of pain medication to administration time, a run chart

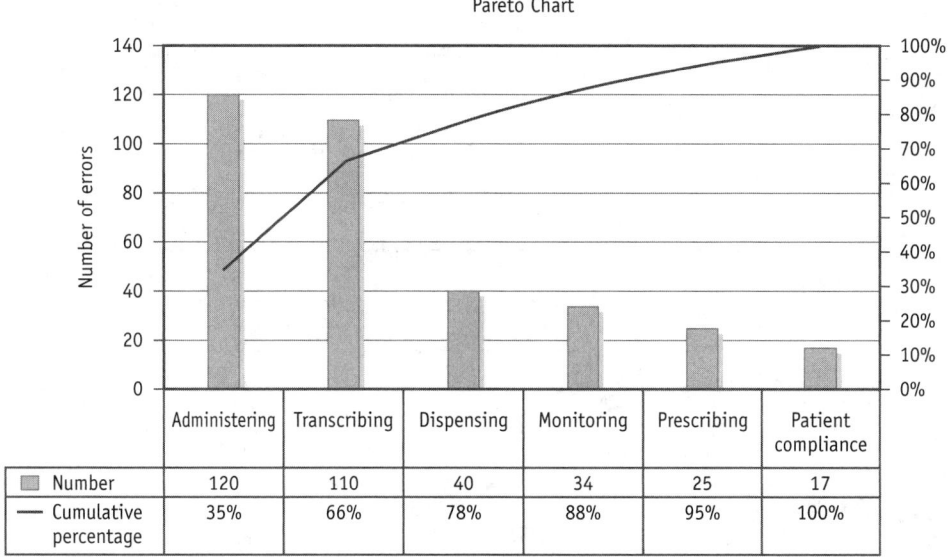

Pareto Chart

	Administering	Transcribing	Dispensing	Monitoring	Prescribing	Patient compliance
▨ Number	120	110	40	34	25	17
— Cumulative percentage	35%	66%	78%	88%	95%	100%

FIGURE 9-4 Pareto chart.

ID	❶	Task Name	Duration	Start	Finish	Predecessors	Resource Names	Apr 1, '12 S M T W T F S	Apr 8, '12 S M
1		**Scope**	**3.5 days**	**Mon 4/2/12**	**Thu 4/5/12**				
2		Determine project scope	4 hrs	Mon 4/2/12	Mon 4/2/12		Management	Management	
3		Secure project sponsorship	1 day	Mon 4/2/12	Tue 4/3/12	2	Management	Management	
4		Define preliminary resources	1 day	Tue 4/3/12	Wed 4/4/12	3	Project Manager	Project Manager	
5		Secure core resources	1 day	Wed 4/4/12	Thu 4/5/12	4	Project Manager	Project Manager	
6		Scope complete	0 days	Thu 4/5/12	Thu 4/5/12	5		4/5	
7		**Analysis/Software Requirements**	**9 days**	**Thu 4/5/12**	**Wed 4/18/12**				
8		**Conduct needs analysis**	**0 days**	**Thu 4/5/12**	**Thu 4/5/12**	6	Analyst	4/5	
9		Scheduling (Angel)	0 days	Thu 4/5/12	Thu 4/5/12			4/5	
10		Clocking System (Kronos)	0 days	Thu 4/5/12	Thu 4/5/12			4/5	
11		ADT (AS400)	0 days	Thu 4/5/12	Thu 4/5/12			4/5	
12		Barcode Scanning	0 days	Thu 4/5/12	Thu 4/5/12			4/5	
13		Charges (DAR)	0 days	Thu 4/5/12	Thu 4/5/12			4/5	
14		Inventory (HSS)	0 days	Thu 4/5/12	Thu 4/5/12			4/5	
15		Accounting	0 days	Thu 4/5/12	Thu 4/5/12			4/5	
16		Patient Abstracting	0 days	Thu 4/5/12	Thu 4/5/12			4/5	
17		Incident Reporting	0 days	Thu 4/5/12	Thu 4/5/12			4/5	
18		Financial (AS400)	0 days	Thu 4/5/12	Thu 4/5/12			4/5	
19		HCAHPS	0 days	Thu 4/5/12	Thu 4/5/12			4/5	
20		Draft preliminary software specifications	3 days	Thu 4/5/12	Tue 4/10/12	10	Analyst		
21		Develop preliminary budget	2 days	Tue 4/10/12	Thu 4/12/12	20	Project Manager		
22		Review software specifications/budget with team	4 hrs	Thu 4/12/12	Thu 4/12/12	21	Project Manager, Analyst		
23		Incorporate feedback on software specifications	1 day	Fri 4/13/12	Fri 4/13/12	22	Analyst		
24		Develop delivery timeline	1 day	Mon 4/16/12	Mon 4/16/12	23	Project Manager		
25		Obtain approvals to proceed (concept, timeline, budget)	4 hrs	Tue 4/17/12	Tue 4/17/12	24	Management, Project Manager		
26		Secure required resources	1 day	Tue 4/17/12	Wed 4/18/12	25	Project Manager		

FIGURE 9-5 Gantt chart.

can be used to show the average number of minutes per day that it took patients to receive pain medication after the request was made. Control charts are run charts with three additional lines: center line (CL), upper control limit (UCL), and lower control limit (LCL). These lines provide a "window" of acceptable performance. **FIGURE 9-6**

shows a control chart for a 60-day period of time. The CL is a horizontal line representing the average for a day. The UCL and LCL are placed 2 or 3 standard deviations above or below the average to create the window. Any point above the UCL or below the LCL would be considered outside the acceptable limits for the process. In

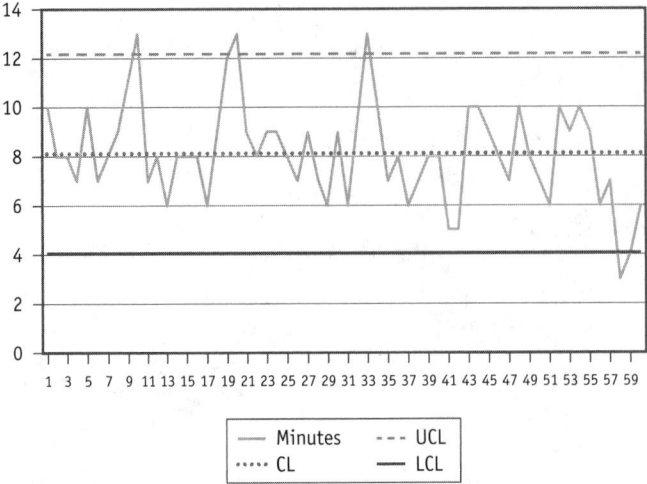

FIGURE 9-6 Control chart.

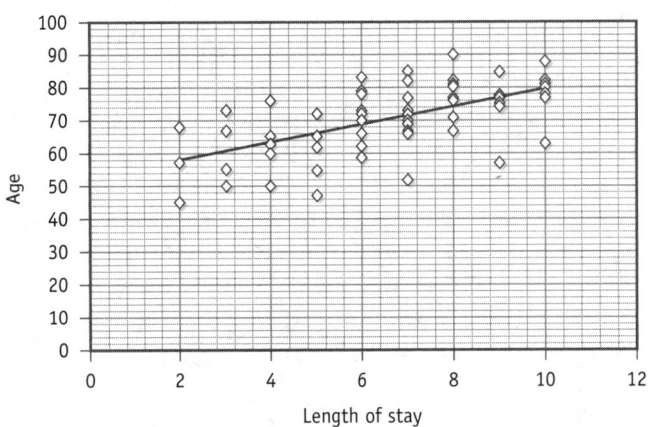

FIGURE 9-7 Scatterplot.

the case of promptness of pain medications, a point below the LCL is actually good.

Scatterplots demonstrate the relationship of two points to one another. Scatterplots are useful when looking for an association or correlation. **FIGURE 9-7** illustrates a scatterplot of patient age and the length of hospital stay. This relationship is positive—in other words, as the age of a person increases, the length of hospital stay increases too. Scatterplots can show an inverse or negative relationship. For example, as a person's age increases, the muscle strength decreases.

A force field analysis is used to analyze the issues surrounding change. Implementation of an EHR represents a large departure from paper systems. When conducting a force field analysis, the health IT team examines the forces driving change and forces restraining the change. If the team can increase the driving forces, change is more likely to occur. A force field analysis is shown in **FIGURE 9-8**. The driving forces are the factors that are likely to move an exercise program for patients with cancer forward, whereas the restraining forces are likely to

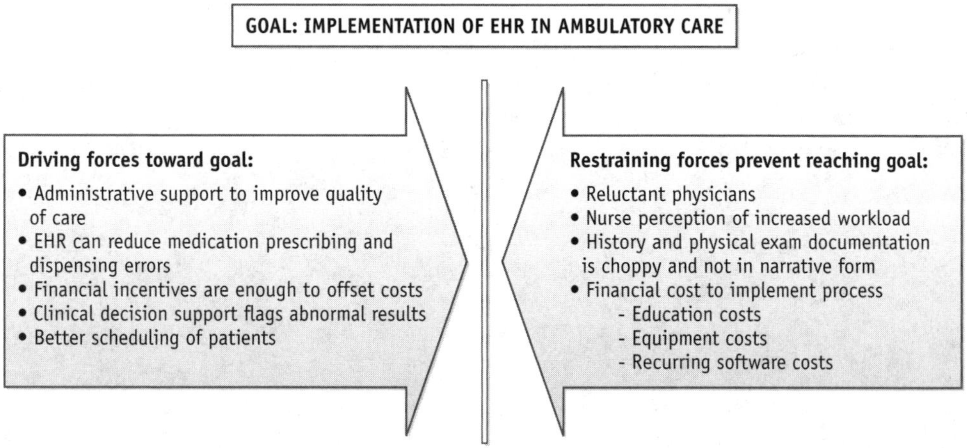

FIGURE 9-8 Force field analysis.

reduce the chances of the exercise program being successful.

A tool that works well for brainstorming and illustrating workflow problems is a cause and effect chart, commonly called a fishbone chart. The problem is illustrated as the head of the fish, and each spine represents a category of causes. In **FIGURE 9-9**, communication with patients who have limited English proficiency is the problem. The causes are identified as time constraints, patient education, hospital interpreter list, Health Insurance Portability and Accountability Act of 1996 (HIPAA) compliance, economics, documentation, health literacy, and telephone language line. Each cause has multiple contributing issues. This data display tool is effective because it conveys a great deal of information in an understandable manner.

▶ Gap Analysis and Workflow Redesign

An initial workflow analysis conducted before health IT is implemented will likely reveal **inefficiencies** that can be improved with workflow redesign. For example, a workflow study of vital sign assessment and documentation in three hospitals demonstrated differences in time based on the type of documentation system in use (Yeung, Lapinsky, Granton, Doran, & Cafazzo, 2012). In hospitals with paper-based systems, nurses documented vital signs immediately on bedside flowsheets, whereas nurses in hospitals with EHRs wrote vital signs on notepaper and later documented them in the patient record. This transcription of vital signs in hospitals with EHRs was redundant and inefficient with regard to time. The delay in documenting in the EHR also made vital signs unavailable to other HCPs. Finally, the transcription of vital signs from paper notes to the electronic record could have introduced errors (also called **defects** in the workflow literature).

The inefficiencies discovered in a workflow analysis could be used as a starting point for redesign (Bowens & Jones, 2010). The inefficiencies represent a gap between the current, inefficient workflow and the future, desired workflow with health IT. A formal report of the gap is called a **gap analysis**. Using the results described earlier (Yeung et al., 2012), a health IT design team would readily understand the need for bedside documentation capabilities in an EHR. The documentation of vital signs needs to be fast and error free, so one solution could be mobile electronic vital sign monitors with wireless communication to a mobile vital sign documentation module in the EHR. This

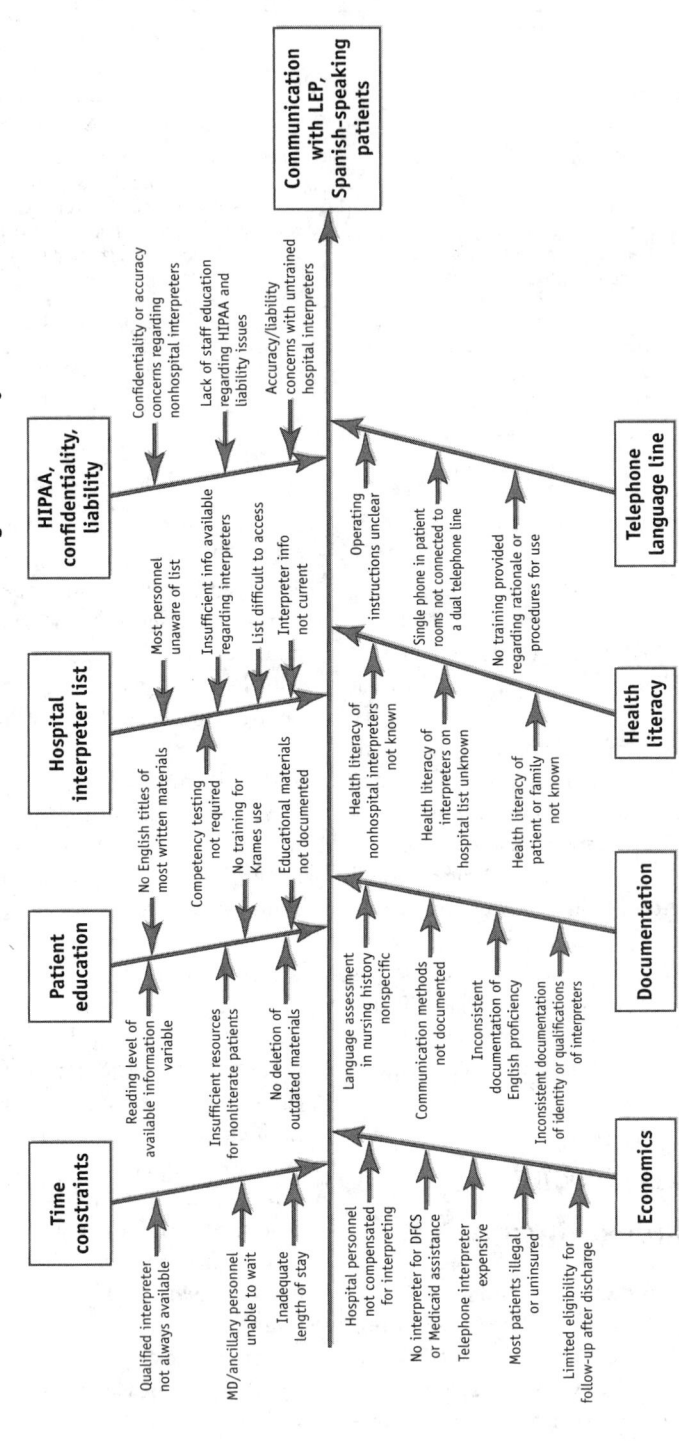

FIGURE 9-9 Cause and effect chart.

solution would eliminate the need to remember vital signs, write them down, and transcribe them later into an EHR. Having identified the gap between current and future workflow, the health IT team can select products that meet the requirements. It is through analysis of workflow that real return on health IT investment can be achieved (Jones et al., 2012).

An area of workflow inefficiency many nurses experience is searching for medication, supplies, and equipment. Health IT systems can be used to maintain appropriate inventory levels of frequently used medications and supplies. Medication systems that store, count, track use, and automatically generate messages for inventory restocking are particularly efficient because the systems remove the requirement for redundant work such as counting narcotics and calling for supplies to be restocked. Systems can reduce the time nurses wait for deliveries of newly ordered medications and supplies. When supplies and medications are readily available via a health IT system, it can reduce the tendency for nurses to stash supplies, a costly practice, in terms of inventory.

Nurses and other HCPs who experience workflow problems after implementation of health IT will often develop **workarounds**, which are unauthorized ways to use health IT (Miller, Fortier, & Garrison, 2011). Miller and colleagues conducted a study of medication administration after implementation of a barcode medication administration system. The approved workflow had eight steps, including review of medication order, bar scan of patient wristband, review of electronic medication administration record (e-MAR), bar scan of medication, resolution of any system alert, administration of medications, confirmation of administration in e-MAR, and review of documentation in charting session. The researchers found that 20% of medications generated alerts requiring additional steps by nurses. Of the medications with alerts, 97% were administered with an override of the system, most of the time without a documented reason. This behavior of administering when

alerts were generated without documenting a reason for administration may represent "alert fatigue," a dangerous consequence of an improperly calibrated alert system. In addition to alert overrides, the researchers found other workarounds categorized as "omission of a process step, performance of an unauthorized step, or performance of steps in improper sequence" (p. 164). These workarounds represent defects in the health IT implementation and should be corrected because of the risk for medication errors (Miller et al., 2011).

Studies of nursing efficiency following implementation of health IT indicate that several work processes can become more efficient: hand offs at the change of shift, medication reconciliation, order processing, and follow up on new orders (Thompson, Johnston, & Spurr, 2009). Processes that can be automated greatly add to nursing efficiency including automatic flow of data from medical devices into the EHR; automated lists of tasks generated from orders; documentation that autopopulates fields with previous entries from the EHR, with options to edit or enter new information; decision support alerts; autocalculation of medications and intravenous fluids; and autofill of documentation from dietary, respiratory, physical therapy, and creation of discharge instructions from physician orders and nursing care plans (Thompson et al., 2009).

▶ Workflow to Improve Care Processes and Organizational Operations

Efficient and Safe Care Processes

For clinical workflow, **clinical decision-support systems (CDSS)** integrated into an EHR can improve the efficiency and safety of care processes. The Office of the National Coordinator for

Health Information Technology (2013) provided the following definition of CDSS:

> Clinical decision support provides clinicians, staff, patients or other individuals with knowledge and person-specific information, intelligently filtered or presented at appropriate times, to enhance health and health care. CDS [clinical decision support] encompasses a variety of tools to enhance decision-making in the clinical workflow. These tools include computerized alerts and reminders to care providers and patients; clinical guidelines; condition-specific order sets; focused patient data reports and summaries; documentation templates; diagnostic support, and contextually relevant reference information, among other tools.

Clinical decision support is developed by understanding clinical workflow at a very granular level. The workflow is mapped using flowcharts and sophisticated logic that continuously monitors and moves workflow based on definitions and preset conditions. For example, a CDSS was developed and tested to improve nurses' early identification of patients who need a rapid response team to prevent deterioration that would result in full code blues and/or transfers to an intensive care unit (Heal, Silvest-Guerrero, & Kohtz, 2017). The authors' CDSS looked for variations from expected physiological measures including respiratory rate, heart rate, oxygen saturation, temperature, and mean arterial blood pressure and provided a score of 0–3. A score over 3 would send an alert to a "crisis nurse" who would consult with the unit nurse and evaluate the patient. The researchers compared two medical-surgical units in the same hospital and found that a significantly higher number of rapid response teams were deployed to the unit with the CDSS as compared to a unit that used nurses' judgment alone. Likewise, the unit with CDSS had fewer transfers to an intensive care unit (Heal et al., 2017). To understand CDSS,

watch a short YouTube video on the Soarian Workflow Engine Congestive Heart Failure workflow at Main Line Health on the companion website for this text.

Health IT adoption does not always mean that the goals of improved care processes are achieved. Bar Code Medication Administration (BCMA) systems provide a perfect example of this phenomenon. Bowers et al. (2015) evaluated the effect of a BCMA on the medication administration practices in a single hospital with three medical-surgical units and three intensive care units. The researchers believed that implementation of BCMA would "increase real-time medication administration documentation, decrease medication administration–related errors, increase Workstation on Wheels (WOW) usage at the bedside for medication administration, and increase the use of the electronic medication administration record (e-MAR) for medication retrieval" (Bowers, 2015, p. 503). They found mixed results: real-time documentation and use of WOW increased as predicted, but errors increased, and the use of the e-MAR remained unchanged. The researchers found that some workflow from the paper system persisted in the intensive care units, particularly related to the use of the e-MAR (Bowers, 2015). This observation indicates that workflow with BCMA and e-MAR in intensive care units was not sufficiently planned to account for the nurses' needs.

Exceptional Patient Experiences and Effective Throughput

The Institute of Medicine's report, *Crossing the Quality Chasm*, defined exceptional patient and family experiences as having six critical characteristics: care that is patient centered, safe, effective, timely, efficient, and equitable (IOM, 2001). The patient experience with care often turns from satisfying to dissatisfying based on the timeliness of being seen for appointments, procedures, or surgery and based on the coordination among different HCPs along the continuum from prevention, acute treatment, to transition to ambulatory care or rehabilitation. (Lee, Moriarty, Borgstrom, & Horwitz 2010). The timeliness, efficiency, and coordination can be expressed as patient throughput, and in the next two sections, these topics are explored with regard to health IT.

Timely and Efficient Care

Patient throughput is the movement of patients from one part of a healthcare delivery system to another. There can be many initiatives aimed to improve patient throughput, but all approaches should use established methods such as Six Sigma or Lean with information technology to yield data, which can inform processes and assess effectiveness of changes in throughput (Walker, Kappus, & Hall, 2016). Other system-wide strategies include the creation of patient placement or transfer center departments that use bed management software to manage where patients are admitted and to notify departments of pending discharges. Bed management software typically have a locator device on beds or patients so messages about locations are automatically generated. Other software solutions improve the scheduling of procedures and surgeries and locate equipment using electronic monitoring. Some systems are worn by staff to locate nurses, to monitor for hourly rounding, to assess hand hygiene, and countless other activities that can be used to understand and improve throughput.

The first efforts aimed at improvements in throughput were focused in emergency departments (EDs) due to long waits and patient dissatisfaction. The admission of patients from EDs to inpatient units, called boarding, can also slow patient treatment and can cause additional delays in EDs. The Joint Commission (TJC) set a standard to reduce boarding time to 4 hours, and most hospitals have responded with improvement campaigns to reduce throughput time from emergency departments to inpatient units (TJC, 2013). One such study was described by Simmons and Goldschmidt (2014) using what they termed a nursing SWAT team to monitor

the electronic medical record (EMR) for admissions from the emergency room to an inpatient unit. Nurses on the SWAT team would then perform the admission regardless of location. When needed, a nurse from the team would accompany a patient to diagnostic or treatment areas. The SWAT team reorganized nursing workflow to accelerate the admission process resulting in a higher number of admissions per month managed by the SWAT team.

Another more common approach to improving patient throughput in emergency departments is the use of "scribes" who document encounters in EMRs for physicians and nurse practitioners. Scribes have been used as workarounds when documentation in EMRs created a slower pace of work for physicians than paper or dictation systems. Studies find that scribes increase the satisfaction of physicians, increase the number of patients seen per hour, and improve revenue; however, the effect on patient length of stay in emergency departments is less clear (Heaton, Castaneda-Guarderas, Trotter, Erwin, & Bellolio, 2016).

Seamless Transitions of Care from Hospital to Outpatient Settings

Patients need care that is coordinated between different healthcare settings so that HCPs carry out plans of care between those transitions. However, such seamless transitions have not been realized even with the investment of federal dollars from the HITECH Act of 2009. As noted earlier in the chapter, problems with interoperability have presented the exchange of data between systems that could have provided access to real-time data, decision support for the healthcare team, and immediate answers to questions about medications or follow-up appointments with primary care providers that could have prevented readmissions (Escobedo, Kirtane, & Berman, 2012). The Office of the National Coordinator, along with other stakeholders conducted an invitational meeting called "Putting the 'IT' in Care TransITions."

At this think-tank meeting, several consensus statements were identified regarding the use of health IT to improve transitions.

- There needs to be a plan of care that spans time and setting, incorporates social and medical factors, reflects patient goals, and is accessible to all care team members;
- Effective and efficient medication reconciliation continues to evade even the most sophisticated providers;
- IT-enabled feedback loops are underdeveloped, but they are critical to ensure safe care and self-management; and,
- Shifting from a hospital-centric model is the most important enabler for the spread and uptake of IT-enabled care transitions solutions. (Escobedo, Kirtane, & Berman, 2012, pp. 60–61)

The most vulnerable to insufficient care transitions are the elderly and those with chronic illnesses. Four critical elements that can improve transitions for these patients include a discharge process including automated plan of care and decision support for after-hospital needs and risk assessment accessible to patients and providers, automated information flow across settings, automated medication reconciliation that integrates providers and pharmacies, and patient/family engagement through portals that include decision support and patient education (Marcotte, Kirtane, Lynn, & McKethan, 2015).

Use of Human Resources

Business process automation in healthcare organizations is most often used for inventory management, billing, human resource management, and other business processes. There are many different human resource management software solutions that are aimed at managing workflow. For example, the assignment of newly admitted patients to nurses on a particular unit of a hospital can be calculated based on a nurse's workload for the past 15 minutes to estimate

an anticipated workload for an entire shift (Sundaramoorthi, Chen, Rosenberger, Kim, & Buckley-Behan, 2010). Other human resource solutions include scheduling transporters and housekeepers at peak times to accelerate patient transfers between departments and prepare rooms after use (Goldberg, & Robbins, 2011). The decision about appropriate human resource deployment requires real-time data that can be nimbly acted upon by leaders whose main concerns are patient throughput.

Logistics and Supply Chain Management

Logistics is a term used to describe the organization of supplies and equipment to place them in the right locations at the right time for use. The term is sometimes used interchangeably with **supply chain management**, but supply chain management typically refers to a system of manufactures or suppliers that is coordinated to move a product from production through distribution to consumers. Regardless of the terms used in health care, the main point is to have equipment and supplies in places where they are needed (Coustasse, Tomblin, & Slack, 2013). Delays or omissions of care can occur when nurses have trouble locating equipment needed for patient care. This lost efficiency can be addressed with technology. Coustasse et al. (2013) conducted a literature review on the most common technology used for hospital logistics: Radio-frequency Identification (RFID). The RFID tags and readers form a net of coverage across a hospital to have real-time information about the location of any tagged supplies or equipment. Studies of RFID deployment in hospitals have shown better control of inventory and reduced unrecovered cost and efficiency in the deployment of supplies and equipment. While only 10% of hospitals in the United States have adopted RFID technologies, the outlook is promising (Coustasse et al., 2013).

▶ Healthcare Provider Roles in Workflow Analysis

Providers who worked with paper systems are likely to experience the profound changes in the clinical processes after health IT is implemented, because they are inexperienced with systems such as EHRs. However, even nurses and other providers who enter the workforce after the implementation of EHRs is widespread will be involved in continuous improvements to health IT and implementation of cutting-edge technology. It is important for nurses to participate in workflow studies by participating in a design team or by being observed and interviewed. Participation in a health IT implementation team represents an opportunity to understand clinical processes and the fit with health IT. **BOX 9-1** provides a case study of workflow analysis involving nurses.

BOX 9-1 Workflow Analysis After Implementation of Computer Provider Order Entry

A study of medication administration workflow was conducted after implementation of computerized provider order entry (CPOE) by Tschannen, Talsma, Reinemeyer, Belt, and Schoville (2011). The researchers used mixed methods to gather data about the workflow of nurses. The first step of the analysis was to map the process of medication administration. Tschannen and colleagues interviewed nurses who worked in the target hospital and found that the process had 17 distinct steps.

Next, Tschannen and colleagues observed nurses as medications were being administered, and they timed each step with a stopwatch. The researchers observed 86 medication administrations for 32 hours over a 30-day period in an adult intensive care unit (ICU) and a pediatric unit. The researchers found the mean time for medication administration in the adult ICU was 8.45 minutes and in the pediatric unit it was 9.92 minutes. Nurses who worked in the pediatric unit spent more time preparing medications because they had to crush or dilute medications for children.

The researchers interviewed nurses to better understand workflow issues. They found four main concerns: "systems issues, variations in standards of care, workflow variability, and changes in communication practices" (p. 407). System issues were related to the screen layout in the e-MAR. The print was small, and nurses had to scroll and click more often than they liked. The computers were also slow and at times would not function. Variations in standards of care concerned the lack of a designated time to check for new medication orders. If a stat dose had been entered by a provider in the CPOE, nurses might not know, and the system did not provide an alert. Duplicate orders were problematic for nurses in the system. The nurses also reported that medication reconciliation was more difficult to perform with CPOE than with paper orders. The most profound change was communication between physicians and nurses. Because physicians entered their own orders, there was little need for discussion. Nurses did find the organization of medications in the CPOE to be better than paper orders because the medications could be grouped by name or route, making review much faster. Observations by researchers corroborated the concerns nurses expressed in interviews.

Check Your Understanding

1. What other data-collection methods could have been used to analyze workflow of medication administration after implementation of CPOE?
2. What charts or graphs could be used to illustrate nurses' workflow or concerns with altered workflow?
3. Which changes in workflow after implementation of CPOE could result in medication errors?
4. Could any of the workflow be automated? If so, which processes would benefit from automation?

TABLE 9-1 Workflow Tools Found Online

Source	Website	Description
U.S. Department of Health and Human Services	https://innovations.ahrq.gov /qualitytools/workflow-assessment -health-it-toolkit	Guide and tools for workflow analysis
Agency for Healthcare Research and Quality (AHRQ)	http://healthit.ahrq.gov/portal/server .pt/community/health_it_tools_and _resources/919/workflow_assessment _for_health_it_toolkit/27865	Workflow Assessment for Health IT Toolkit
AHRQ	http://healthit.ahrq.gov/portal /server.pt/community/health _it_tools_and_resources/919/time _and_motion_studies_database/27878	Time and Motion Studies Database. Formatted, blank access database available for free download. User manual is provided.
AHRQ	https://healthit.ahrq.gov/health-it -tools-and-resources/evaluation -resources/health-it-evaluation-toolkit -and-evaluation-measures-quick -reference	Health IT Evaluation Measures: Quick Reference Guides. This is a collection of tools with advice about methods of data collection that can be used to assess and then compare performance and outcomes before and after implementation of health IT.
AHRQ	http://healthit.ahrq.gov/portal/server .pt/community/health_it_tools _and_resources/919/health_it_survey _compendium/27874	Health IT Survey Compendium. This is a searchable database of survey tools for use in the preliminary stage of health IT adoption through reevaluations of health IT impact.
Soarian Workflow Engine	http://www.youtube.com /watch?feature5player_ embedded&v=ZC4b4dEusEY	Video demonstrating clinical decision-support workflow with congestive heart failure.

▶ Summary

Implementation of health IT requires analysis of workflow, which is a detailed examination of the care processes. Analysis of workflow should be directed by an implementation team that includes a nurse informaticist. The implementation team uses many methods to study workflow and communicate the results of the analysis. The most common of these are task analysis, interviews, flowcharts, and process mapping (see **TABLE 9-1**). After understanding current workflow and finding gaps to the future, desired workflow, product review, and selection can be targeted to health IT that fills the workflow gaps. High priority should be given to health IT that automates clinical or business processes to improve efficiency and productivity.

References

Boone, E. (2010). EMR usability: Bridging the gap between nurse and computer. *Nursing Management, 41*(3), 14–16.

Bowens, F. M. A., & Jones, W. A. (2010). Health information technology: Integration of clinical workflow into meaningful use of electronic health. *Perspectives in Health Information Management, 7*, 1–15.

Buchini, S., & Quattrin, R. (2012). Avoidable interruptions during drug administration in an intensive rehabilitation ward: Improvement project. *Journal of Nursing Management, 20*(3), 326–334. doi: 10.1111/j.1365-2834.2011 .01323.x

Carayon, P. (Ed.). (2012). *Handbook of human factors and ergonomics in health care and patient safety* (2nd ed.). Boca Raton, FL: CRC Press, Taylor & Francis Group.

Choi, J., & Kim, H. (2012). A workflow-oriented framework-driven implementation and local adaptation of clinical information systems: A case study of nursing documentation system implementation at a tertiary rehabilitation hospital. *CIN: Computers, Informatics, Nursing, 30*(8), 409–414; quiz 415–406. doi: 10.1097 /NXN.0b013e3182512ffd

Cornell, P., Herrin-Griffith, D., Keim, C., Petschonek, S., Sanders, A. M., D'Mello, S., . . . Shepherd, G. (2010). Transforming nursing workflow, part 1. *Journal of Nursing Administration, 40*(9), 366–373. doi: 10.1097/NNA .0b013e3181ee4261

Cornell, P., Riordan, M., Townsend-Gervis, M., & Mobley, R. (2011). Barriers to critical thinking workflow interruptions and task switching among nurses. *Journal of Nursing Administration, 41*(10), 407–414. doi: 10.1097/NNA .0b013e31822edd42

Coustasse, A., Tomblin, S., & Slack, C. (2013). Impact of radio-frequency identification (RFID) technologies on the hospital supply chain: A literature review. *Perspectives in Health Information Management*, 1–17.

Dasgupta, A., Sanger, S. S., Jacob, S. M., Frost, C. P., Dwibedi, N., & Tipton, J. (2011). Descriptive analysis of workflow variables associated with barcode-based approach to medication administration. *Journal of Nursing Care Quality, 26*(4), 377–384.

Effken, J. A., Brewer, B. B., Logue, M. D., Gephart, S. M., & Verran, J. A. (2011). Using cognitive work analysis to fit decision support tools to nurse managers' work flow. *International Journal of Medical Informatics, 80*(10), 698–707. doi: 10.1016/j.ijmedinf.2011.07.003

Elganzouri, E. S., Standish, C. A., & Androwich, I. (2009). Medication administration time study (MATS): Nursing staff performance of medication administration. *Journal of Nursing Administration, 39*(5), 204–210.

Escobedo, M., Kirtane, J., & Berman, A. (2012). Health information technology: A path to improved care transitions and proactive patient care. *Generations, 36*(4), 56–62

Goldberg, A. J., & Robbins, S. B. (2011). Portion control opportunities: Real time gains for hospital patient throughput. *Journal of Healthcare Management, 56*(5), 293–297.

Heal, M., Silvest-Guerrero, S., & Kohtz, C. (2017). Design and development of a proactive rapid response system. *CIN: Computers, Informatics, Nursing, 35*(2), 77–83. doi: 10.1097/CIN.0000000000000292

Healthcare Operations Management Solutions. TeleTracking. (n.d.). Retrieved from http://www.teletracking.com

Heaton, H. A., Castaneda-Guarderas, A., Trotter, E. R., Erwin, P. J., & Bellolio, M. F. (2016). Effect of scribes on patient throughput, revenue, and patient and provider satisfaction: A systematic review and meta-analysis. *American Journal of Emergency Medicine, 34*(10), 2018–2028. doi: 10.1016/j.ajem.2016.07.056

Helmons, P. J., Wargel, L. N., & Daniels, C. E. (2009). Effect of bar-code-assisted medication administration on medication administration errors and accuracy in multiple patient care areas. *American Journal of Health-System Pharmacy, 66*(13), 1202–1210. doi: 10.2146/ajhp 080357

Healthcare Information and Management Systems Society. (2005). What is interoperability? Retrieved from http://about:reader?url=http%3A%2F%2Fwww.himss .org%2Flibrary%2Finteroperability-standards%2Fwhat -is-interoperability

Holden, R. J., Scanlon, M. C., Patel, N. R., Kaushal, R., Scoot, K. H., Brown, R. L., . . . Karsh, B. T. (2011). A human factors framework and study of the effect of nursing workload on patient safety and employee quality of working life. *BMJ Quality & Safety, 20*(1), 15–24. doi: 10.1136/bmjqs.2008.028381

Institute of Medicine. (1999). *To err is human: Building a safer health system.* Washington, DC: National Academies Press.

Institute of Medicine. (2001). *Committee on Quality of Health Care in America. Crossing the quality chasm: A new health system for the 21st century.* Washington, DC: National Academies Press.

Institute of Medicine. (2011). *Health IT and patient safety: Building safer systems for better care.* Washington, DC: Committee on Patient Safety and Health Information Technology, Board on Health Care Services.

Joint Commission. (2013). *The "patient flow standard" and the 4-hour recommendation joint commission perspectives*, 33. Retrieved from http://www.jointcommission.org /assets/1/18/S1-JCP-06-13.pdf

Jones, S. S., Heaton, P. S., Rudin, R. S., & Schneider, E. C. (2012). Unraveling the IT productivity paradox—lessons for health care. *New England Journal of Medicine, 366*(24), 2243–2245.

Kjeldskov, J., Skov, M. B., & Stage, J. (2010). A longitudinal study of usability in health care: Does time heal? *International Journal of Medical Informatics, 79*(6), e135–e143. doi: 10.1016/j.ijmedinf.2008.07.008

Kohle-Ersher, A., Chatterjee, P., Osmanbeyoglu, H. U., Hochheiser, H., & Bartos, C. (2012). Evaluating the barriers to point-of-care documentation for nursing staff. *CIN: Computers, Informatics, Nursing, 30*(3), 126–133.

Lee, A. V., Moriarty, J. P., Borgstrom, C., & Horwitz, L. I. (2010). What can we learn from patient dissatisfaction? Analysis of dissatisfying events at an academic medical center. *Journal of Hospital Medicine: An Official Publication of the Society of Hospital Medicine, 5*(9), 514–520. doi: 10.1002/jhm.861

Lee, S., & McElmurry, B. (2010). Capturing nursing care workflow disruptions: Comparison between nursing and physician workflows. *CIN: Computers, Informatics, Nursing, 28*(3), 151–161.

Marcotte, L., Kirtane, J., Lynn, J., & McKethan, A. (2015). Integrating health information technology to achieve seamless care transitions. *Journal of Patient Safety, 11*(4), 185–190.

McGonigle, D., & Mastrian, K. (2012). *Nursing informatics and the foundation of knowledge.* Burlington, MA: Jones & Bartlett Learning.

Miller, D. F., Fortier, C. R., & Garrison, K. L. (2011). Bar code medication administration technology: Characterization of high-alert medication triggers and clinician workarounds. *Annals of Pharmacotherapy.* doi: 10.1345/aph.1P262

National Institute for Health Care Management Foundation. (2005). *Steps in a basic workflow analysis.* Retrieved from http://nihcm.org/pdf/AHRQ-QandA.pdf

Office of the National Coordinator for Health Information Technology. (2013). *Clinical decision support.* Retrieved from http://www.healthit.gov/policy-researchers-implementers/clinical-decision-support-cds

Page, A. (Ed.), Committee on the Work Environment for Nurses and Patient Safety, Board on Health Care Services. (2004). *Keeping patients safe: Transforming the work environment of nurses.* Washington, DC: National Academies Press.

Simmons, C., & Goldschmidt, K. (2014). A nursing SWAT team: Using the EMR to improve patient throughput. *Journal of Pediatric Nursing, 29*(6), 705–708. doi: 10.1016/j.pedn.2014.08.007

Sundaramoorthi, D., Chen, V. C., Rosenberger, J. M., Kim, S. B., & Buckley-Behan, D. F. (2010). A data-integrated simulation-based optimization for assigning nurses to patient admissions. *Health Care Management Science, 13*(3), 210–221.

Thomas, R. (2006). Information-based transformation: The need for integrated, enterprisewide informatics. *Healthcare Financial Management, 60*(9), 140–142.

Thompson, D., Johnston, P., & Spurr, C. (2009). The impact of electronic medical records on nursing efficiency. *Journal of Nursing Administration, 39*(10), 444–451. doi: 10.1097/NNA.0b013e3181b9209c

Thune, J., Alexander, L., Roberts, P., & Enzi, M. (2015). Where is HITECH's $35 billion dollar investment going? Retrieved from http://healthaffairs.org/blog/2015/03/04/where-is-hitechs-35-billion-dollar-investment-going/

Trbovich, P. (2014). Five ways to incorporate systems thinking into healthcare organizations. *Biomedical Instrumentation & Technology, 4831–4836.* doi: 10.2345/0899-8205-48.s2.31

Tschannen, D., Talsma, A., Reinemeyer, N., Belt, C., & Schoville, R. (2011). Nursing medication administration and workflow using computerized physician order entry. *CIN: Computers, Informatics, Nursing, 29*(7), 401–410. doi: 10.1097/NCN.0b013e318205e510

Unertl, K. M., Johnson, K. B., & Lorenzi, N. M. (2012). Health information exchange technology on the front lines of healthcare: Workflow factors and patterns of use. *Journal of the American Medical Informatics Association, 19*(3), 392–400. doi: 10.1136/amiajnl-2011-000432

U.S. Department of Health and Human Services. (2009). HITECH Act. Retrieved from http://www.healthit.gov/policy-researchers-implementers/hitech-act-0

Varpio, L., Kuziemsky, C., MacDonald, C., & King, W. J. (2012). The helpful or hindering effects of in-hospital patient monitor alarms on nurses: A qualitative analysis. *CIN: Computers, Informatics, Nursing, 30*(4), 210–217. doi: 10.1097/NCN.0b013e31823eb581

Walker, C., Kappus, K., & Hall, N. (2016). Strategies for improving patient throughput in an acute care setting resulting in improved outcomes: A systematic review. *Nursing Economics, 34*(6), 277–288.

Watkins, N., Kennedy, M., Lee, N., O'Neill, M., Peavey, E., Ducharme, M., & Padula, C. (2012). Destination bedside: Using research findings to visualize optimal unit layouts and health information technology in support of bedside care. *Journal of Nursing Administration, 42*(5), 256–265. doi: 10.1097/NNA.0b013e3182480918

Yeung, M. S., Lapinsky, S. E., Granton, J. T., Doran, D. M., & Cafazzo, J. A. (2012). Examining nursing vital signs documentation workflow: Barriers and opportunities in general internal medicine units. *Journal of Clinical Nursing, 21*(7/8), 975–982. doi: 10.1111/j.1365-2702.2011.03937.x

Promoting Patient Safety with the Use of Information Technology

Stephanie Norman-Lenz, MSN, RN
Crayton Fargason, Jr., MD, MBA
Joni Hall, MSN, RN
Yeow Chye Ng, PhD, RN

LEARNING OBJECTIVES

1. Provide an overview of the major information technologies (ITs) that have the potential to impact the safety of care.
2. Describe the manner in which these technologies are deployed in order to improve patient safety.
3. Review the nursing impact of such technology deployments.
4. Describe the data and connectivity requirements that are needed to implement these safety strategies.
5. Discuss common points of failure experienced when these technologies are implemented.

KEY TERMS

Alert fatigue
Clinical decision-support
systems (CDSS)
Clinical microsystem
Commission

Errors
Knowledge-based error
Omission
Out-of-range alarms
Patient safety

Point of care
Rule-based error
Slip
System fault alarms

▶ Chapter Overview

The focus of this chapter is the use of health information technology (health IT) deployed to improve patient safety. More specifically, the primary focus is on technologies that directly impact nursing workflow and practice. The need for improvement in health IT is not a new issue, but it gained national attention after reports by the Institute of Medicine in 1999 and 2011.

The Healthcare Information and Management Systems Society (HIMSS) defines information as "data to which meaning has been assigned, according to context and assumed conventions" (HIMSS, 2010, p. 62). Furthermore, it defines an information system as one that "takes input data, processes it, and provides information as output" (HIMSS, p. 63). The information infrastructure at a patient's bedside is a more sophisticated environment than it was a generation ago when much of the clinical documentation was completed on paper. While many new tools are available to address patients' healthcare needs, not all advances in technology have improved outcomes, and many have resulted in increased healthcare costs (Lighter, 2013). In addition, many of the promised patient safety benefits of health IT are yet to be completely realized.

▶ Health IT Used in Patient Care

One can view information technology operating at multiple levels. The area where changes in health IT are most visible to nurses is at the sharp end or **point of care**, whether in a hospital room or an exam room in a clinic. The point of care (shown in Zone 1 of **FIGURE 10-1**) can contain a vast array of medical devices and technology to manage and properly document patient care. The electronic health record (EHR) has evolved over time to include elements such as electronic orders and results, electronic medication administration record (e-MAR), and healthcare provider (HCP) documentation. Computerized provider order entry (CPOE) is another important workflow crossing many functional and professional domains that has been incorporated into the EHR. Moving outward from the bedside point of care, the next area of consideration is the hospital unit or clinic (Zone 2 in Figure 10-1). The first and second zones establish a **clinical microsystem**, which is considered to be a small group of people who work to provide care to a group of patients (The Dartmouth Institute, 2013). These clinical microsystems are often embedded in larger organizations such as hospitals, multi-specialty practices, or other outpatient settings, which form the third zone of the diagram. The fourth zone of the diagram depicts information exchange across organizations such as a health system with hospitals, clinics, home health, and outpatient services. This fourth zone also includes communication with patients using portals and with other care providers using some form of health information exchange. At each of these zones, IT tools can be deployed to improve patient safety. The tools employed at different zones often have different connectivity and data infrastructure requirements associated with them and varying impact on nursing workflow.

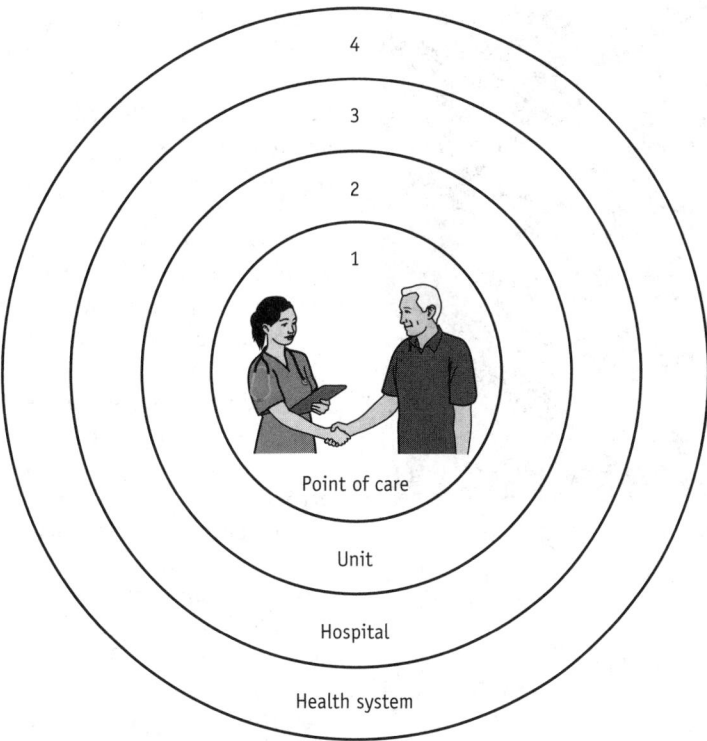

FIGURE 10-1 Zones in health care.

▶ Patient Safety at the Point of Care

Initiating Care

Errors may occur. HCPs do not intentionally commit errors. Nonetheless, errors may equate to individuals being harmed while receiving care. HIMSS defines **patient safety** as "freedom from unacceptable risk of harm" (HIMSS, 2013, p. 89). Most errors result from deficiencies in systems of care, and the generation of errors in general can be conceptualized using Reason's Swiss cheese model (Reason, 2000). Reason defines **errors** as risks that pass through gaps in protective barriers that normally defend patients from harm. The probability of errors increases when the number of holes in barriers increase and/or the number of barriers decrease (Reason, 1990).

So, the probability of errors can be reduced by adding protective barriers (adding additional slices of cheese to the process), or by minimizing the safety gaps (holes in the cheese) at a given layer (see **FIGURE 10-2**). IT is often envisioned as a means of providing additional protective barriers; however, achieving reduction in risk depends on far more than technology.

Healthcare services are ultimately delivered by people, and the delivery of care is therefore influenced by the limitations of humans. Reason's (1990) model recognizes several human sources of error that have implications for the safety of care delivered to patients. One type of error, a **slip**, is an instance in which a person knows the correct actions, yet at the time care is delivered, an incorrect action is taken (Reason, 1990). A colloquial example of this would be placing a carton of milk in the kitchen cabinet instead of the refrigerator. The analogous example in health

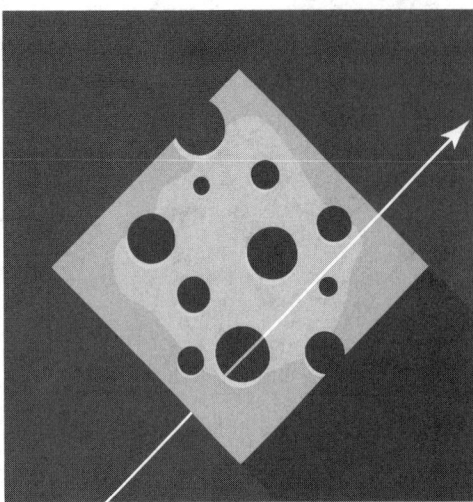

FIGURE 10-2 Swiss cheese model of medical errors.
© alya_haciyeva/Shutterstock

care would be grabbing the wrong breastmilk from a refrigerator and giving it to a patient. A second type of error is a **rule-based error**. This is when a good rule is applied in the wrong situation. Making a right turn when the traffic light is red after a complete stop is a good rule, but it should not be applied if it leads to driving the wrong direction on a one-way street. Likewise, penicillin may be the antibiotic of choice in the treatment of streptococcal pharyngitis, however it is not the appropriate agent if the patient is allergic to penicillin. Finally, **knowledge-based errors** occur when an individual does not possess the information needed to determine the appropriate action. An example of this might be the simultaneous administration of two intravenous (IV) medications that a provider does not realize are chemically incompatible. **Clinical decision-support systems (CDSS)** are often deployed within clinical information systems to minimize the risk of these types of errors.

Other concepts that help in discussions of safety are **commission** and **omission**. HIMSS defines error as: "An act of commission (doing something wrong) or omission (failing to do the right thing) that leads to an undesirable outcome or significant potential for such an outcome"

(HIMSS, 2013). An act of commission would be administering penicillin to a patient with a known allergy to penicillin. When an opportunity to perform an action that could benefit a patient is missed, an error of omission has occurred. For example, failure to rescue a patient in septic shock because of delayed recognition is an example of an error of omission (Schmid, Hoffman, Happ, Wolf, & DeVita, 2007). Each of the human vulnerabilities identified by Reason (1990) can lead to acts of commission or acts of omission.

Additional layers of protection and checks within each layer can help decrease the risk of slips, rule-based errors, and knowledge-based errors by HCPs. CDSS generate reminders when an action is necessary (preventing acts of omission), and warn providers of potentially inappropriate actions (preventing acts of commission). Nurses may view such health IT aides as essential, yet they are often unaware of the limitations and risks associated with the adoption and implementation of such tools. The discussion that follows focuses on how failure can occur despite the use of health IT, as well as describes how information systems can improve safe care delivery.

There have been many technological advances to improve patient safety at the point of care. Examples include physiologic monitors, alarms, smart medication pumps, electronic handheld communication devices, barcode medication administration, and radiofrequency identification (RFID). These technologies are cross-mapped in **TABLE 10-1** to the potential error types discussed previously.

Physiologic monitors are ubiquitous. They are designed to prevent errors of omission that may result if staff do not respond promptly to significant changes in a patient's physiologic condition. These technologies offer other advantages. For example, electronic capture of bedside parameters linked to the EHR allows immediate access to information for multiple providers in various locations (even away from the bedside). Such availability may improve the safety and efficiency of patient care.

TABLE 10-1 Devices at the Bedside

Device	Location	Minimal Level of Data Integration	Type of Error Addressed
Physiologic monitors	Bedside	Device/unit centric	Omission: inattentive slips
Smart pumps	Bedside	Local data sets residing in device "brain"	Commission: slips, rule-based errors, knowledge-based errors
Location monitoring	Unit or institution	Unit-based or centrally integrated information	Omission: inattentive slips
Barcoding devices	Unit	Centrally integrated with e-MAR	Commission: slips
Embedded sensors	Institution	Centrally integrated information	Omission: inattentive slips

e-MAR, electronic medication administration record

Alarms in Physiologic Monitoring

The patient's physiologic condition can be monitored noninvasively and invasively. Noninvasive outputs of bedside monitors can generate graphical (waveforms) and numeric displays by means of leads or probes attached to the patient. Examples of noninvasive parameters that can be monitored are blood pressure, heart rate, respiratory rate, body temperature, and pulse oximetry. Before the implementation of electronic physiologic monitoring, many of these parameters were determined manually. Consider pulse oximetry, for example: Prior to the advancement of pulse oximetry, staff directly monitored oxygen saturation. The monitoring individuals had to be vigilant and skilled in estimating oxygen levels based on clinical observation. Even skilled observers may have disagreed (O'Donnell, Kamlin, Davis, Carlin, & Morley, 2007). Pulse oximetry eliminates problems with observer error. However, accurate pulse oximetry readings require the detection of adequate pulsations. Inadequate detection of pulsations can lead to erroneous readings. This type of detection problem is common in the critically ill patient with poor perfusion. Active patients (children, for example) can also disrupt the quality of the signal received by the device, leading to false alerts. When these false alerts occur frequently, staff members experience **alert fatigue**. This fatigue introduces a "cry wolf" bias in staff: Pulse oximeter alarms in the absence of any problem with oxygen saturation are ignored. Errors of omission can occur when meaningful alerts are subsequently ignored due to fatigue with false positive alerts.

Like pulse oximeters, most monitoring technologies have basic requirements for successful use. When these conditions are not met (e.g., a poorly perfused patient with pulse oximetry monitoring), more sophisticated, noninvasive technologies are sometimes available. For example, staff might use near-infrared spectroscopy (NIRS) to monitor tissue oxygenation in the cases where patients have decreased pulsatile flow. NIRS can accurately evaluate oxygen status even when a pulsatile waveform is not present (Boas et al., 2001).

In some cases, limitations of noninvasive approaches necessitate the use of invasive monitoring tools. In complex cases, providers rely on information from more invasive types of monitoring such as intracranial pressure (ICP), cerebral perfusion pressure (CPP), central venous pressure (CVP), invasive blood pressure (IBP), or invasive cardiac monitoring. While invasive monitoring provides valuable information, its use increases the risk of harming patients. For example, insertion of a central line to monitor CVP could increase the risk of a catheter-associated bloodstream infection.

Most bedside physiologic monitoring devices produce nearly continuous streams of data, which remain in the local monitor during the patient's stay. The bedside nurse can pull samples from this continuous data stream into nursing computerized documentation on a regular basis (depending on orders). Both invasive and noninvasive monitors can also generate alarms and alerts by comparing the input received from the patient with predefined parameters that are either manually entered by the caregiver or derived from algorithms programmed in the device. Such algorithms often correct for factors such as the patient's age. Examples of additional alerts often encountered by nursing staff are **out-of-range alarms** and **system fault alarms**:

- *Out-of-range alarms* are triggered when a patient's value is above or below a set parameter. These high and low limits can be set manually by the nursing staff or can be set to a default determined by institutional policy.
- *System fault alarms* are triggered when there is an ineffective reading potentially due to displaced leads or other system malfunction(s).

As with any technology, alarms should not take the place of licensed caregivers. Rather, they are designed to aid in the decision-making process. Indeed, overreliance on such devices often contributes to errors of omission. Physiologic monitoring must be validated with the physical assessment of the patient. Success with the use of this type of monitoring depends on many factors, including proper placement of electrodes for noninvasive monitoring; accurate calibration of devices, proper setup, and maintenance for invasive monitoring.

▶ Beyond the Initial Point of Care

Need for Connectivity

When data from devices is captured in clinical documentation there is usually an interest in propagating this information beyond the bedside. For information generated by medical devices to be meaningful beyond the point of care, there must be some connection to a larger information network. Connection to a larger information infrastructure also allows more sophisticated modulation of the information returned to the provider at the point of care. Links to this larger information network can be accomplished by hardwired or wireless connections. The hardwired connections are generally more reliable, but less portable. Wireless connections offer portability, but often incur the risk for disruption by interference or signal decay.

The benefits of connectivity are typically realized initially within the clinical microsystem. Central monitoring stations for managing cardiac rhythms are one example of such connectivity. Generally, these central stations are hardwired to bedside devices. Central monitoring stations receive real-time hemodynamic monitoring feeds from multiple patients at any given time. Having specialty trained staff monitor signals adds a new layer that decreases the risk of inattentive omissions (failure of a bedside provider to see and recognize a dangerous rhythm). The stations also decrease the risk of knowledge-based errors. Typically, these stations are staffed with skilled technicians who are trained to monitor rhythms. This level of constant attentiveness by an expert trained in cardiovascular rhythms would be expensive to duplicate at every patient bedside.

Recently, wireless technology has facilitated unit-based information sharing. Not only are these devices useful for communication (via voice or text), but they are also being used to access patient data away from the point of care. Consider, for example, the use of smartphones. With an appropriate software interface, smartphones can communicate patient physiologic alarms to staff away from the point of care (Mosa, Yoo, & Sheets, 2012). Such tools are gaining popularity due to their capability to propagate alarms generated at the bedside not only to the assigned nurse, but other members of the care team. The rules that govern the alert distribution can and often should be adjusted. The goal is to decrease the risk of omission errors caused when nurses are too busy or too far removed from the patient's physical location to audibly hear the bedside alarm. Typically, cascade alarms are configured so that if the original alarm is sent to the assigned nurse and is not acknowledged within a period of time, the alarm will retrigger to other HCPs in the patient's care area.

When using technology that sends or receives patient-specific information, it is crucial that the intended associations are properly connected. Association with the appropriate patient should be ensured. Association in this context means electronically connecting the patient's chart to the appropriate component (e.g., connecting the bedside monitor to the patient's EHR in order to record the vital signs). Visual cues make this easy to accomplish with wired connections, but less obvious when one seeks to "associate" bedside monitors with handheld devices. Two issues arise: (1) making the right association and (2) being aware of an interrupted association. Making the right association is important when propagating patient alarms or pulling patient-specific information into the EHR for documentation purposes. Often two levels of association are required—identifying the correct patient and identifying the correct episode of service within the patient record. Errors occur when the wrong patient is selected (a risk when more than one patient record is open at a time) or when the wrong episode is selected (observations entered on the wrong patient encounter within a record). Likewise, if a nurse believes that his or her smartphone is associated with a device alarm, but the association does not exist, alarms will be missed. In this case, the nurse will be following an implied rule ("all alerts will be forwarded to my smartphone") that is not applicable at that moment, which can result in an error of omission.

Documentation in Electronic Records

Data are entered (or electronically imported) and stored, ideally with contextual information that can generate knowledge to improve care. The preceding section discussed data generated by medical devices. These data can be pulled into the EHR rather than manually entered. A link must be made between the correct patient's physiologic monitor and the associated care event within the EHR. This information should be "validated" by staff prior to saving it into the permanent record. Additionally, nurses or other healthcare staff may enter data manually into the permanent record. Connecting to a larger network allows for data storage beyond the level of a single medical device. With wired connections, transmission of data from the point of care to data storage is very reliable, so data loss is not generally a concern. Wireless connections, on the other hand, can experience variable connectivity, which in turn may impact data integrity. If a wireless connection is interrupted, data may be dropped or delayed, which in turn could lead to lost or corrupted data.

Professionals enter much of the data generated at the point of care manually, and intermittently. A common example is the entry of the nurse's physical assessment into the EHR. Several issues become important when manual, intermittent processes are utilized. Humans routinely make mistakes when entering information manually into systems. Such errors may reduce the clarity of records but may also initiate an error that cascades and injures a patient. For example, if a nurse documents the wrong weight into the flowsheet for a dialysis patient, the prescriber may alter the therapy based on the erroneous weight. The relationship and/or the difference between the clinical event and the documentation of the event is more visible and receives more scrutiny in an EHR. For example, time stamps are ubiquitous in electronic records and are generated with great precision in computerized records. Small inconsistencies in time stamps become very noticeable and thus more problematic in the EHR. Decision rules that have algorithms based on time stamps may be negatively impacted by entry errors.

A subtler problem is the loss of information when data or actions at the microsystem level are not "saved" in the central data repository, either because the appropriate save sequence was not followed or because an unexpected disruption of service interfered with saving the information. When information is entered in the EHR, it exists in a local temporary memory until the information is loaded into more permanent electronic storage. While the item may appear to have been saved at the point of care, it may not be recognized at the central data repository when connectivity problems occur or there was a lack of adherence to the proper save sequence.

In order to give data meaning, data elements must have definitions assigned to them. While this is a complex topic, and largely outside the scope of this chapter, there is one important implication that all nurses should remember. Data entry, or documenting, in the EHR, must be done in standardized formats for data to be easily reused in the future. Achieving appropriate data context depends not just on computer systems, but also on thoughtful planning and integration with nursing workflow and practice. For example, in pediatrics dose/weight calculations are essential to safe medication management. To make sure such calculations are performed appropriately, the organization must adopt a convention that defines the type of values that are permissible in the weight field. Entering pounds when kilograms are called for can be extremely hazardous.

▶ Integrating Health IT and Patient Safety Goals

Informed Medication Administration

The first of the 2013 National Patient Safety Goals published by the Joint Commission was to improve the accuracy of patient identification by using at least two patient identifiers when providing care, treatment, and services (Joint Commission, 2013). In addition, although number of rights to medication administration have augmented over the years, five rights remain at the core of medication safety: ensuring the right patient, right medication, right dose, right route, and right time. Bar Code Medication Administration (BCMA) can aid in compliance by automating components of the workflow related to these rights. The U.S. Food and Drug Administration (FDA) has recognized patient safety benefits of BCMA. In 2004, the FDA issued a rule requiring barcodes on thousands of human drugs and biological products, leading prescription drug manufacturers to place barcodes on most of the drugs used in hospitals (FDA, 2004).

The typical workflow for BCMA begins with the caregiver scanning the patient's armband, which positively identifies the patient and associates them with medications ordered for them within the EMR. Next, the caregiver scans the medication they intended to administer. If the scanned patient, the scanned medication, and the electronic order (with corresponding schedule) are not consistent, a notification will fire, notifying the RN of the potential error. Once all the medications have been scanned and administered, there is an electronic completion that occurs, updating the electronic medication administration record in real time.

When implemented properly, there are three levels of safety associated with BCMA. Level 1 (assuring the five rights of medication administration) is the simplest layer and serves as the foundation to the automated double check of the prescribed medication order. This layer may also include nursing work lists, alerts for missed doses, and a reference to the hospital's formulary. Level 2 is more involved and incorporates educational tools such as medication reference libraries. These libraries can benefit the nursing staff and patients. Information on medications can be accessed and printed on demand for patient education. In addition, calculation tables are integrated within this phase that allow the nurse to reference dosing information. Level 3 provides clinical decision support tools. This level presents alerts and warnings specific to the medication regimen within the context of the individual patient condition (Yang, Brown, Trohimovich, Dana, & Kelly, 2002). Examples of warnings generated at this level are those that are triggered upon reaching a patient-specific maximum cumulative dose (with, for example, certain chemotherapy agents), medications that fall into the look-alike/sound-alike or high-risk categories, and medications that may require clinical actions. Additionally, this level can incorporate order reconciliation and near-miss reports (Yang et al., 2002).

While barcoding assists in timely documentation of medication administration and has the potential to decrease medication errors by as much as 86%, hospitals in the process of implementing this technology must take a serious look at the workflow and limitations of the technology when setting up the system (Patient Safety Authority, 2008). Most medications come barcoded from the manufacturer, which allows for a reliable scan when the original packaging is utilized. A problem does arise when repackaging is necessary. This is often seen with suspensions in pediatric institutions. There is an opportunity for error when the pharmacist must print a new barcoded label to place on the altered manufacture-distributed medication.

"Smart" IV pumps are another technology that can be used to improve the safety of medication practice. IV pumps have not always been smart! For many years, nurses simply dialed in a rate for the medication to be administered and pushed "start." Unfortunately, this approach was not error proof. Estimates suggest there are 1.5 million preventable adverse drug events (ADEs) reported each year, of which 7,000 result in death (Agius, 2012). One-third occur at the point of order initiation, another third during the transcription and dispensing stage, and the remaining third occur during the actual administration of the medication (Agius, 2012). Ninety percent of hospitalized patients receive an IV medication as a part of their treatment plan. The delivery of IV medications is associated with more errors than other delivery routes (Husch et al., 2005).

The first step in the evolution of smart pumps is endowing them with a "brain." Smart pumps are IV devices that house a library of medications along with their corresponding concentrations and safe dose ranges. If the nurse mistakenly enters a dose that exceeds limits programmed into the pump, the pump will alert the nurse of the potentially dangerous dose. The alert can be programmed with soft-stop and hard-stop alerts. A soft-stop alert only warns HCPs that something is out of the ordinary but does not keep them from executing the intended action. Hard-stop alerts, on the other hand, warn the HCP that their anticipated plan is not actionable and will stop them from moving forward in their current execution. The library of medications on the pump can be tailored to a condition (often location) in which the pump will be utilized. For example, if a patient is admitted to an acute care unit, it is possible to prevent the nurse caring for the patient from accessing the library for vasoactive drips. Programming for the administration of vasoactive drips can be limited to the intensive care unit setting. However, an override function can be created so that floor nurses have access to the features under certain situations (e.g., code event).

Bedside smart IV pumps not only facilitate delivery of medications; they also provide data on the care process (the administration rate of a fluid over time) and the behavior of providers (data on nursing keystrokes during programming and the nurse response to alerts). Just as the drug catalog stored in the smart pump's memory, data on the care-delivery process are stored on the device for a period and can be downloaded for examination (if a negative event occurs, for example).

Of course, smart pumps do not stay smart if their brains are not updated or if there are errors in the programming the device. Updates generally occur on an intermittent basis, usually when the pump is not actively engaged in the delivery of patient care. While the technology of smart pumps is appealing and can facilitate reduction of ADEs, they should not take the place of critical thinking skills or manual verification steps. Proper training is essential to ensure competency in programming the device. For pumps to be smart, they must be intelligently used.

While smart pumps have proven their effectiveness in patient care, manual programming is still required. Because manual pump programming lends itself to error, some institutions have implemented smart pump integration. This technology associates the smart pump to the patient and their medication orders. It is often used in conjunction with BCMA. The typical nursing workflow for smart pump integration is for the RN to scan the patient, then scan the IV medication(s), and lastly scan the associated IV pump the medication will be administered from. In doing this, all five rights of medication administration have been addressed, and the IV pump is automatically programmed based on the order. To ensure that validation has been done, the RN must verify the programming information prior to starting the infusion. While there is limited research on the benefits of smart pump integration, possible benefits could include decreased opportunity for programming-based errors and increased nursing productivity associated with IV infusions (Vanderveen, 2014). Further investigation regarding possible risks

(such as passive verification) associated with this technology should be conducted (see **BOX 10-1**).

▶ Where, Oh Where, Has My Patient Gone?

The use of barcoding in health care extends beyond medication management. In fact, barcodes are one of several technologies used at the institutional level (Zone 3 of Figure 10-1) to improve materials flow and also improve the safety of care delivery. Often operating room (OR) supplies are managed and documented in the EHR with the use of barcodes. The barcodes typically capture details about the particular supply, such as the name, lot number, and expiration date. Because information associated with surgical devices and supplies can be traced back to the surgical event, this information is extremely useful when an adverse event occurs following a surgery. Expiration date tracking within the OR setting is not only useful for patient safety but also can help with inventory management. In addition, should an adverse event related to a device be discovered at a future date, the information captured and linked to the surgical procedure can be used to facilitate "recalls" or patient notification of risk.

Barcoding is merely a "static" accounting for materials that is not conducive to tracking and monitoring the flow of materials across the physical environment of an organization. Some healthcare organizations use RFID to give more detailed tracking information related to patient care, patient movement, and supply management. With RFID technology, an automated wireless data-collection process designed to capture location and movement of identified objects is possible (Radio-frequency identification, 2005). This type of system is made up of four parts: a computer chip "sensor," antennas to transmit data, a computing device "reader," and software to analyze the data. As sensors move in and out of antenna range, nearby readers detect radio wave signals transmitted from tags. The radio wave signals are converted to digital or audio signals

BOX 10-1 Case Study

The hospital notes occurrence of an increased number of hypoglycemic episodes in its adult medical/surgical patients, along with many complaints from patients regarding extended wait times for meal services. A system-wide evaluation of root causes for the issues revealed that while nurses were giving correct dosages of rapid- and short-acting insulins before meals, patients were experiencing delays in room deliveries by food services, leading to episodes of hypoglycemia in patients who were not in specialized care units. Other causes for the hypoglycemic events included reduction in caloric intake by the hospitalized patients (compared to food intake in the home setting), duplication of insulin orders in the CPOE, and persistent use of sliding-scale insulin (SSI) due to healthcare professionals' lack of familiarity with basal/bolus regimens and the need to match insulin dosages with carbohydrate intake and premeal correction factors. The hospital administration decided to create a multidisciplinary committee, including representatives from all departments in the hospital, to address the problem of hypoglycemic episodes. The committee worked to support the integration of multiple mechanisms, using health IT, to reduce the incidence of inpatient hypoglycemic episodes.

The first task of the hospital was the upgrade of their EHR to add the use of a touch-screen management system with the capability to scan and track room food service delivery processes. Carlos, an experienced medical/surgical floor nurse, was appointed to participate in the team designated to design and launch a new electronic response charting pathway with the goal to produce the desired outcome of on-time meal delivery to prevent episodes of hypoglycemia in patients treated on medical/surgical floors.

Carlos understood the need for accuracy in the collection and aggregation of data regarding nutritional services in patients to improve patient safety. He worked as a trainer for staff in multiple units and departments, coaching them on the need to use preprogrammed entries in the database fields, appearing as drop-down boxes, so that use of free text was avoided and staff charting was more efficient and easier. Additional capabilities in the charting pathway offered clinical staff the opportunity to review food types given to the patient by nutritional services (also entered using predesignated choices). Food service delivery staff were also taught to scan the patient's ID band and their personnel badges in the meal delivery process. By using the electronic charting pathway, clinical staff were able to verify the delivery of meals to patient rooms before administering mealtime insulin therapy.

Analysis of the charting pathway implementation by the multidisciplinary committee revealed unanticipated benefits for patient safety as a result of its use. For example, the pathway could also be implemented for patients who were administered other medications for which food consumption (or the lack of it) was needed. Cross-checking for food allergies in patients was an additional example of how the charting pathway could be used to improve nutritional services and patient satisfaction.

Check Your Understanding

1. How could use of the electronic charting pathway be used in other ways to improve patient safety such as appropriate medication use and HCP education?
2. What other types of data could be collected from health IT tools to improve patient safety?
3. How can the use of health IT tools to improve patient safety lead to increases in patient satisfaction? Healthcare professional satisfaction? Healthcare professional safety?

(i.e., alarms) for a user to interpret or transmit to another device (such as a computer) for analysis (Roark & Miguel, 2006). The success of RFID depends on the reliability of the distributed network that registers the movement of tags through the environment.

With tracking information, one can better facilitate direct patient care. For example, RFID can be used to prevent retention of foreign bodies within the OR. An example of this is RFID-enabled surgical sponges that are counted automatically when dropped into a "smart" bucket. If any sponges are missing at the end of the surgical case, a handheld wand can alert the surgical team to the location of the misplaced sponge (Feldman, 2011).

In addition to tracking information on patient care, RFID is also used to better monitor the flow of patients throughout the hospital (Zone 3, Figure 10-2). One area of interest related to patient flow and RFID is infant abduction, which remains a major concern in nurseries and pediatric care environments. Affixing an RFID sensor to the infant's ID bracelet allows for the capability of an alarm to sound if the baby is moved out of the care area, adding an

additional level of protection against abductions. Likewise, the same type of technology can be used in psychiatric and geriatric units where elopement and wandering are a risk (Kamel Boulos & Berry, 2012; **FIGURE 10-3**).

Similarly, the management of supplies, equipment, and human resources can use RFID functionality. Expensive medical equipment can be tagged with an RFID sensor to prevent loss or theft. RFID-tagged wheelchairs and stretchers have the capability to be "visible" to staff on an electronic facility map, streamlining patient transport between units and ancillary departments. Hospitals can save time and resources by knowing exactly where equipment is at the precise time it is needed. In some organizations, RFID technology is used to track human resources. By affixing an RFID sensor to the employee name badge, senior management can better determine staff allocation in specific areas (Kamel Boulos & Berry, 2012). This same technology can help with employee hand hygiene compliance. Receiving sensors are placed on the wall-mounted sanitizers within the proximity of a patient room. If the employee enters the room (RFID sensor is attached to the employee badge) without

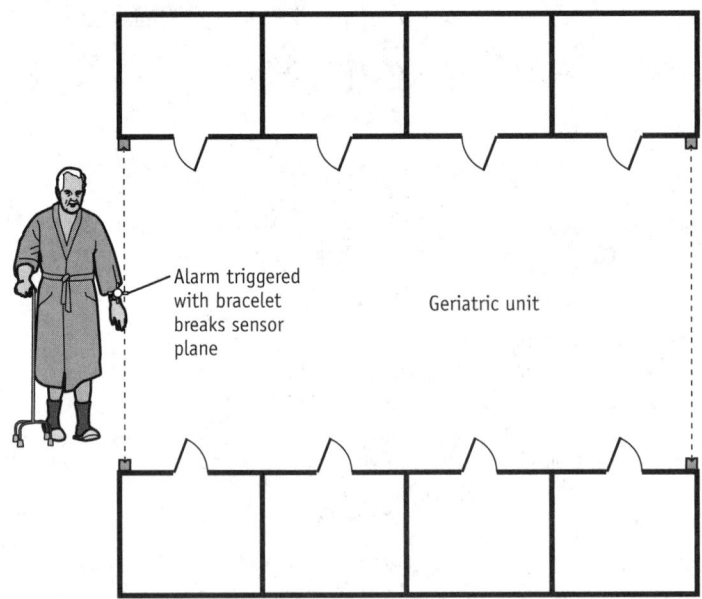

Alarm triggered with bracelet breaks sensor plane

Geriatric unit

FIGURE 10-3 RFID in the geriatric unit.

stopping at the wall-mounted hand sanitizer, the lack of compliance is recorded.

▶ Safety of Medical Devices

Issues in Device Design

As described earlier in this chapter, medical devices can be effective in reducing the risk of harm to patients. However, there are issues of device safety that cannot be overlooked. The U.S. Food and Drug Administration (FDA, 2012) has the responsibility for regulating the approval and recall of medical devices. Because of this regulatory responsibility, the FDA has guidelines for medical device design, testing, and error reporting. Human factors are an important aspect to consider in the design and use of medical devices. Medical devices should be designed for use by particular HCPs or by patients and their families. If people other than the intended users operate the device, the device may be unsafe. For example, ventilators are typically designed for use by physicians, respiratory therapists, and nurses. However, a patient who becomes ventilator-dependent may be sent home on a ventilator. The family will then become the user, and unintended, unsafe use errors can occur if the technology does not account for the varying needs of this type of user. Second, medical devices should be tested in laboratory and clinical environments that are similar to the ones in which the device will ultimately be used. However, medical devices are often used in settings beyond the intended environment. Varying lighting conditions, noise levels, and distractions are often not accounted for within testing environments. The less-than-optimal characteristics of real-world medical environments can lead to use errors and unsafe patient outcomes. Lack of consistent interface design among a class of medical devices can complicate the problem. For example, if bladder ultrasound devices have different pathways to guide nurses through measurement of urine in the bladder and a hospital unit has three bladder ultrasound devices made by different manufacturers, use errors can occur.

The FDA regulates the use of medical devices through safety communications, post-market surveillance studies, recalls, and mandatory medical device error reporting through the Medical Product Safety Network (MedSun). It is the responsibility of all HCPs to understand the risks of using medical devices and to report any device malfunction or contribution to patient harm to the FDA. The FDA issues email alerts to notify HCPs when a recall has been issued. These alerts are freely available to anyone who subscribes to the alert system on the FDA website (http://www.fda.gov).

Implications of EHR Downtime

HCPs have become accustomed to EHRs delivering patient health data at the click of a button. Despite the many safety benefits of EHRs, technical issues, including system downtime, can slow or halt the delivery of critical patient health data to HCPs. Downtime is defined as a period during which all or part of an organization's health IT is unavailable (Wang et al., 2016). EHR downtime can be either planned or unplanned. *Planned downtimes* are scheduled in advance for system upgrades and maintenance. They are expected. *Unplanned downtimes* can be caused by system failures, power outages, or natural disasters (Fahrenholz, Smith, Tucker, & Warner, 2009). They occur at unexpected times. Recent studies show that EHR downtime can lead to a disruption in the continuity of care, delay diagnosis and treatment, increase patient length of stay, and ultimately place patients at greater risk of harm (Hanuscak, Szeinbach, Seoane-Vazquez, Reichert, & McCluskey, 2009; Oral, Cullen, Diaz, Hod, & Kratz, 2015; Sittig, Gonzales, & Singh, 2014). Unfortunately, downtimes are not unusual in healthcare organizations.

The patient safety risks posed by EHR downtime are multifaceted. One major risk is the workflow disruption experienced by HCPs (Oral et al., 2015). The current era is one in which many HCPs have never relied on paper documentation to record or deliver care. To facilitate care without access to the electronic system and familiar workflow processes that are EHR dependent, HCPs may omit pertinent documentation, perform redundant work, or even worse, resort to unsafe work-arounds (Campbell, Sittig, Guappone, Dykstra, & Ash, 2007). Incomplete documentation can impair clinical decision making and lead to poor patient outcomes. Without access to the EHR, HCPs also lose the patient safety benefits of functions such as clinical decision support systems, e-MAR, and barcode medication administration systems. In a study by Hanusack et al. (2009), the most significant medication error that occurred within a 12-month period was directly related to CPOE/e-MAR downtime. This happened despite having backup systems and downtime protocols in place. Additionally, a downtime medication error was directly linked to increased length of stay for one patient. e-MAR-related downtime risks include delayed drug therapy, overdosing, and missed doses.

Delay in the delivery of critical laboratory results is another potential patient safety risk associated with an EHR downtime. HCPs rely on the prompt delivery of critical laboratory results from hospital laboratory systems to EHRs. Interfaces are often required to achieve this functionality. Any system failure that slows the delivery of laboratory results can delay HCPs' ability to diagnose critical conditions and intervene appropriately. During downtimes, laboratory personnel must often resort to manual processes for the delivery of results. Resorting to manual processes increases the workload on laboratory personnel and can significantly slow the reading and delivery of results (Oral et al., 2015). Wang et al. (2016) found that for five laboratory test types, downtime leads to significant increases in laboratory turnaround time (the time from test performance to the time results were available to be read by a clinician). The study also found that during one downtime event, clinician read times for potassium and hemoglobin labs were five and six times longer than those of a control group. Similar delays with cytology, pathology, or PACS results can lead to delayed diagnoses and treatment delays.

Healthcare organizations can mitigate the patient safety risks of EHR downtime by devising comprehensive downtime policies and procedures. In 2014, the Office of the National Coordinator for Health Information Technology (ONC) published nine SAFER Guides (Safety Assurance Factors for EHR Resilience) to assist healthcare organizations with the mitigation of the risks introduced by using EHRs. The SAFER Guides provide EBP-based self-assessment checklists that cover recommended practices surrounding EHR implementations. The *SAFER Self-Assessment: Contingency Planning* guide covers downtime practices. Phase 1 of the guide covers duplication of hardware, verification of adequate generator power supply, availability of paper forms to replace electronic documentation, patient data backup, and development of downtime policies and procedures for before, during, and after downtime (Ash, Singh, & Sittig, 2014). Phase 2 provides recommended practices for staff training on downtime and recovery procedures. New-hire training and recurring refresher courses are instrumental in ensuring that all essential HCPs have a thorough understanding of current downtime procedures (Fahrenholz et al., 2009). Downtime drills are an example of recurring education that serves as both an effective test of HCPs' knowledge of downtime processes and an opportunity to bridge any existing education gaps in a nonpunitive environment (Kashiwagi et al., 2016; Nelson, 2007). Phase 2 of the guide also covers the development of downtime communication independent of the computing infrastructure, written policies and procedures for downtime and recovery periods, and having a user interface on downtime systems that is easily distinguished from that of the live EHR environment. Phase 3, the monitoring phase, provides recommendations for testing and monitoring strategies for both the prevention and navigation of system downtime (Ash et al., 2014). A comprehensive downtime strategy, such as that suggested by the SAFER Guides, is a healthcare organization's best tool to mitigate the potential adverse patient safety effects of EHR downtime.

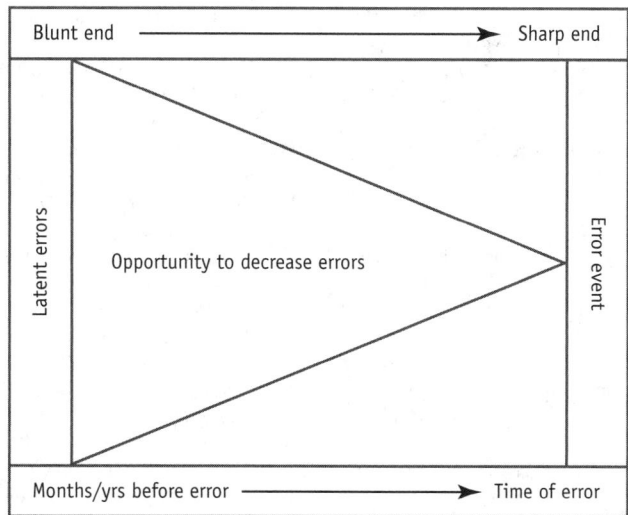

FIGURE 10-4 Human factors and medical device use.

▶ Summary

Organizations seek to improve quality while decreasing costs. Continuous advances in health IT provide tools to assist nurses and other HCPs in achieving these goals. This chapter has focused on care delivery and the potential benefits of adapting health IT at the various levels of care. It has not addressed how HCPs and organizations must mobilize to ensure that the technologies put into place actually improve care delivery. As noted earlier, the point of care is the sharp end of care. Using time as the key variable, **FIGURE 10-4** shows the relationship between the sharp end of care and the blunt end. Decisions about technology adoption are made at the blunt end of the process. If adoption is to improve care, such decisions must take into consideration the impact of new tools on the entire sociotechnologic system. In addition, proactive planning for the instances when technology is not available is essential to ensuring there are not unintended consequences of system downtime. The complexity of the current healthcare environment requires everyone, including nurses, to ensure patients are well taken care of and protected against harm throughout their medical journey.

References

Agius, C. R. (2012). Intelligent infusion technologies: Integration of a smart system to enhance patient care. *Journal of Infusion Nursing, 35*(6), 364–368. doi: 10.1097 /NAN.0b013e3182706423

Ash, J., Singh, H., & Sittig, D. (2014). *SAFER Guides: Safety assurance factors for EHR resililence.* Retrieved from https://www.healthit.gov/safer/guide/sg003

Boas, D. A., Gaudette, T., Strangman, G., Cheng, X., Marota, J. J., & Mandeville, J. B. (2001). The accuracy of near infrared spectroscopy and imaging during focal changes in cerebral hemodynamics. *Neuroimage, 13*(1), 76–90. doi: 10.1006/nimg.2000.0674

Campbell, E. M., Sittig, D. F., Guappone, K. P., Dykstra, R. H., & Ash, J. S. (2007). Overdependence on technology: An unintended adverse consequence of computerized provider order entry. *AMIA Symposium Proceedings,* 94–98.

Carayon, P. (2012). Work system design in health care. In *Handbook of human factors and ergonomics in health care and patient safety* (2nd ed., pp. 65–79). Boca Raton, FL: CRC Press.

Carayon, P., Hundt, A., Karsh, B., Gurses, A., Alvarado, C., Smith, M., & Brennan, P. (2006). Work system design for patient safety: The SEIPS model. *Quality and Safety in Health* Care, *15*(suppl. 1), i50–i58.

Dartmouth Institute. (2013). *Clinical microsystems.* Retrieved from http:// www.clinicalmicrosystem .org/about/background/

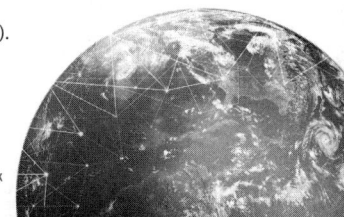

Fahrenholz, C. G., Smith, L. J., Tucker, K., & Warner, D. (2009). Plan B: A practical approach to downtime planning in medical practices. *Journal of AHIMA, 80*(11), 34–38. Retrieved from http://library.ahima.org/doc?oid=95715#.WGbFNzt_ehh

Feldman, D. L. (2011). Prevention of retained surgical items. *Mount Sinai Journal of Medicine, 78*(6), 865–871. doi: 10.1002/msj.20299

Hanuscak, T. L., Szeinbach, S. L., Seoane-Vazquez, E., Reichert, B. J., & McCluskey, C. F. (2009). Evaluation of causes and frequency of medication errors during information technology downtime. *American Journal of Health-System Pharmacy, 66*(12), 1119–1124. doi:10.2146/ajhp080389

Healthcare Information and Management Systems Society. (2013). *HIMSS dictionary of healthcare information technology terms, acronyms and organizations* (3rd ed.). Chicago, IL: Author.

Husch, M., Sullivan, C., Rooney, D., Barnard, C., Fotis, M., Clarke, J., & Noskin, G. (2005). Insights from the sharp end of intravenous medication errors: Implications for infusion pump technology. *Quality and Safety in Health Care, 14*(2), 80–86. doi: 10.1136/qshc.2004.011957

Institute of Medicine. (1999). *To err is human: Building a safer health system.* Washington, DC: National Academies Press.

Institute of Medicine. (2011). *Health IT and patient safety: Building safer systems for better care.* Washington, DC: Committee on Patient Safety and Health Information Technology, Board on Health Care Services.

Joint Commission. (2013). *Hospital: 2013 national patient safety goals.* Retrieved from http://www.jointcommission.org/hap_2013_npsg/

Kamel Boulos, M. N., & Berry, G. (2012). Real-time locating systems (RTLS) in healthcare: A condensed primer. *International Journal of Health Geographics, 11*, 25. doi: 10.1186/1476-072x-11-25

Kashiwagi, D. T., Sexton, M. D., Graves, C. E. S., Johnston, J., Callies, B. I., Yu, R. C., & Thompson, J. M. (2016). All CLEAR? Preparing for IT Downtime. *American Journal of Medical Quality, 8*, 1–5. doi: 10.1177/1062860616667546

Lighter, D. E. (2013). *Basics of health care performance improvement: A lean six sigma approach.* Burlington, MA: Jones & Bartlett Learning.

Mosa, A. S., Yoo, I., & Sheets, L. (2012). A systematic review of healthcare applications for smartphones. *BMC Medical Informatics and Decision Making, 12*, 67. doi: 10.1186/1472-6947-12-67

Napper, C., Battles, J., & Fargason, C. (2003). Pediatrics and patient safety. *The Journal of Pediatrics, 142*(4), 359–360.

Nelson, N. C. (2007). Downtime procedures for a clinical information system: A critical issue. *Journal of Critical Care, 22*(1), 45–50. doi: 10.1016/j.jcrc.2007.02.004

O'Donnell, C. P. F., Kamlin, C. O. F., Davis, P. G., Carlin, J. B., & Morley, C. J. (2007). Clinical assessment of infant colour at delivery. *Archives of Disease in Childhood: Fetal and Neonatal Edition, 92*(6), F465–F467.

Oral, B., Cullen, R. M., Diaz, D. L., Hod, E. A., & Kratz, A. (2015). Downtime procedures for the 21st century: Using a fully integrated health record for uninterrupted electronic reporting of laboratory results during laboratory information system downtimes. *American Journal of Clinical Pathology, 143*(1), 100–104.

Patient Safety Authority. (2008). Medication errors occurring with the use of bar-code administration technology. *Pennsylvania Patient Safety Advisory, 5*(4), 122–126.

Radio-frequency identification: Its potential in healthcare. (2005). *Health Devices, 34*(5), 149–160.

Reason, J. (1990). *Human error.* New York, NY: Cambridge University Press.

Reason, J. (2000). Human error: Models and management. *The Western Journal of Medicine (0093–0415), 172*(6), 393.

Roark, D. C., & Miguel, K. (2006). RFID: Bar coding's replacement? *Nursing Management, 37*(2), 28–31.

Sittig, D. F., Gonzalez, D., & Singh, H. (2014). Contingency planning for electronic health record-based care continuity: A survey of recommended practices. *International Journal of Medical Informatics, 83*(11), 794–804.

Schmid, A., Hoffman, L., Happ, M. B., Wolf, F., & DeVita, M. (2007). Failure to rescue: A literature review. *Journal of Nursing Administration, 37*(4), 188–198.

U.S. Food and Drug Administration. (2004). Bar code label requirement for human drug products and biological products. Final rule. *Federal Register, 69*(38), 9119–9171.

U.S. Food and Drug Administration. (2012). *Overview of medical device regulations.* Retrieved from http://www.fda.gov/Training/CDRHLearn/ucm162015.htm#overview

Wang., Y, Coiera, E., Gallego, B., Concha, O. P., Ong, M. S., Tsafnat, G., . . . & Magrabi, F. (2016). Measuring the effects of computer downtime on hospital pathology processes. *Journal of biomedical informatics, 59*, 308–315. doi: 10.1016/j.jbi.2015.12.016.

Yang, M., Brown, M., Trohimovich, B., Dana, M., & Kelly, J. (2002). The effect of bar-code-enabled point-of-care technology on medication administration errors. In R. Lewis (Ed.), *The impact of information technology on patient safety* (pp. 37–56). Chicago, IL: Healthcare Info and Management Systems.

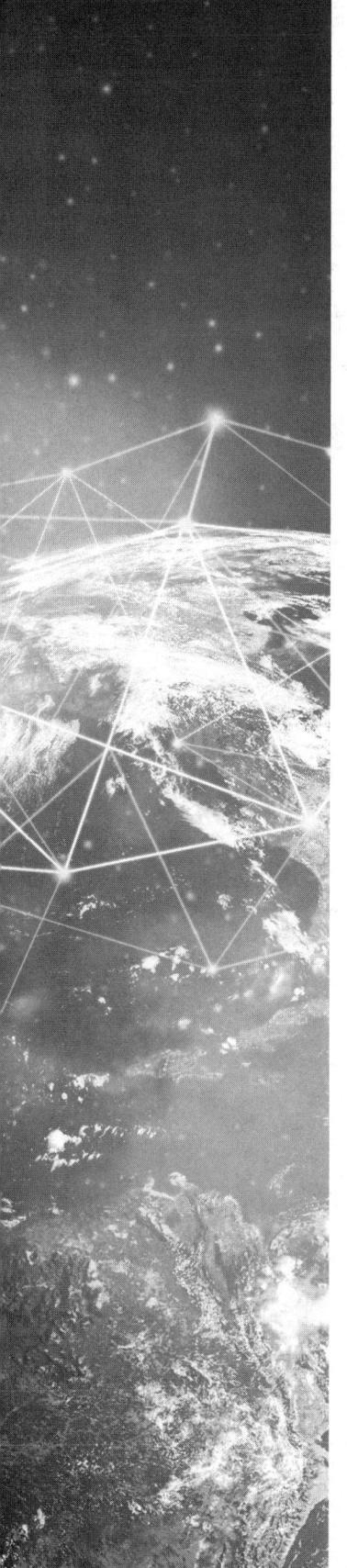

SECTION III

Use of Clinical Informatics Tools in Care Delivery Systems

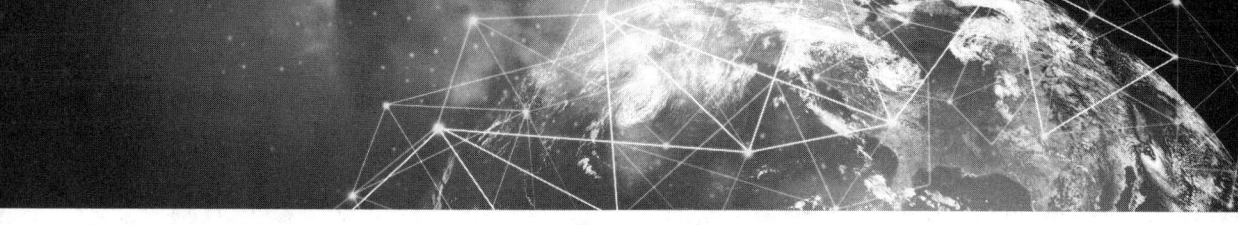

CHAPTER 11

The Electronic Health Record

Susan Alexander, DNP, ANP-BC, ADM-BC
Donna Guerra, EdD, MSN, RN

LEARNING OBJECTIVES

1. Define and describe the electronic health record (EHR) and its common features.
2. Review the benefits of EHR use in daily practice.
3. Describe the impact of the EHR on tasks such as data management and the support of evidence-based practice.
4. Review the challenges of EHR use including interoperability, effects on workflow patterns, system and system-related expenses, performance, and security concerns.
5. Examine the role of the nurse in the use of EHR systems.

KEY TERMS

Access control tools
Clinical vocabulary
Computerized provider order
   entry (CPOE)
Decryption
Electronic health record (EHR)
Electronic medical record (EMR)

Encryption
End user
Health maintenance
Interface
Interoperability
Penetration testing
Point of care data entry

Recovery capabilities
Remote access
Security risk analysis
Superusers
System downtime
Virtual private network
   (VPN)

▶ Chapter Overview

Any nurse who has spent valuable time working with the traditional paper chart can appreciate the many features of the **electronic health record (EHR)**. The ability to document nursing activities at the point of care, retrieve data quickly, and access clinical decision support within an EHR system can streamline nurses' daily work. There are other important potential benefits of EHR use, particularly in improving patient care, which have been recognized and supported by the federal government. In 2004, the need for computerization of health records was addressed by President George W. Bush in his State of the Union Address which quickly gained bipartisan support. The Health Information Technology for Economic and Clinical Health (HITECH) Act, which was designed to promote the adoption and meaningful use of health information technology, was signed into law on February 17, 2009. The HITECH Act provides the Department of Health and Human Services with the authority to establish programs to improve the quality, safety, and efficiency of health care by promoting health IT, including EHR systems and electronic health information exchange (U.S. Department of Health and Human Services, n.d.a). As a result of the HITECH Act, healthcare providers and facilities can receive incentive payments for the adoption and meaningful use of EHR systems.

Current estimates from the National Electronic Health Records Survey (NEHRS) in 2015 suggest that EHR use in provider offices likely exceeds 78%, while the Office of the National Coordinator for Health Information Technology reported that 96% of hospitals have adopted certified EHRs. Collective incentive payments to healthcare providers and hospitals exceeded $35 billion to date in 2016 (Healthit.gov, 2016).

As the use of EHRs continues to increase in health care, it is important for the nurse to become familiar with the features and capabilities of the systems. This chapter begins with a description of the benefits and features of EHRs, along with the problems that have been identified in using EHR systems. Issues of security, reliability, and accuracy will also be reviewed. Finally, the chapter concludes with a description of the nurse's role in preparing for and implementing the EHR, delivering care, and evaluating outcomes, and the nurses' perceptions on interaction with EHR systems (Emanuel, 2012).

▶ Definitions and Descriptions

It is helpful to understand that EHR and **electronic medical record (EMR)** may be referred to interchangeably, but there are differences in the ways these terms are defined. According to the Healthcare Information and Management Systems Society (HIMSS), an EHR is a "a longitudinal electronic record of patient health information generated by one or more encounters in any care delivery setting" (HIMSS, 2012–2013). An EMR is defined as an electronic version of a patient's paper chart with medical information from one provider practice or healthcare facility (Healthit.gov, 2016).

Many students are experienced in the creation and management of electronic documents, but an EHR is more than the exchange of a paper chart into an electronic file. With optimum use, the EHR is a robust database, with an almost endless capacity for customization, that can be adapted to the needs of the patient, the healthcare provider (HCP), and the healthcare organization. EHRs are designed to collect many types of data, ranging from patient demographics to radiology images, and contain features such as secure online messaging systems and order entry systems (**TABLE 11-1**). The data that are collected can then be made available to multiple providers across healthcare settings, however remote, through a system of shared networks. EHR system features can also be adapted to meet the needs of single-provider office practices or multiuser sites with remote locations. Systems that are designed for use in outpatient and inpatient care delivery settings and that meet the criteria for a minimum level of accuracy, reliability, security,

TABLE 11-1 Basic Features of Many Practice and Hospital-Based EHR Systems

EHR Feature	Example
Charting	<ul><li>Note templates that are both predesigned and customizable</li><li>Patient "dashboards" containing multiple types of information such as:<ul><li>List of current medications</li><li>Advance directives</li><li>Past medical history</li><li>Social history</li><li>Growth charts</li><li>Current vital signs</li></ul></li></ul>
Medication Management	<ul><li>Current and historical medication lists</li><li>Medication allergies and intolerances</li><li>Preferred pharmacies</li><li>E-prescribing capabilities</li><li>Computerized provider order entry</li></ul>
Scheduling	<ul><li>Single and multiple provider appointments</li><li>Appointments for multiple locations and varieties (groups vs. individuals)</li><li>Automatic appointment reminders for patients and providers</li></ul>
Labs	<ul><li>Most recent lab tests</li><li>History of all lab tests</li><li>Trends in lab results</li><li>Integration with in-house and reference labs for results via embedded interfaces</li></ul>
Referrals	<ul><li>Immediate referrals to providers in the EHR system</li><li>Instant fax with confirmation to providers outside the EHR system</li><li>Secure messaging to providers outside the EHR system</li></ul>
Billing/Coding	<ul><li>Creation of a superbill using elements from the note (ICD9 and CPT codes)</li><li>Streamlined billing using integrated vendors</li></ul>
Reporting/ Surveillance Capabilities	<ul><li>Customizable reports using various data elements such as:<ul><li>ICD9 codes</li><li>CPT codes</li><li>Medications</li></ul></li></ul>
Health Maintenance	<ul><li>Age-based templates for capturing recommended preventative health services (e.g., immunizations and colorectal cancer screenings)</li><li>Gender-based templates for capturing gender-specific health needs (e.g., mammograms and bone densitometries)</li><li>Disease-based templates for tracking clinical practice guidelines used in chronic disease management (e.g., eye and foot examinations for patients with diabetes mellitus)</li></ul>

and interoperability, can obtain a designation for quality from the Certification Commission for Health Information Technology (CCHIT).

Under the HITECH Act, a hospital, HCP, or critical access hospital that adopts a certified EHR technology and uses it to achieve specified objectives can qualify for incentive payments from the Centers for Medicare and Medicaid Services (CMS). Referred to as "Meaningful Use Criteria," the sets are a group of core and menu objectives that are specific to the hospital or the HCP and must be met in order to receive incentive payments. Benefits of meaningful use of EHRs include the maintenance of complete and accurate information about patients, improved access to information for providers, and the empowerment of patients to take a more active role in their health (U.S. Department of Health and Human Services, n.d.a). Meaningful use criteria and objectives have evolved in stages

over the last several years (**FIGURE 11-1**). Nurses have an essential role in aiding healthcare facilities and other healthcare professionals to meet meaningful use criteria of EHR systems.

▶ Benefits of Using EHRs

When fully functional, an EHR has many benefits for nurses that can make daily tasks easier. The features of EHR systems offer automation of manual repetitive tasks, streamlined documentation, and access to information (Table 11-1). After the nurse enters a personalized username and password, **point of care data entry** allows the nurse to capture the activities of care as they occur, be it the administration of medications, assessment of vital signs, physical exam, updating of medical histories, or other nursing duties (**FIGURES 11-2, 11-3, 11-4**). The data that are

Stage 1 2011–2012 Data capture and sharing	Stage 2 2014 Advance clinical processes	Stage 3 2016 Improved outcomes

Stage 1: Meaningful use criteria focus on:	Stage 2: Meaningful use criteria focus on:	Stage 3: Meaningful use criteria focus on:
Electronically capturing health information in a standardized format	More rigorous health information exchange (HIE)	Improving quality, safety, and efficiency, leading to improved health outcomes
Using that information to track key clinical conditions	Increased requirements for e-prescribing and incorporating lab results	Decision support for national high-priority conditions
Communicating that information for care coordination processes	Electronic transmission of patient care summaries across multiple settings	Patient access to self-management tools
Initiating the reporting of clinical quality measures and public health information	More patient-controlled data	Access to comprehensive patient data through patient-centered HIE
Using information to engage patients and their families in their care		Improving population health

FIGURE 11-1 Stages of meaningful use criteria.

Data from HealthIT.gov. (n.d.). Meaningful use regulations. Retrieved from http://www.healthit.gov/policy-researchers-implementers/meaningful-use

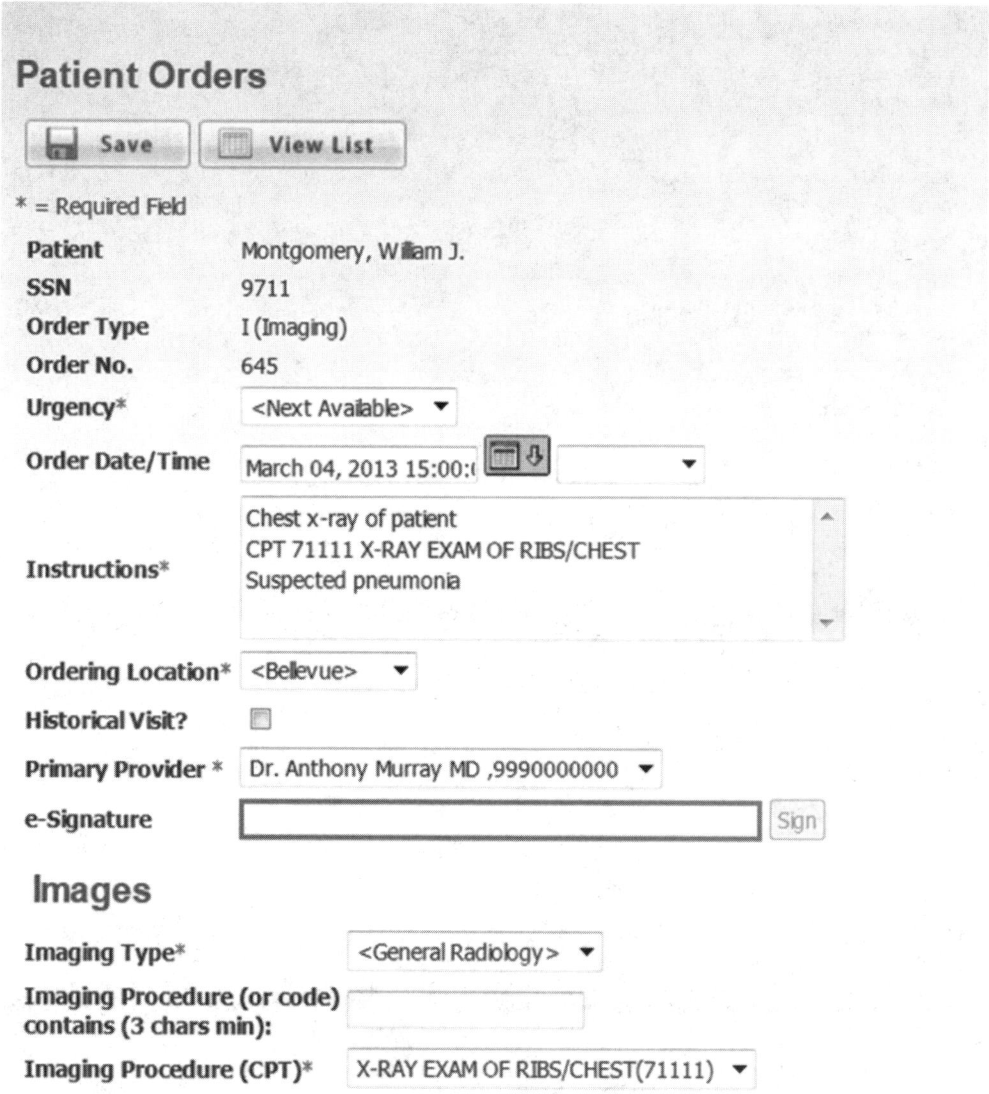

Patient Orders

[**Save**] [**View List**]

* = Required Field

Patient	Montgomery, William J.
SSN	9711
Order Type	I (Imaging)
Order No.	645
Urgency*	\<Next Available\> ▼
Order Date/Time	March 04, 2013 15:00:0

Instructions*
```
Chest x-ray of patient
CPT 71111 X-RAY EXAM OF RIBS/CHEST
Suspected pneumonia
```

Ordering Location*	\<Bellevue\> ▼
Historical Visit?	☐
Primary Provider *	Dr. Anthony Murray MD ,9990000000 ▼
e-Signature	[Sign]

Images

Imaging Type*	\<General Radiology\> ▼
Imaging Procedure (or code) contains (3 chars min):	
Imaging Procedure (CPT)*	X-RAY EXAM OF RIBS/CHEST(71111) ▼

FIGURE 11-2 Computerized provider order entry screen.
Courtesy of DataWeb Incorporated.

entered into the EHR are captured in a structured, coded format, and saved. These data can easily be retrieved for later quantitative analysis or use in clinical decision support. For example, a nurse working at the bedside in a healthcare facility or practice could get access to a patient's chart from more than one location, for easier and more accurate charting. EHRs often include decision support tools, alerts, and reminders that can help to reduce medication errors and adverse events. Drug–drug interactions and intravenous drug incompatibility information are common components of EHR systems. Another good example is patient medication allergies and intolerances. Once this information is entered, it can populate many different fields, so that anyone who is prescribing or administering medications to the patient will automatically be

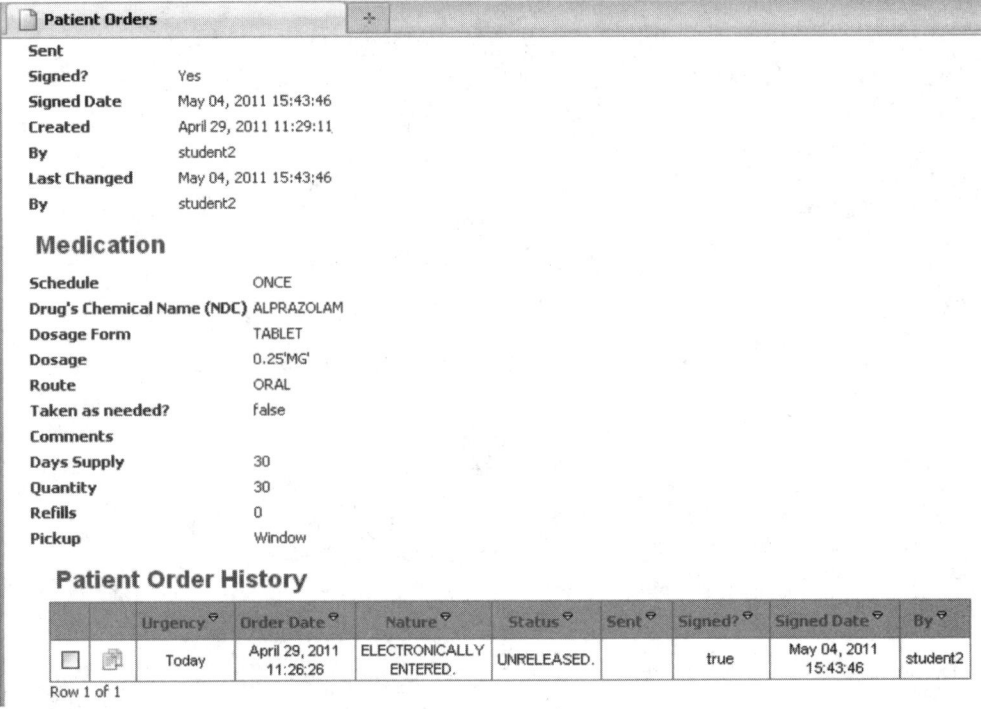

FIGURE 11-3 Medication order entry screen.

Courtesy of DataWeb Incorporated.

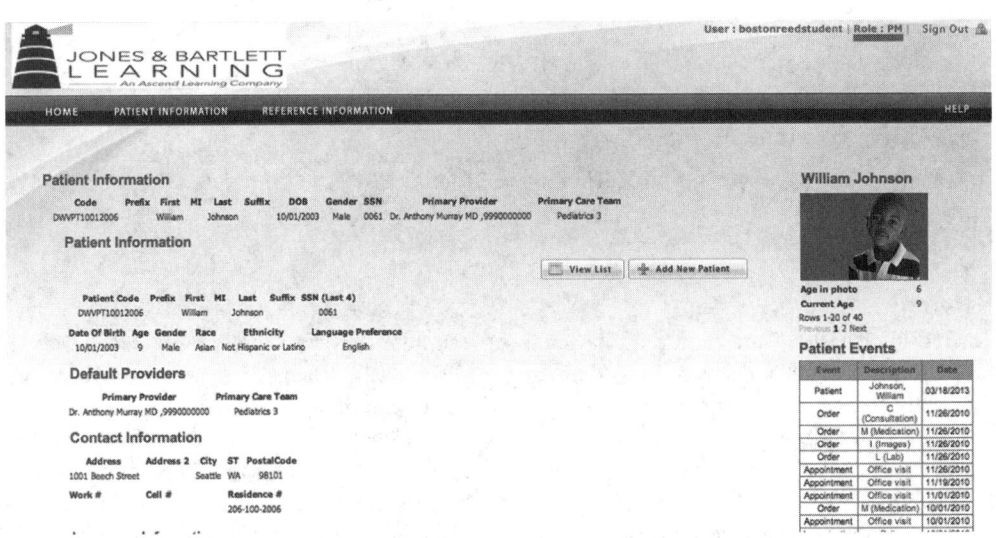

FIGURE 11-4 Patient demographics screen.

Courtesy of DataWeb Incorporated; © Jaimie Duplass/Shutterstock (photo)

given an alert if an incompatible drug is used. In an EHR, documentation of care that is provided is legible, so that time is not wasted in attempting to decipher the handwritten notes or orders of another HCP, and interfaces with labs ensure that results populate the chart automatically for review.

In addition to their benefits for direct nursing care, EHR systems can indirectly assist the work of the nurse by providing benefits available to other staff in healthcare facilities. The rapid access to patient-related data that is possible when an EHR is used can simultaneously support many HCPs and ancillary staff, such as medical coding specialists, lab personnel, and billing departments. Information retrieval is almost immediate, and the record may be continuously updated as HCPs and other staff enter information related to patient care. In some care settings, the EHR may be available using remote workstations, enabling access to patient data without having to be in the physical location. This can be a great benefit for HCPs and staff who need access to patient charts for aspects of their jobs but do not necessarily have to be on-site. Busy HCPs who are working in offices several miles away can access the EHR to get up-to-date information on hospitalized patients without leaving their office.

Healthcare facilities are increasingly accountable for care that patients receive during their stays in such facilities. Hospital Compare (https://www.medicare.gov/hospitalcompare) is a consumer-oriented website created through the efforts of Medicare and the Hospital Quality Alliance. Hospitals are required to report data on their performance in caring for patients with the most common conditions requiring admission to a hospital for treatment, including pneumonia, acute myocardial infarction, heart failure, pneumonia, and surgeries. Consumers can then select multiple hospitals and compare the performance of those hospitals using the performance data submitted to the website by each hospital. In reviewing a database of performance measures related to pneumonia, acute myocardial infarction, and heart failure from 2,021 hospitals, those facilities that maintained a basic EHR system

(operational electronic patient record, clinical data repository, and decision support) realized a 2.6% improvement in quality of care scores for heart failure management (Jones, Adams, Schneider, Ringel, & McGlynn, 2010).

Collection, Aggregation, and Reporting of Data

In addition to caring for individual patients, nurses often work in positions that require the aggregation and review of data to guide policy or practice, such as infection and quality control. In the past, this could be a time-intensive process necessitating the collection of data from stacks of paper charts, entry of data into a statistical analysis software package for analysis, and generation of final reports for review. The use of EHR systems has simplified this process. Data collection takes place at the point of care, as the nurse or other HCP enters the relevant data points into the EHR. The reporting features of the EHR system can then be used to rapidly generate needed reports, using multiple data points such as medications, diagnoses, or procedures.

There is evidence to demonstrate that public health initiatives can benefit from the timely data gleaned from EHR systems. BioSense 2.0 is a web-based application, administered by the Centers for Disease Control and Prevention (CDC) that can provide a real-time picture of any health condition, anywhere in the country. It pulls together information on emergency department visits and hospitalization from sources including the Department of Veterans Affairs and the Department of Defense. Civilian hospitals with EHR systems that meet Stages 1 and 2 criteria for meaningful use can also contribute data to the BioSense 2.0 program. Analysis of data that are contributed to the BioSense 2.0 tool can help public health officials to track health issues as they evolve, offer detailed insight into the health of communities, and support national, state, and local responses to health threats. Updates on evolving issues pertinent to national health, including the 2009–2010 H1N1 flu pandemic, the 2010 Gulf Oil Spill, and the 2011 U.S. heat wave, were transmitted to state and local health officials, via the program website and social media tools such as Facebook and Twitter, so that responsive protocols could be implemented (Gould, Walker, & Yoon, 2017)

Decision Support and Potential for Evidence-Based Practice

EHR systems have the ability to embed evidence such as clinical practice guidelines and best practice protocols to assist nurses in making clinical decisions. EHRs can rapidly facilitate the translation of research into practice and influence decisions that nurses and other HCPs make at the actual point of care. Weaver, Warren, and Delaney (2005) describe three case studies in which EHR systems were used to generate evidence-based knowledge to guide nursing practice:

■ Case Study 1: Querying practice to generate best practice evidence
  • Embedding of the Braden Pressure Sore risk assessment tool into the admission assessment for a hospital in Naples, Florida, resulted in a total pressure ulcer rate of 4.8%, half the national average.
■ Case Study 2: Adoption of a clinical information system to teach evidence-based practice in an undergraduate nursing program
  • Faculty at the University of Kansas School of Nursing, in conjunction with Cerner Corporation, use the Simulated e-Health Delivery System (SEEDS) to combine education on pathophysiology, assessments, and plan of care development for virtual patients with evidence-based practice content.
■ Case Study 3: Bench informatics-embedding evidence-based nursing protocols into front line clinical workflows
  • The University of Iowa College of Nursing, in partnership with Cerner Corporation, is developing a method to translate evidence-based nursing protocols and

guidelines into both the reference features and point of care decision support tools in EHR systems for nurses at the bedside.

Other mechanisms to support evidence-based decision making by nurses in multiple care settings may include the use of standing order sets. Such order sets can allow nurses to carry out specific protocols of patient care prior to examination or approval by an HCP. Order sets are frequently used for the management of common disorders found in both hospital and ambulatory care settings, such as pneumonia, diabetes, and chest pain. A study of office-based practices across the United States reviewed the implementation of standing orders sets using the **health maintenance** reminder feature in an EMR for health screenings, immunizations, and diabetes care. Findings from the study revealed statistically significant improvements in osteoporosis screening, pneumococcal vaccination for adults older than 65 years and younger adults at high risk, tetanus/diphtheria and zoster vaccinations, and measurement of urinary microalbumin in patients with diabetes (Nemeth, Ornstein, Jenkins, Wessell, & Nietert, 2012).

▶ Challenges of EHR Use

Despite the many benefits associated with EHR systems, challenges related to widespread implementation continue to be bothersome in health care. The lack of **interoperability**, the economic aspects of system adoption and maintenance, and threats to performance and security may prevent installation or full utilization of an EHR and its features in many delivery settings. Practical solutions that address these challenges do exist. If possible, healthcare facilities and providers should develop plans to address anticipated challenges prior to installation or expansion of EHR systems.

Lack of Interoperability

In the manufacturing world, a silo is a structure that is capable of storing bulk materials for later use. Informatics science has modified the term, using it to designate an information storage system that is incapable of reciprocal operations with other, similar systems. Though an EHR typically has a substantial capacity for information storage, it should not serve only to accumulate data for later use. HIMSS defines *interoperability* as "the ability of different information technology systems and software applications to communicate, exchange data, and use the information that has been exchanged" (2010, p. 190). Ideally, an EHR system acts as a hub for the flow of information to improve care for the patient, from many different sources in a healthcare setting, including reference labs, specific areas within the facility (emergency departments, operating rooms, or critical care units), or outside HCP practices. The point at which the separate systems meet and communicate is called the **interface**. The phenomenon of communicating health-related information across multiple platforms and care delivery settings is known as *interoperability*, and it has been notoriously difficult to achieve between various EHR systems and components. Many reasons on the failure to achieve interoperability in health care have been proposed.

A significant reason for the lack of interoperability among EHR systems is the need for a common **clinical vocabulary**, or a common terminology that can be used globally in all computerized health information systems. This need was addressed by the U.S. Institute of Medicine report (2003), *Patient Safety: Achieving a New Standard for Care*:

> If health professionals are to be able to send and receive data in an understandable and usable manner, both the sender and the receiver must have common clinical terminologies for describing, classifying, and coding medical terms and concepts. Use of standardized clinical terminologies facilitates electronic data collection at the point of care; retrieval of relevant data, information, and knowledge; and reuse of data for multiple purposes

(e.g., disease surveillance, clinical decision support, patient safety reporting). (pp. 37–38)

Encouraging the use of a common clinical vocabulary in EHR systems is one way to improve the interoperability of systems. SNOMED CT is a comprehensive, multilingual clinical healthcare terminology developed by the International Health Terminology Standards Development Organisation (IHTDSO). Already used in more than 50 countries around the world, SNOMED CT contains 311,000 active concepts organized into hierarchies, which can then be integrated into software applications to consistently represent the clinical activities of health care (International Health Terminology Standards Development Organisation, n.d.). As a member country of the IHTSDO, the United States is eligible to distribute the SNOMED CT language in multiple formats free of charge via the National Library of Medicine (https://www.nlm.nih.gov/healthit/snomedct/).

Other issues that prevent full interoperability of EHR systems include both the reluctance to share data among system developers, known as *vendors*, and the lack of unique identifiers for each patient. The highly competitive market for EHR systems and their proprietary software make many companies reluctant to develop the interface tools necessary to share data between systems. However, recent recommendations from HIMSS support the development of standards and criteria that will encourage vendors to build robust interoperability into systems to facilitate the exchange of information across healthcare delivery settings, disaster response, and public health initiatives (HIMSS, 2010). The use of financial incentives to encourage vendors to produce EHR systems with greater interoperability has been suggested as an additional strategy (Hoffman & Podgurski, 2012).

The exchange of healthcare information across systems could also be assisted by the use of unique patient identifiers to prevent errors associated with mismatching of patient identities. Though HIMSS acknowledges the need for correct linkage of patients to their data is key to achieving quality health care with EHRs, privacy and security concerns have prevented Congress from successfully passing legislation that will address the issue. At this time, the accurate pairing of patient identifiers and healthcare data is managed within an EHR system (Hillestad et al., 2008).

Change in Workflow Patterns

The adoption and implementation of an EHR system often poses a significant change to the daily workflow patterns of staff, which can be a source of stress for the facility and HCPs, be it a small medical practice or a multisite healthcare organization. Despite the promises of ongoing EHR use in improving patient care and reducing errors, the failure to consistently engage clinicians in decision making about usability aspects of systems can result in unintended consequences that lead to patient harm. Research regarding the impact of **computerized provider order entry (CPOE)** features on the number and character of patient care errors has demonstrated that the use of CPOE can inadvertently increase the need for coordination of activities among clinicians and result in errors (Cheng, Goldstein, Geller, & Levitt, 2003; Harrington & Kennerly, 2011). The source of errors may be due to the assumptions inherent in the construction of CPOE features by designers. Cheng et al. (2003) found that the use of CPOE gave HCPs the freedom to place patient care orders at many locations within the facility, even at points far away from traditional patient care areas. While this change in work flow processes can reduce conversations at the bedside between staff and HCPs, and be more convenient for HCPs who need to enter patient care orders, it can also be a source of miscommunications or errors.

In reviewing the implementation of CPOE in multiple facilities, Campbell, Sittig, Ash, Guappone, and Dykstra (2006) identified new sources of potential causes of patient care mistakes: juxtaposition errors (selection of an item adjacent to an intended choice), desensitization to alerts, confusing presentation of order options,

and system design issues (poor organization and display of data). Yet there are strategies that EHR system users and developers can take to minimize sources of error. The appointment of ongoing clinician champions to maintain performance improvement (PI) processes and the establishment of a multidisciplinary PI group should regularly review processes and errors, as they occur, and communicate with facility leadership so that durable solutions can be designed. This approach was identified in studies of patient errors that occurred after implementation of emergency department information systems and could be extrapolated to facility areas (Farley et al., 2013). Additionally, Farley et al. (2013) call attention to the need for EHR vendors to distribute patient safety improvements to all installation sites.

In the past, entry of information into a chart was often the responsibility of a single person in an office or on a hospital unit. This clerk, or secretary, had the full responsibility of familiarity with the system, along with transcription of medical and nursing orders. More recently, responsibilities for data entry have expanded, and the skill sets of HCPs in many care delivery settings now include familiarity of working with an EHR system, in addition to their clinical knowledge. Systems with poor usability can serve as sources of frustration for a busy HCP and increase the potential for error in the entry of documentation data. Examples of data entry errors include the insertion of information into incorrect fields, transposition of numbers, and the copying and pasting of narratives from previous encounters, which may no longer be accurate (Hoffman & Podgurski, 2012).

System and System-Related Expenses

The initial and ongoing fees for EHR systems represent a significant financial investment for healthcare facilities and providers. Evidence related to the expenses associated with the implementation and ongoing maintenance of systems is limited and often conflicting. The direct expenses of an EHR system can vary according to its features, data storage (either on-site with in-house servers or remotely via cloud-based applications), and system maintenance. There are also indirect costs that are associated with implementation that are often harder to quantify, such as hardware equipment and personnel salaries associated with implementation and maintenance of system operations (DeSimone, 2016; Eastaugh, 2013; Healthit.gov, 2014).

A study by Fleming, Culler, McCorkle, Becker, and Ballard (2011) found that implementation of an EHR for an average five-physician practice had an estimated total cost of $162,000 and $85,000 in maintenance expenses during the first year of use. Elements of implementation considered in the cost estimation included (Fleming et al., 2011):

- Hardware costs (Computers, printers, scanners, wireless Internet connections, switches, and cables)
- Software and maintenance costs (software licensing, hosting, technical support, and networking)
- Nonfinancial costs (implementation team, "opportunity cost"—time spent learning the system and adjusting work practices instead of time spent seeing patients)
  - Network implementation team (time the team spent on development before launching the system)
  - Practice implantation team (time practice employees spent in training and workflow redesign)
  - End users (time end users spend in learning and integrating the system into the practice)

Hospitals have a similar cost breakdown for EHR implementation with relationship to the costs of hardware, software, maintenance and personnel time dedicated to the project. According to Orszag (Congressional Budget Office, 2008), the total cost of implementation of an EHR system in a hospital could average $4,500 per bed. Similarly, the hospital would also have a yearly maintenance cost as well as system specialists' salaries and opportunity cost of HCPs

learning to use the system and integration of workflow in the care of patients.

Preparing a budget for EHR adoption and implementation is a process specific for each organization that requires much planning to be successful. Initially, it may be best for facilities to prioritize implementation in areas that stand to create the greatest impact on patient care and organizational revenues, such as a pharmacy information system. Incremental approaches can distribute the financial burden over a lengthier period of time (U.S. Department of Health and Human Services, n.d.b). Adoption of an EHR system is no guarantee of an increase in return on financial investment. In a survey analysis of 49 community practices in Massachusetts, 27% reported a positive return on investment by using strategies such as increasing the numbers of patients seen daily by providers and a reduction in the number of rejected claims for billing (Adler-Milstein, Green, & Bates, 2013).

The website, Healthit.gov, has a variety of resources available to assist HCPs and practices in planning for implementation and meaningful use of EHR systems. Regional extension centers (RECs) are available in every part of the United States to offer education, outreach, and technical assistance. The RECs help providers in specific geographic areas to select, successfully adopt, and use certified EHR systems in a meaningful way (http://www.healthit.gov/providers-professionals/regional-extension-centers-recs#listing). The National Learning Consortium, an ongoing collection of resources contributed by field staff from the Office of the National Coordinator for Health IT (ONC) outreach programs, is also available for health information technology (health IT) professionals, HCPs, and other staff who are working to implement health information technology (http://www.healthit.gov/providers-professionals/about-national-learning-consortium).

There are other strategies that office-based practices and hospitals can employ to save on start-up and annual maintenance costs. For smaller facilities, web-based EHR systems can be economic alternatives to satisfy the need for information systems. In a web-based system,

HCP or hospitals pay a monthly subscription fee to vendors to access EHR systems rather than purchasing permanent systems. Users can then access the EHR system from any computer via the Internet, without having to purchase dedicated servers and the extra hardware and software needed to work with those servers. Known as an application service provider (ASP) or Software as a Service (SaaS), the concept of providing cloud-based access to software records is becoming more widespread in healthcare delivery systems. Though there are drawbacks to the use of the cloud- or web-based systems, such as slower response times to retrieve information, particularly if the healthcare facility has a slow bandwidth, they remain a viable alternative to reduce the expenses of installing and maintaining EHR systems.

Performance and Security Concerns

Issues of system performance and security maintenance are critical for healthcare facilities that use EHR systems. Frequent reports of stolen healthcare data can be found in the news media. While unprotected EHR systems can be vulnerable to hackers, laptops with both unencrypted and encrypted information have been taken from employees of healthcare organizations (Walker, 2013). In another case, a thumb drive that was used to back up one hard drive from another on the campus of the Oregon Health and Science University Hospital was inadvertently taken home by an employee in a briefcase, which was later removed from the employee's home during a burglary (Oregon Health and Science University, 2012). Even more disturbing are accounts of the targeting of healthcare data by hackers for use in identity theft and commercial ventures (Hall, 2013). To protect electronic health care information, it is essential that employees, HCPs, and facility leaders understand their role in maintaining the privacy, security, and confidentiality of the information.

The Health Insurance Portability and Accountability Act (HIPAA) Security Rule requires that facilities take specific measures to safeguard

electronic protected health information so that its confidentiality, integrity, and security is ensured (U.S. Department of Health and Human Services, 2013). Safety measures to protect information are often built into EHR systems, such as **access control tools** like user-specific passwords and personal identification numbers. Stored information frequently undergoes **encryption**, meaning that health information cannot be interpreted by anyone unless it is translated by an authorized person who has a specialized key for **decryption** of the information. To further comply with HIPAA Security Rules, organizations must have physical safeguards in place that limit access to its facilities, particularly workstations, and policies for the secure use of electronic media. Technical safeguards are requirements that limit access to electronic health information to authorized personnel, ensure that electronic health information is not improperly altered, destroyed, or transmitted, and that the facility has the procedural mechanisms in place to generate audit trails of access to electronic health information if needed. Facilities that use in-house servers to store data generated in their EHR system employ additional daily data backup, so that data can be recovered in case of the failure of a system or loss of power. Remote storage of data, or transmission of data to be stored at a site away from the physical location of the EHR system, is another strategy that healthcare facilities use to keep healthcare data safe and retrievable.

Healthcare organizations should regularly assess the security of their EHR systems. A **security risk analysis** compares present security measures in the EHR to those that are legally required to safeguard patient information, and the analysis can help in identifying high-priority threats and vulnerabilities. The security risk analysis is the initial step in creating an effective action plan for addressing threats and weaknesses of the system. Toolkits that guide organizations of all sizes in conducting risk assessments are available online (National Institute of Standards and Technology, 2017). The Office for Civil Rights, Department of Health and Human Services, maintains an online list of breaches affecting

500 or more individuals. Theft or less, hacking/IT, and unauthorized access/disclosure are common reasons for these breaches (U.S. Department of Health and Human Services, 2017).

In addition to regular risk analyses, other approaches to assess the security of patient care information must be used. **Penetration testing** is a method that has been used in other areas of electronic information management to assess the security of systems. It can be conducted by information technology personnel within the healthcare facility or by external providers. The results of penetration testing reveal gaps in the system's security that can make it vulnerable to attackers. Results can be used to further improve the action plan to prevent breaches and loss of patient information.

Clinicians are increasingly using home devices to access EHR systems remotely from their homes or offices. Known as **remote access**, this activity can pose special risks to the security of EHR systems. Data tampering and theft can occur by hackers' exploitation of weaknesses in the perimeter protection of the network and at the home or office locations. The use of a **virtual private network (VPN)** can reduce risks because the remote user accesses the EHR network through the VPN, which uses a tightly configured firewall. VPNs encrypt data between computers and the Internet, providing security even on unsecured public networks and mobile devices. The process generates little activity on the Internet that could be detected and exploited by hackers. Despite the security of VPNs, home computers may be subject to risk due to operation outside the protection of organization control. Multilevel passwords, user authentication of devices, restricted access, audit trails, and the use of biometrics to access EHRs can help to improve the security of VPNs.

A further issue of concern for healthcare facilities in using EHR systems is unplanned **system downtime** and **recovery capabilities**. Downtime can occur for reasons as simple as short-term power outages, or can be prolonged if natural disasters, such as floods, affect healthcare facilities. Regardless of the size of the facility,

mechanisms to retrieve necessary data to carry on normal operating procedures, and to prevent the loss of data when downtime occurs suddenly, must be in place. Battery-powered backups that plug directly into the server can be one option; facilities can also choose to use automated remote backups at sites located away from the healthcare facility campus. Recovery capabilities of EHR systems vary considerably, and it is important to remember that once power is restored to a system, a time period of several minutes or more may be necessary in order for it to return to full operation. Commonly, the reactivation of interfaces within the system may take several minutes. During this time, the system can be vulnerable to crashes if overwhelmed with an excessive number of users attempting to get back online. The appointment of a single person who can communicate to staff with instructions on system access can be valuable in rapid restoration of system use.

▶ Role of the Nurse and the EHR

The roles and responsibilities of the nurse related to EHR systems should begin in pre-licensure education. Conceptual understanding and practical experience, while increasing the pre-licensure nurse's level of comfort in working with EHR systems, can foster improvements in understanding how components of EHRs work together to create outcomes for patients and HCPs. Unfortunately, the literature suggests that academic programs do not sufficiently prepare students for using EHRs in the clinical setting. Students are unaware of the types of patient errors that can result from the use of EHR systems, and even those students with a greater degree of comfort with technology have been reported as experiencing difficulties in using EHRs (Borycki, Joe, Bellwood, & Campbell, 2011). Strategies to reduce barriers to EHR use in the academic programs may include using faculty members who have prior experience with EHR to integrate its use into the curriculum of pre-licensure programs (Borycki et al., 2011).

Ultimately, nurses are likely the largest group of HCPs to use EHRs (Strudwick & Hall, 2015). As primary **end users** of EHRs, nursing competency includes clinical practice skills as well as fundamental informatics knowledge (Furlong, 2015). Effective end user training is essential in healthcare facilities to ensure that nurses are competent in using EHRs to complete the daily clinical care of patients. While nurses in professional practice can be expected to achieve a minimum level of competence with use of EHR systems, it is likely that nurses who seem to have a special flair for working with the system will also emerge.

Often referred to as **superusers**, these nurses tend to display a positive attitude toward EHR use, are willing to take the time for extra training, and serve as a resource for others in the use of the system (**FIGURE 11-5**). Superusers lead other staff and HCPs in the implementation and ongoing use of EHR systems and are crucial to the success of EHR systems in healthcare facilities. Superusers can facilitate the initial and ongoing training of employees in healthcare facilities regarding EHR use, which has been identified as an important factor in both successful implementation and in continued use (Ash & Bates, 2005).

Nurses' Perceptions of EHR Systems

With more than three million registered nurses in the United States, some consideration of their opinions on the use of EHR systems must be given, if continued expansion and success of the systems can be expected (U.S. Bureau of Labor Statistics, 2010). For the implementation of EHR systems to succeed, nurses need to be convinced that the benefits of electronic records will outweigh the benefits of paper records. There is evidence that nurses' attitudes toward EHR implementation is changing. Positive attitudes on EHR use are more frequent, particularly in nurses who report more prior computer experience (Huryk, 2010). A positive attitude from administration creates a more positive attitude in staff, and this can be fostered by continued training opportunities with frequent facility-specific examples of how EHRs are used to improve patient care (Huryk, 2010). Adequate training time, and sessions that are staggered according to technological ability, are also mechanisms that can improve nurses' positive perceptions of EHR implementation (Huryk, 2010).

Care Delivery and Surveillance

It is important to note that the point of EHR implementation is the improvement of patient care, and not simply the automation of manual documentation. Technology should be viewed as a way to facilitate and enable positive change in how health care is delivered (Kinser, 2011). EHR allows the capture of care transactions, data storage of this information, and clinical decision support that drives nursing actions based on the patient's current condition or diagnosis. Clinicians can also more easily see patients' clinical progress and data (IOM, 2012). Nurses can use EHRs as a tool to guide practice by taking advantage of patient data trends and clinical decision support embedded in the system. A case study example is provided in **BOX 11-1** to

---

Are you a superuser?
• Can you maintain a positive attitude during times of technological stress? • Do you have the patience to train others, answer questions, and take calls when you least expect them? • Are you committed to the successful use of an EHR at your healthcare organization?

FIGURE 11-5 Are you a superuser?

BOX 11-1 Case Study

Margaret is the unit manager of a 24-bed intensive care unit (ICU). The unit has seen a rise in the number of central venous catheter-related bloodstream infections (CRBSIs) over the last three months. Margaret held a meeting with the ICU nursing staff, and together they have set a goal to have zero CRBSIs for the next three months. Margaret has enlisted the help of the infection control nurse and the hospital nurse informaticist to implement a performance improvement program to reduce CRBSIs.

The infection control nurse has provided Margaret with central venous catheter (CVC) care bundles to be used as a tool to support the unit's efforts to implement evidence-based practices to eliminate CRBSIs. Together, the infection control nurse and Margaret educate the ICU staff and other providers on the use of the bundles to incorporate these evidence-based practices into the workflow of the ICU. The insertion bundle includes such clinical interventions as proper hand hygiene, strict barrier and antiseptic precautions, and site selection with (CVC) insertion. In addition, a maintenance bundle has also been implemented to include a daily assessment of CVCs for necessity, insertion site and dressing integrity, dedicated port usage for parenteral infusions, and strict aseptic techniques for CVC access.

To further support the compliance of the staff with the CVC bundle, the nurse informaticist has incorporated specific insertion checklists into the EHR with preselected drop-down menus for the nurses to use when performing point-of-care documentation during the insertion of CVCs. Additionally, a specific tool with a similar drop-down menu concept was created in the EHR for the nurses to document CVC assessments per shift. Any variations in the recommended practices for CVC maintenance required a free text entry by the nurse. Discontinuation of CVCs was documented with reasons for removal recorded. If patients had more than one CVC, each line was identified by number and documented separately.

At the end of the first month, Margaret collected surveillance data of CVCs via audit reports within the EHR. Data revealed that compliance with the CVC insertion bundle was only 75%, and compliance with the daily CVC maintenance bundle was only 90%. The unit also had one positive CRBSI reported during the month. Using data collected from the EHR audit reports, Margaret reinforced clinical education with the ICU staff and providers, encouraging full engagement of the performance improvement project. At the end of the three-month period, Margaret again used the EHR audit reports to assess the progress of the ICU's efforts to decrease CRBSIs. Compliance with the CVC insertion bundle increased to 99%, and the daily CVC maintenance bundle improved to 100%. As a result, the ICU had a reduction in reported CRBSIs to zero for the second and third month.

illustrate the way in which an EHR can drive nursing practice.

The Institute of Medicine (IOM, 2006) has proposed that by 2020 clinical decisions in health care should be driven by best evidence and supported by accurate, timely, and up-to-date information (O'Brien, Weaver, Settergren, Hook, & Ivory, 2015). When nurses use EHRs to document patient care in "real time" or at the "bedside," the information is captured at the point of care, and is not delayed until the end of the shift when information may be forgotten, or inaccurate.

The multiple features of EHR systems, such as clinical decision support, can make it simple for the nurse to identify and facilitate the delivery of care for patients. Additionally, EHRs can be used to track one or more conditions or treatments in patients. In one study of medical practices who used a common EHR tool, records revealed that

TABLE 11-2 Success Strategies for Projects Involving EHR Systems

Select the leader	The leader is responsible for summarizing the baseline performance of the organization, and how the project can be implemented in order to improve patient care.
Find the vision	With input from other staff, the leader clarifies the vision for the project implementation and sustainability.
Choose measurement criteria	Select a realistic set of performance measurements that can be assessed regularly throughout the project implementation, and used to indicate successes and areas for improvement.
Support the vision	Though transition can be difficult, remember the need to work together toward the common vision.
Empower the patients	Use the features available in many EHR systems, such as patient education tools, to assist patients in taking an active role in their care.
Remember the ultimate goal	Improving the quality of care for each patient is the purpose of the project.

an estimated 89.5% of female patients ($>/=40$ years) associated with one practice were found to have received annual mammograms. An examination of the strategies used to achieve this remarkable goal revealed that the project leader, a licensed vocational nurse within the practice, used the health maintenance feature of the EHR system to identify and contact females who needed to be scheduled for mammograms (**TABLE 11-2**) (Feifer et al., 2007).

Increased Time for Documentation

Nursing documentation often varies little from patient to patient in terms of the forms that are used. Standardized care plans, assessments, admission/registration forms, and medication lists may be used for each patient. Nurses will often access and review similar sets of documentation, in the same physical location, several times throughout the course of a day's work. For this reason, electronic documentation can make the work of nurses more efficient. Although nursing documentation is classified as a patient intervention in the Nursing Intervention Classification (NIC), many nurses do not regard documentation as a true patient-care activity.

In a systematic review of studies examining the impact of EHR implementation on the amount of time nurses spent in documentation, six studies demonstrated a reduction in the average time spent in documentation, ranging from 2.1–45.1% (Poissant, Pereira, Tamblyn, & Kawasumi, 2005). However, further review of the studies suggested that location of the computer terminals could affect nurses' efficiency in documentation. Two of the studies found that the use of bedside terminals increased the amount of time needed for documentation (7.7% and 39.2%, respectively) (Poissant et al., 2005). Specific strategies for integration of computer-assisted documentation into the daily workflow of nurses to improve efficiency and effectiveness can be found in **TABLE 11-3**.

> **TABLE 11-3** Don't Let the Computer Be an Intruder! Five Strategies for Making the Computer Work for You When the Terminal Is in the Room
>
> - **The patient comes first.** When you walk into the room, address the patient and the patient's family first. Introduce yourself and assess the patient's needs. After you finish your preliminary care, explain that you are going to move to the computer terminal, laptop, or other device to continue your care.
>
> - **Positioning is everything.** The computer is a tool and not the focus of attention. The terminal should be placed in a position between you and the patient, so that you can change your focus between the screen and the patient with a slight turn of the head.
>
> - **Focus, focus, focus.** Changing your attention from the patient to the computer screen, while maintaining rapport with the patient or family, may seem difficult at first. Don't worry; this is a skill that will improve with practice, as your comfort in using the EHR system and computer terminal increases.
>
> - **The computer is never the patient.** Do not walk into a patient's room and begin to use the computer without addressing the patient. Always explain what you are about to do.
>
> - **Use the power of the system for you and your patient.** EHR systems have a variety of features that can be used to enhance patient care at the bedside or in the exam room. Investigate graphing functions that can be used to display trends in lab results, vital signs, or other measures that could serve as teaching moments for patients. Many EHRs also have embedded patient education tools that can be downloaded and printed for on-demand use.

Modified from Mehallow, C. (n.d.). Communication tips for nurses when electronic health records enter the exam room. Retrieved from http://career-advice.monster.com/in-the-office/workplace-issues/nurse-communication-tips-ehr/article.aspx. Reprinted by permission of Monster.com.

▶ Summary

The expansion and growth of EHRs is expected to continue, and it is the nurse who can play a key role in optimizing use of systems to improve outcomes for patients and healthcare facilities. Preparing nurses for integral roles in the design, selection, and implementation of EHR systems begins with exposure to systems in prelicensure education and continued training in the clinical setting. Nurses can offer unique perspectives on the workflow of common tasks, such as assessments and medication administration, that designers can integrate into EHR systems, improving function and reducing the risk for patient errors.

Not every nurse will become an EHR superuser, but all can achieve a level of competence with system use if facility administrators and peers provide adequate training and support. Demonstration of skill in EHR use is essential if nurses are to have a part in developing policy and systems for future use.

References

Adler-Milstein, J., Green, C. E., & Bates, D. W. (2013). A survey analysis suggests that electronic health records will yield revenue gains for some practices and losses for many. *Health Affairs, 321*, 3562–3570.

Ash, J., & Bates, D. W. (2005). Factors and forces affecting EHR system adoption: Report of a 2004 ACMI discussion. *Journal of the American Medical Informatics Association, 12*(1), 8–12.

Borycki, E., Joe, R. S., Bellwood, P., & Campbell, R. (2011). Educating health professionals about electronic health records (EHR): Removing the barriers to adoption. *Knowledge Management & E-Learning: An International Journal, 3*(1), 51–62.

Campbell, E. M., Sittig, D. F., Ash, J. S., Guappone, K. P., & Dykstra, R. H. (2006). Types of unintended consequences related to computerized provider order entry. *Journal of the American Medical Informatics Association, 13*(5), 547–556.

Cheng, C. H., Goldstein, M. K., Geller, E., & Levitt, R. E. (2003). The effects of CPOE on ICU workflow: An observational study. *AMIA Symposium Proceedings, 150*–154.

Congressional Budget Office. (2008, July 24). *Testimony of Peter R. Orszag, director: Evidence on costs and benefits of health information technology.* Washington, DC: U.S. House of Representatives Ways and Means Committee, Subcommittee on Health. Retrieved from http://www.cbo.gov/sites/default/files/cbofiles/ftpdocs/95xx/doc9572/07-24-healthit.pdf

DeSimone, D. M. (2016). EHRs, communication, & litigation– the high cost of all 3! *The Oklahoma Nurse*, 10–12.

Emanuel, E. (2012). Results of HITECH Act: "Nothing short of spectacular." Retrieved from http://www.ihealthbeat.org/articles/2012/3/7/ezekiel-emanuel-results-of-hitech-act-nothing-short-of-spectacular.aspx

Eastaugh, S. R. (2013). The total cost of EHR ownership. *Healthcare Financial Management, 67*(2), 66–70.

Farley, H. L., Baumlin, K. M., Hamedani, A. G., Cheung, D. S., Edwards, M. R., Fuller, D. L., . . . Pines, J. (2013). Quality and safety of implementation of emergency department information systems. *Annals of Emergency Medicine, 62*(4), 399–407.

Feifer, C., Nemeth, L., Nietert, P. J., Wessell, A. M., Jenkins, R. G., Roylance, L., & Ornstein, S. (2007). Different paths to high quality care: Three archetypes of top performing practice sites. *Annals of Family Medicine, 5*(3), 233–241. doi: 10.1370/afm.697

Fleming, N. S., Culler, S. D., McCorkle, R., Becker, E. R., & Ballard, D. J. (2011). The financial and nonfinancial costs of implementing electronic health records in primary care practices. *Health Affairs, 35*(12), 481–489.

Furlong, K. (2015). Learning to use an EHR: Nurses' stories. *Canadian Nurse, 111*(5), 20–24.

Gould, D. W., Walker, D., & Yoon, P. W. (2017). The evolution of Biosense: lessons learned and future directions. *Public Health Reports, 132*(1), 7S–11S.

Hall, S. D. (2013). *Stolen health data increasingly sought after for commercial ventures.* Retrieved from http://www.fiercehealthit.com/story/stolen-health-data-increasingly-sought-after-commercial-ventures/2013-03-25

Harrington, L., & Kennerly, D. (2011). Safety issues related to electronic medical record (EMR): Synthesis of literature from the last decade, 2000–2009. *Journal of Healthcare Management, 56*(1), 31–43.

Healthit.gov (2014). How much is this going to cost me? Retrieved from https://www.healthit.gov/providers-professionals/faqs/how-much-going-cost-me#footnote-1

Healthit.gov (2016). Benefits of EHRs: What is an electronic medical record (EMR)? Retrieved from https://www.healthit.gov/providers-professionals/electronic-medical-records-emr

Hillestad, R., Bigelow, J. H., Chaudhry, B., Dreyer, P., Greenberg, M. D., Meili, R.D., . . . Taylor, R. (2008). *Identity crisis: An examination of the costs and benefits of a unique patient identifier for the United States health care system.* Santa Monica, CA: Rand Corporation. Retrieved from http://www.rand.org/content/dam/rand/pubs/monographs/2008/RAND_MG753.sum.pdf

Healthcare Information and Management Systems Society. (2010). *Dictionary of healthcare information technology terms, acronyms and organizations* (2nd ed.). Chicago, IL: Author, Appendix B, p. 190.

Healthcare Information and Management Systems Society. (2012–2013). *Electronic health records.* Retrieved from http://www.himss.org/library/ehr/?navItemNumber =13261

Hoffman, S., & Podgurski, A. (2012, Spring). Big bad data: law, public health, and biomedical databases. *Journal of Law, Medicine, and Ethics*, 50–60.

Huryk, L. A. (2010). Factors influencing nurses' attitudes towards health information technology. *Journal of Nursing Management, 18*, 606–612.

Institute of Medicine. (2003). *Patient safety: Achieving a new standard for care.* Washington, DC: National Academies Press.

Institute of Medicine. (2006). Roundtable on value and science driven healthcare. Retrieved from http://www.nationalacademies.org/hmd/~/media/Files/Activity%20Files/Quality/VSRT/Core%20Documents/Background.pdf

Institute of Medicine. (2012). *Health IT and patient safety: Building safer systems for better care.* Washington, DC: National Academies Press.

International Health Terminology Standards Development Organisation. (n.d.). About SNOMED CT. Retrieved from http://www.ihtsdo.org/snomed-ct/snomed-ct0/

Jones, S. S., Adams, J. L., Schneider, E. C., Ringel, J. S., & McGlynn, E. A. (2010). Electronic health record adoption and quality improvement in U.S. hospitals. *American Journal of Managed Care, 16*, SP64–SP71.

Kinser, D. E. (2011). Connecting end-users to the EMR–the "last 100 feet." Retrieved from http://s3.amazonaws.com/rdcms-himss/files/production/public/HIMSSorg/Content/files/EDI_ConnectingEndUsersEMR_Last100Feet.pdf

National Institute of Standards and Technology. (2017, July 13). HIPAA Security Rule Toolkit. Retrieved online from: https://scap.nist.gov/hipaa/

Nemeth, L. S., Ornstein, S. M., Jenkins, R. G., Wessell, A. M., & Nietert, P. (2012). Implementing and evaluating electronic standing orders in primary care practice: A PPRNet study. *Journal of the American Board of Family Medicine, 25*(5), 594–604.

O'Brien, A., Weaver, C., Settergren, T., Hook, M. L., & Ivory, C. H. (2015). EHR documentation. *Nursing Administration Quarterly, 39*(4), 333–339.

Oregon Health and Science University. (2012). OHSU contacts patients about data stolen during burglary. Retrieved from http://www.ohsu.edu/xd/about/news_events/news/2012/07-31-ohsu-contacts-patients-a.cfm

Poissant, L., Pereira, J., Tamblyn, R., & Kawasumi, Y. (2005). The impact of electronic health records on the time efficiency of physicians and nurses: A systematic review. *Journal of the American Medical Informatics Association, 12*(5), 505–516.

Strudwick, G., & Hall, L. M. (2015). Nurse acceptance of electronic health record technology: A literature review. *Journal of Research in Nursing, 20*(7), 596–507.

U.S. Bureau of Labor Statistics. (2010). *Occupational outlook handbook*. Retrieved from http://www.bls.gov/ooh/Healthcare/Registered-nurses.htm

U.S. Department of Health and Human Services. Office of the National Coordinator for Health Information Technology. (n.d.*a*). Policymaking, regulation, and strategy. What is meaningful use? Retrieved from http://www.healthit.gov/policy-researchers-implementers/meaningful-use

U.S. Department of Health and Human Services. Office of the National Coordinator for Health Information Technology. (n.d.*b*). Answer to your question: How much is this going to cost me? Retrieved from http://www.healthit.gov/providers-professionals/faqs/how-much-going-cost-me

U.S. Department of Health and Human Services. (2013). Modifications to the HIPAA Privacy, Security, Enforcement, and Breach Notification Rules Under the Health Information Technology for Economic and Clinical Health Act and the Genetic Information Nondiscrimination Act; Other Modifications to the HIPAA Rules (to be codified as CFR Pts. 160 & 164). *Federal Register* 5567.

U.S. Department of Health and Human Services, Office of Civil Rights. (2017). Breach Portal: Notice to the Secretary of HHS, Breach of Unsecured Protected Health Information. Retrieved from https://ocrportal.hhs.gov/ocr/breach/breach_report.jsf

Walker, D. (2013). Laptop stolen from California health care provider exposing data of 1,500. Retrieved from http://www.scmagazine.com/laptop-stolen-from-calif-health-care-provider-exposing-data-of-1500/article/298999/

Weaver, C. A., Warren, J. J., & Delaney, C. (2005). Bedside, classroom, & bench: Collaborative strategies to generate evidence-based knowledge for nursing practice. *International Journal of Medical Informatics, 74*, 989–999.

CHAPTER 12

Clinical Decision-Support Systems

Gennifer Baker, DNP, RN, CCNS
Dorothy Alford, MSN, RN, CEN, CHI
Jane M. Carrington, PhD, RN

LEARNING OBJECTIVES

1. Identify the typical parts of a clinical decision-support system.
2. Understand how clinical decision-support systems can improve patient safety.
3. Discuss a nurse's responsibility when using clinical decision-support systems embedded in electronic health records and other health information technologies.

KEY TERMS

Artificial intelligence	Data quality and validity	Reasoning engine
Clinical decision rules	Knowledge base	Standardized or controlled data
Clinical decision-support systems (CDSSs)	Natural language processing (NLP)	

▶ Chapter Overview

This chapter introduces **clinical decision-support systems (CDSSs)**, beginning with the underpinnings of CDSS and user-technology interfaces. CDSSs and their integration into professional practice issues are also presented. The chapter provides a detailed description of CDSSs including data capture, quality and validity of the data, applications, clinical reasoning, and alert fatigue. Examples are provided to increase understanding.

▶ Introduction

The American Recovery and Reinvestment Act of 2009 (ARRA) set a mandate for technology to increase patient safety and reduce healthcare costs (Civic Impulse, 2017). Implementation and adoption of the electronic health records (EHR) is included in the technology requirements, along with the use of computerized provider order entry (CPOE), electronic prescribing, drug–drug and drug–allergy interaction checks, active medication lists, trending of patient vital signs, and **clinical decision rules** (Centers for Medicare & Medicaid Services [CMS], 2010). To meet the criteria for implementation of clinical decision rules, the EHR must have a functioning CDSS.

Nurses and other healthcare providers (HCPs) collect and manage vast amounts of patient information each shift (Kannampallil et al., 2013; Moore & Fisher, 2012). In addition, HCPs have to recall evidence-based practice standards for allergies, medications, laboratory data, and so forth. A quick scan of patient rooms, hospital units, intensive care units, and outpatient settings reveals many types of medical devices including cardiac monitors, pulse oximeters, syringe pumps, and intravenous (IV) fluid pumps; many of these devices have CDSSs embedded in their operating systems. These CDSSs function in efficient ways to alert HCPs when a patient's physiological parameters are outside the accepted normal ranges.

A CDSS contained in an EHR uses principles of **artificial intelligence** and information science to provide active knowledge systems combined with patient data to generate clinical, patient-specific advice (Demner-Fushman, Chapman, & McDonald, 2009). This definition has several implications. First, a computer can be trained to provide clinical advice that is patient specific. Second, patient information can be organized in such a manner as to fit the data structure required for computer logic. Finally, CDSSs are capable of providing advice to guide patient-care decisions (Demner-Fushman et al., 2009).

▶ Clinical Decision-Support Systems

A CDSS provides the HCP with intelligently filtered information that can guide clinical practice at appropriate times (Hebda & Czar, 2009). When applied to all phases of clinical practice, CDSS can positively influence care delivery by adding efficiency to processes and enhancing the safety parameters embedded in the tools utilized by the HCPs. CDSSs contain reference information, order sets, reminders, alerts, and condition-specific or patient-specific information accessible to HCPs when this information is critical to decision making (Ash et al., 2012). Within the EHR, the discrete information entered by the HCP or information automatically uploaded from the different equipment with an interface to the EHR can be analyzed and trended to provide a clinical picture of the patient. The information presented can trigger a parameter set within the EHR through CDSS that can alert HCPs to perform an intervention or place an order for an intervention for the patient. For example, a patient's laboratory result for potassium is low. The HCP sees a pop-up alert: "K+ < 2.5 mEq." The alert informs the HCP that the patient's potassium level needs to be elevated prior to starting the patient on a planned treatment. Because of the alert, the HCP will order a potassium infusion, supplements, and/or check for the influence of diuretics. The CDSS provides essential information and enhances patient safety in a complex and chaotic environment. This safety feature is one reason CDSSs are included as part of the meaningful use criteria in the ARRA.

▶ Data Capture

CDSSs are designed to use clinical information in providing advice for the HCP. Stated another way, CDSSs are a form of artificial intelligence (AI) whereby a computer has been "trained" to perform human behavior. There are three essential elements to most CDSSs: **knowledge base**, **reasoning engine**, and a *mechanism to communicate* with the end user (Wright et al., 2009). Data are entered into the CDSS as part of the routine documentation process. For example, data such as patient age, gender, symptoms, diagnosis, medications, vital signs, and assessment data are entered into the EHR, seamlessly populating the CDSS in a standardized or controlled manner.

An important element of CDSS is the standardized or controlled data recognized by the reasoning engine of the CDSS. **Standardized or controlled data** are accepted laboratory values, vital signs, and preaccepted items from a drop-down menu. This implies that free text is not recognized by the CDSSs; therefore, it does not contribute to the decision making of the system or alert.

The reasoning engine functions as a series of logic schemes for eventual output (Wright et al., 2009). Using the Bayesian network, for example, the reasoning engine will work to determine the likelihood of an event occurrence (Sim et al., 2001). The system might use "if-then" logic, for example, "if the K+ level is < 2.5 mEq, then alert." The knowledge base informed the reasoning engine of the preadopted K+ value and uses evidence-based practice guides from the literature, expert opinion, and preadopted normal values to link with the

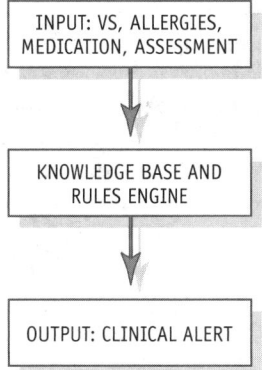

FIGURE 12-1 Architecture of CDSSs.

Data from Berner, E. S., & Ball, M. J. (1998). *Clinical decision support systems: Theory and practice.* New York, NY: Springer, 35.

reasoning engine (Sim et al., 2001). The reasoning engine and knowledge base are simultaneously interchanging information to preestablished rules. Finally, the output is possibilities provided by rank of probability based on results from the reasoning engine and knowledge base (Sim et al., 2001). **FIGURE 12-1** illustrates this using a clinical example.

▶ Data Quality and Validity

The familiar adage "garbage in-garbage out" is especially relevant with CDSSs. The CDSS can potentially threaten the safety of patients if the data entered as input and knowledge base lack quality and validity. Assuming the rules are written correctly, the threat to **data quality and validity** is data entry into the EHR. Berner, Kasiraman, Yu, Ray, and Houston (2005) examined 178 transcriptions of standardized patient visits to test the data quality and CDSS function. Focusing on the GI Risk Score, developed by Singh and licensed by Stanford University, data from the study suggest that missing data or incomplete documentation had an impact on the decision rule and CDSS, potentially threatening patient safety (Singh, Ramey, Triadafilopoulus, Brown, & Balise, 1998).

A variety of clinical situations contribute to missing data. A chaotic and complex work environment and poor workflow contribute as HCPs rush through documentation. Another contributing factor could be the constraints put on HCPs by the standardized response required by the system. For example, Carrington (2012) reported results from a study where nurses were interviewed to elicit their perceptions of the usefulness of standardized nursing languages to communicate a sudden change in patient condition. Researchers reported that nurses perceived standardized nursing languages as constraining, which fostered inaccurate patient information.

A possible solution is using natural language processing to include free text from the electronic documentation to inform the rules engine and trigger an alert. **Natural language processing (NLP)** is a method of taking free text from progress notes, nursing documentation, discharge summaries, or radiology reports, for example, and analyzing it for patterns and added meaning to create added rules and generate more individualized patient-specific alerts (Demner-Fushman et al., 2009). Natural language processing is considered a method that will increase alert sensitivity or the ability to detect subtle data elements describing patient status.

This is an exciting area of research in health care and CDSSs.

▶ CDSS Applications

CDSSs are often purchased from vendors of information systems such as EHR, CPOE, electronic medication administration records (e-MAR), or the Bar Code Medication Administration (BCMA). Other CDSSs are designed for specific purposes by information analysts and HCPs such as physicians and nurses at the hospital or health system level. Refer to **TABLE 12-1** for a list of applications with a brief description.

CDSS Architecture

The strength of CDSSs lies within their architecture. CDSSs are very efficient in how they take patient information and generate an alert. This capability is due to the science of machine learning or teaching the computer how to "think." Moreover, the reasoning engine requires two patient data points at minimum to construct a rule (Spooner, 2007). This requirement implies

TABLE 12-1 CDSS Applications		
Application	**Role**	**Example**
Computerized Provider Order Entry (CPOE)	1. Medication incompatibilities 2. Dosing and patient weight 3. Medication and laboratory values 4. Medications and allergies	1. Patient is on a medication that is incompatible with another. 2. For a patient weight, the dose or frequency is inappropriate. 3. For a particular medication, a laboratory value is too high/low, or unknown. 4. Known patient allergy and medication.
Allergies	1. Allergies to medications 2. Allergies to intravenous nutrition	1. See above. 2. Element in intravenous solution and patient allergy.
Diagnostics	1. Patient diagnostics 2. Laboratory values 3. Vital signs	Link these patient information points for diagnosis support.

that elements included in routine patient care documentation are enough to create rules and generate alerts for safe care. Requiring only two data points to generate an alert further suggests that the alert could fire sooner than having the system wait for 3, 4, or 10 data points, which may not be entered at the same time or in the same area in the EHR.

▶ Clinical Reasoning

Nurses and other HCPs collect, process, and filter vast amounts of data to assemble an accurate picture of the patient. The average human would not be able to accurately manage the quantity of data spread over multiple patients. The strengths of CDSSs, as previously mentioned, are the ability to assist with the process of managing patient data and to provide alerts for decision making.

Identification of Key Decision Points and Information Needs

Construction of key decision points and information needs are necessary to build a solid CDSS. Points to consider encompass a model constructed of clinical knowledge and problem-solving behavior. Building a CDSS to address a specific patient population or to provide a means of alert in a particular practice setting would not replace a clinician's competence but rather be considered as a complementary tool in practice.

Clinicians know that CDSSs lack the ability to reason beyond the programmed logic. For example, CDSSs may recognize an aberrant laboratory value, but CDSSs would not "know" to consider that the aberrant value was the result of processing errors, such as dilution or hemolysis. Alerts are constructed from rules and knowledge, but some HCPs resist the alert, believing a machine could not "know" more than the HCP or that the HCP knows the whole patient situation required for decision making (Alexander, 2006).

Building Intelligence into EHRs

The knowledge base in CDSSs is derived from research literature that is considered best evidence. The knowledge base must be updated and maintained when research evidence shows new findings important for patient care. Keeping up with the evidence can be challenging for an organization because of the fast pace of research and its dissemination across thousands of journals in health care. Moreover, Healthcare organizations typically do not employ HCPs with expertise in evidence-based practice. The success of a CDSS depends on involving HCPs who can apply evidence to practice and informaticists who customize EHRs.

Clinician use of a CDSS can improve clinical practice when the system is built to generate information automatically rather than requiring the clinician to seek the information within the system. Systems built to combine tasks, such as order entry and charting, would more likely be viewed as user friendly compared to systems that stand alone on specific tasks. Systems built with stops to force the clinician to acknowledge an alert or chart the reason for circumventing it are more likely to assist in the clinician's practice success than those allowing the clinician to pass with no alert charting acknowledgment (Kawamoto, Houlihan, Balas, & Lobach, 2005).

▶ Professional Practice

As part of professional practice, nurses must use CDSSs that are part of health information technology. Nurses can also participate in the development or customization of CDSSs, because the systems are composed of knowledge bases, algorithms, and clinical decision rules. Any of these parts must be refined to reflect the most effective care for patients possible. Nurses can work with information analysts on committees or on governing boards for CDSSs to bring about change in CDSSs. In fact, nurses may select an advanced role as an informaticist with more education and work with analysts in information system departments. Several principles for effective use of CDSSs are shown in **BOX 12-1**.

Alert Fatigue

Despite the clinical assistance provided by CDSSs, alerts can also be disruptive. Imagine trying to enter orders for a patient and having three alerts trigger to remind you about allergies, laboratory values, medications, and/or diet and treatments or diagnostics. Multiply the alerts by the number of patients in a shift, and eventually, alert fatigue begins. Defined as simply disrupting clinical workflow, alert fatigue can result in dismissed alerts (quickly clicking to remove the alert) without taking the information into account (Kesselheim, Cresswell, Phansalkar, Bates, & Sheikh, 2011). Alert fatigue has contributed to clinicians' resistance to CDSSs when it interferes with their workflow (Huryk, 2012; Jaspers, Smeulers, Vermeulen, & Peute, 2011; Kleeberg, Levick, Osheroff, Reider, & Teich, 2011). **BOX 12-2**

BOX 12-1 Effective Use of CDSS

- Recognize that alerts are presented in context to increase patient safety. This means that an alert should be taken seriously and not ignored without a sound rationale.
- Use the alerts to support patient care, but not to replace critical thinking and advanced human reasoning.
- Incorporate CDSSs into workflow. If an alert appears while entering patient information in the EHR, prepare for the added information and readily incorporate that information into decision making.
- Recommend changes in practice (change to the CDSS logic) based on the research literature. Should a new practice standard be discovered in the literature, follow the appropriate procedures to communicate the suggestion to nursing leadership and eventually add it to the CDSS's knowledge base.

BOX 12-2 Case Study

James is a nurse in the Cardiothoracic Intensive Care Unit (CICU), where a new EHR system was integrated three months ago, including CDSSs to support common clinical decisions and activities within the CICU. CDSSs and their alerts are offered for drug dosage calculations, potential drug–drug interactions, lab values, drug-allergy interactions, and others. While James tries to address each alert as it arises, he finds the frequent alerts to be an increasing source of frustrations, leading him to identify mechanisms to circumvent the CDSSs, and override the alert systems. For example, the CDSSs trigger alerts regarding the use of nephrotoxic medications in all patients, regardless of their renal function. In caring for a patient during one shift, James overrides the alert for a patient who is scheduled to receive tobramycin, an aminoglycoside antibiotic associated with a risk for nephrotoxicity. He does not review the patient's labs related to renal function before giving the dose of medication, and as a result the patient's renal function declines quickly, leading to a nephrology consult for possible dialysis. Fortunately, the patient's renal function later returns to normal ranges several hours later, but James is worried that a similar patient-care situation could occur in the future.

Check Your Understanding

1. What strategies can be implemented within the design of the CDSS rules in the EHR system to minimize alert fatigue?
2. How could examples from other industries be used in health care to improve attention and impact of alerts in CDSSs?
3. Should providers be able to customize alerts for their clinical needs? Why or why not?

provides a case study about implementation of CDSS and alert fatigue.

Slowly implementing rules in the CDSS in practice can minimize alert fatigue (Kuperman et al., 2007). For example, rules for medications with the highest frequency of errors or the highest risk for patient safety can be implemented first. Over time, the number of rules can be increased with appropriate alerts. The number of rules that can be supported by the knowledge base will be largely dependent on the vendor and the software supports. For any given EHR, the number of rules and alerts will vary.

▶ Summary

CDSSs consist of input from the EHR, reasoning engine, knowledge base, and an output in the form of a clinical alert. CDSSs are designed to assist in managing clinical data to increase patient safety. Despite the impact on increasing patient safety, CDSSs also have had an impact on nursing practice. Issues with the user-technology interface consist of alert fatigue and dependence challenges. However, if used as designed and incorporated within the workflow, CDSSs can have a positive influence in nursing practice and ultimately increase patient safety.

References

Alexander, G. L. (2006). Issues of trust and ethics in computerized clinical decision support systems. *Nursing Administration Quarterly, 30*(1), 21–29.

Ash, J. S., McCormack, J. L., Sittig, D. F., Wright, A., McMullen, C., & Bates, D. W. (2012). Standard practices for computerized clinical decision support in community hospitals: A national survey. *Journal of the American Medical Informatics Association, 19*(6), 980–987. doi: 10.1136/amiajnl-2011-000705

Berner, E. S., Kasiraman, R. K., Yu, F., Ray, M. N., & Houston, T. K. (2005). Data quality in the outpatient setting: Impact on clinical decision support systems. *American Medical Informatics Association Symposium Proceedings,* 41–45.

Carrington, J. M. (2012). The usefulness of nursing languages to communicate a clinical event. *CIN: Computers, Informatics, Nursing, 30*(2), 82–88.

Centers for Medicare and Medicaid Services. (2010). Medicare and Medicaid EHR incentive program. Retrieved from http://www.cms.gov/Regulations-and-Guidance/Legislation/EHRIncentive-Programs/Downloads/MU_Stage1_ReqOverview.pdf

Civic Impulse. (2017). H.R. 1—111th Congress: American Recovery and Reinvestment Act of 2009. Retrieved from https://www.govtrack.us/congress/bills/111/hr1

Demner-Fushman, D., Chapman, W. W., & McDonald, C. J. (2009). What can natural language processing do for clinical decision support? *Journal of Biomedical Informatics, 42,* 760–772.

Hebda, T., Czar, P. (2009). *Handbook of informatics for nurses & healthcare professionals* (4th ed.). Upper Saddle River, NJ: Pearson.

Huryk, L. A. (2012). Information systems and decision support systems: What are they and how are they used in nursing? *American Journal of Nursing, 112*(1), 62–65.

Jaspers, M. W., Smeulers, M., Vermeulen, H., & Peute, L. (2011). Effects of clinical decision-support systems on practitioner performance and patient outcomes: A synthesis of high-quality systematic review findings. *Journal of the American Medical Informatics Association, 18,* 327–334.

Kannampallil, T. G., Franklin, A., Mishra, R., Almoosa, K. F., Cohen, T., & Patel, V. L. (2013). Understanding the nature of information seeking behavior in critical care: Implications for the design of health information technology. *Artificial Intelligence in Medicine, 57*(1), 21–29. doi: 10.1016/j.artmed.2012.10.002

Kawamoto, K., Houlihan, C. A., Balas, E. A., & Lobach, D. F. (2005). Improving clinical practice using clinical decision support systems: A systematic review of trials to identify features critical to success. *BMJ,* 1–8. doi: 10.1136/bmj.38398.500764.8F

Kesselheim, A. S., Cresswell, K., Phansalkar, S., Bates, D. W., & Sheikh, A. (2011). Clinical decision support systems could be modified to reduce "alert fatigue" while still minimizing the risk of litigation. *Health Affairs, 30*(12), 2310–2317.

Kleeberg, P., Levick, D., Osheroff, J., Reider, J., & Teich, J. (2010). *HIMSS clinical decision support and meaningful use frequently asked questions.* Retrieved from http://www.himss.org/files/HIMSSorg/content/files/MU_CDS_FAQ_FINAL_April2010.pdf

Kuperman, G. J., Dobb, A., Payne, T. H., Avery, A. J., Gandhi, T. K., Burns, G., . . . Bates, D. W. (2007). Medication-related clinical decision support in computerized provider order entry systems: A review. *Journal of the American Medical Informatics Association, 14*(1), 29–40.

Moore, A. N., & Fisher, K. (2012). Healthcare information technology and medical-surgical nurses: The emergence of a new care partnership. *CIN: Computers, Informatics, Nursing, 30*(3), 157–163.

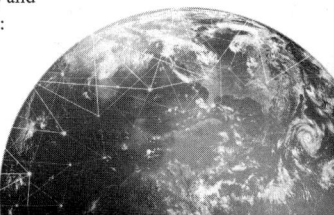

Sim, I., Gorman, P., Greenes, R. A., Haynes, R. B., Kaplan, B., Lehmann, H., & Tang, P. C. (2001). Clinical decision support systems for the practice of evidence-based medicine. *Journal of the American Medical Informatics Association, 8*(6), 527–534.

Singh, G., Ramey, D. R., Triadafilopoulus, G., Brown, B. W., & Balise, R. R. (1998). GI score: A simple self-assessment instrument to quantify the risk of serious NSAID-related GI complications in RA and OA. *Arthritis Rheumatology, 41*(suppl.), S75.

Spooner, S. A. (2007). Mathematical foundations of decision support systems. In E. S. Berner (Ed.), *Clinical decision support systems* (2nd ed., pp. 23–43). New York, NY: Springer.

Wright, A., Sittig, D. F., Ash, J. S., Sharma, S., Pang, J. E., & Middleton, B. (2009). Clinical decision support capabilities of commercially-available clinical information systems. *Journal of the American Medical Informatics Association, 16*(5), 637–644. doi: 10.1197/jamia.M3111

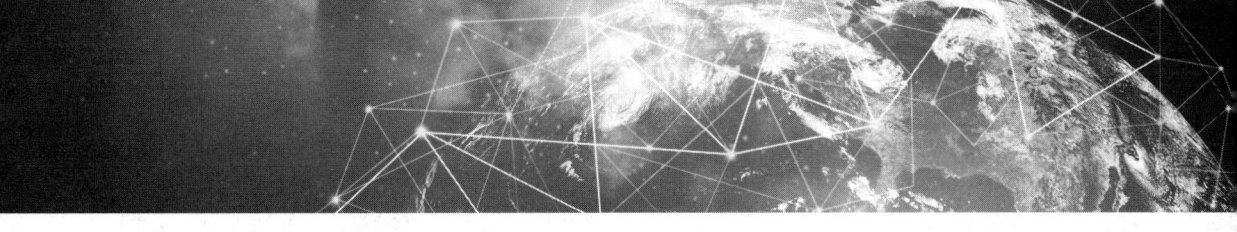

CHAPTER 13

Telehealth Nursing

Marsha Howell Adams, PhD, RN, CNE, ANEF, FAAN
Darlene Showalter, DNP, RN, CNS
Kimberly D. Shea, PhD, RN

LEARNING OBJECTIVES

1. Differentiate between the terms telehealth, telehealth nursing, and telemedicine.
2. Discuss the history of telehealth.
3. Describe the domains of telehealth applications.
4. Understand the relevant legal, policy, and ethical considerations associated with telehealth.
5. Distinguish the utilization of telehealth by populations and/or geographical location.

KEY TERMS

Asynchronous
Digital era
Internet era
Mobile health (mHealth)
Real-time applications (live
   video synchronous)
Remote patient monitoring (RPM)

Store and forward
   applications
Synchronous
Telecommunications
Telecommunications era
Teleconferencing
Teleconsultation

Telehealth
Telehealth nursing
Telemonitoring
Telepresence
Telerehabilitation
Teletrauma
Televisit

▶ Chapter Overview

In this chapter, the concept of telehealth and its definitional variations are explored and differentiated. Also, telehealth applications and the utilization of those applications with different populations and geographical locations are discussed. The chapter provides an overview of the health policy and legal and ethical principles associated with telehealth practice.

▶ Introduction

In *Crossing the Quality Chasm*, a landmark publication by the Institute of Medicine (now known as the National Academy of Medicine), it stated, "information technology must play a central role in the redesign of the health care system if a substantial improvement in quality is to be achieved" (IOM, 2001, p. 16). The free flow of information between healthcare providers and patients is necessary for the transformation of the healthcare system; this flow of information requires information technology.

Telehealth, the process of using technological communication systems in the assessment and management of patients, is an evolving area of nursing practice. The goal of telehealth is to use the many communication technologies that are presently available to expand the provision of healthcare services to locations and populations who are in need of those services, thereby increasing accessibility and decreasing costs. As the definition indicates, telehealth can be used for many different communication purposes and serves as a general "umbrella" that contains numerous services, many of which are designated by the prefix "tele" (e.g., telemonitoring, teleradiology, telenursing, telemedicine, televisits). Telehealth enables health expertise to be available regardless of the patient's ability to physically visit the healthcare services provider.

It is estimated that telehealth will grow at a rate of 4.8%, increasing the telehealth market to approximately $20 billion by 2019 (Iafolla, 2015). The growth in telehealth usage is due to increased consumer demand, strategic pricing options, and cost-efficient protocols supported by the Medicare Access and CHIP Reauthorization Act of 2015 (MACRA) legislation, which supports transparency and innovation in health systems and Medicare payment management.

In 2016, Becker's Health IT and Chief Information Officer Review reported on the growth of telehealth, stating that the most popular modes of delivery were telephone (59%), email (41%), and text messages (29%). The usage of video-based telehealth had increased from 7% in 2015 to 22% in 2016, and the highest telehealth usage was in the range of 25–34 years of age. Individuals over 55 years of age were least likely to engage in telehealth, although more than half of the individuals interviewed in that age range had accessed their healthcare provider via telephone (Cohen, 2016).

Advancements in technology and capacity for communication are allowing vast quantities of information to be sent and received quickly, closing gaps in access to health services created by disabilities and geography. Technology for information transmission has been evolving rapidly and consistently for more than a century, and will continue to evolve as computer and information sciences provide more abilities and knowledge. It is and will continue to be important for healthcare providers to keep up to date with technology and implement it appropriately in their workflow.

▶ Definition of Terms

According to the Institute of Health Care Improvement (IHI), telehealth can have a strong impact on meeting the triple aim of improving population health, providing accessibility and reliability, and decreasing healthcare costs (n.d.). Telehealth is defined by the Health Resources and Services Administration (HRSA) as the "use of electronic information and telecommunications technologies to support long-distance clinical health care, patient and professional health-related education, public health and health administration" (2012). The Center for Connected Health Policy (CCHP) defines telehealth as a "collection of means or methods for enhancing health care, public health, and health education delivery and support using telecommunications technologies" (n.d.). Telemedicine is an older term used to describe clinical diagnosis using technology. **Telehealth nursing** is defined as "the practice of nursing delivered through various telecommunications technologies including high speed Internet, wireless, and satellite and televideo communications" (National Council of State Boards of Nursing [NCSBN], 2014).

These definitions provide the basis for this chapter and guide an examination of the components of telehealth, telehealth nursing, and the implications for the nursing profession. Although the American Telemedicine Association (ATA) considers *telemedicine* and *telehealth* to be interchangeable terms, the use of telehealth encompasses all the health services (not only medical) that can be provided remotely. Other organizations including the CCHP and the American Association of Ambulatory Care Nurses (AAACN) support the use of the term, telehealth because it encompasses a greater scope of health services. **TABLE 13-1** lists the different terms associated with telehealth.

▶ The History of Telehealth

Healthcare providers, unless living with the sick or injured patient, have always had the obstacle of distance to surmount. While the proliferation of telehealth systems and technologies may be an emerging trend, the need to urgently assess patients is not a new problem. As recently as 40 years ago, hospitals began extending care to patients in remote geographical areas by exchanging medical information via electronic communication. Novel efforts at introducing and sustaining telehealth practice have occurred commonly over the last hundred years. In 1880, shortly after the invention of the telephone, attempts were made to transmit heart and lung sounds to an expert trained in auscultation of the organs. However, poor quality in the transmission of the sounds made the assessments virtually useless, and the

effort failed. Other more successful uses for phone lines were later identified. Einthoven, the father of electrocardiography, wrote an article in 1906 about remote transmission of electrocardiogram (EKG) tracings using a string galvanometer to register the human EKG. Alternative telecommunications technologies, such as radio, were also utilized in the development of telehealth. In the 1920s, ships at sea were connected to public health physicians at shore stations via radio. In April 1924, *Radio News Magazine* published a futuristic story of children having their throats examined remotely by a physician. With the rapid spread of telecommunications networks that began in the 1960s came the development and proliferation of a number of different methods for the transmission of video telehealth.

Bashshur (2002) discusses three major eras that shaped the development of telehealth. Contributions from the telecommunications era (1970s–1980s), the digital era (late 1980s), and the Internet era (1990s–present) have built a complex, omnipresent, global communication environment. The **telecommunications era** was characterized by television and broadcast technologies. The **digital era** integrated computerized information that could transmit voice and video data at higher speeds. The **Internet era** has enabled telehealth services such as videoconferencing, remote access to patient data and information, and rapid communication between patients and providers. Most importantly, telehealth continues to enable the provision of healthcare services to areas that would otherwise be drastically underserved. Telehealth is the product of this continued technological development, and it is still being used to address the issues of rising healthcare costs, limited providers, and a lack of access to care in rural and underserved areas.

One example from the beginning of the telehealth movement comes from the Nebraska Psychiatric Institute, which installed closed-circuit television (CCTV) during its construction in 1955 for use as a teaching tool for medical residents and a monitoring tool for the nursing staff (Mallisee & von Rosenberg, 1965). By observing sessions

TABLE 13-1 Terms Used in Describing Telehealth Concepts

Term	Definition
Telepresence	Technologies allowing individuals to feel as if they were present, to appear to be present, or to have an effect at a place other than their true location (ATA, n.d.).
Telecommunications	Communication over a distance by cable, telegraph, telephone, or other broadcasting mechanism. Telecommunications networks include a transmitter that takes information and converts it to a signal. The signal is then carried by a medium to a receiver, where it is translated into usable information for the recipient. Telecommunications networks and the practice of telehealth were established well before the advent of the wireless networks that are present in today's society; however, the ability to move the signal from transmitter to receiver in a wireless fashion has enabled the field of telehealth to grow exponentially.
Televisit	An encounter involving a patient and a healthcare provider that is enabled by telecommunications technologies. Determining the goal for the visit is the first step in deciding which type of televisit to use. The types of televisits include teleassessment (active and engaging remote assessment), telemonitoring (minimally intrusive detection using sensors and measurement devices), telesupport (encounter is to provide support for patients and/or providers), telecoaching (support and instruction for a prescribed therapy are conveyed), and teletherapy (engage in interactive therapy) (Winters & Winters, 2007).
Teleconferencing	Interactive electronic communication between multiple users at two or more sites that facilitates voice, video, and/or data transmission systems: audio, graphics, computer, and video systems (ATA, n.d.).
Teleconsultation	Consultation between a provider and specialist at a distance using either store and forward telehealth or real-time videoconferencing (ATA, n.d.).
Telemonitoring	Patient data such as blood pressure, weight, and pulse are transmitted to the healthcare providers so that they can keep track of a patient remotely.

between patients and physicians, residents in psychiatry were able to develop more advanced techniques of psychotherapy. Nurses used CCTV to assist in monitoring areas of maximum security within the hospital. Vocational counselors at the institute later used CCTV for long-distance patient interview sessions at remotely located state hospitals.

In 1967, collaboration between Logan International Airport and Massachusetts General Hospital (MGH) resulted in the establishment of the Logan International Airport Medical Aid Station. At the aid station, employees in the airport and airline travelers could receive medical care from MGH physicians via a two-way audiovisual microwave circuit. The aid station was staffed continuously by nurses, while physicians were present during the 4 hours of each day that were determined to be peak passenger-use times. Nurses triaged each patient who visited the station, identifying those who needed further medical care. The National Aeronautics and Space Administration (NASA) also played an important part in the development of telehealth in the 1960s with the initiation of space exploration. Physiological data from the astronauts were collected by space suits and spacecraft and transmitted to medical staff on the ground for monitoring during missions.

In the 1970s, healthcare providers in remote Alaskan villages, often nurses and nurses' aides, used high-frequency radio and satellite systems to connect with physicians and obtain remote care for residents. Consisting of fixed blocks of time available 3 days per week, healthcare providers relied on two-way voice and video technologies that allowed the transmission of electrocardiogram, electronic stethoscope, and slow-scan video for X-rays. Though project participants were glad to have video capability, the quality of color images was poor, and therefore limited to black-and-white photos, and the transmission of video images required expensive equipment. Due to limited bandwidth, video transmissions frequently failed. Lessons learned from the project were later used in larger projects created to serve the people of Alaska, including creation of the Alaska Telemedicine Project (Hudson & Ferguson, 2011). Remote transmission of complex images has experienced problems resulting from limited bandwidth, connection speed, bit rates, and complications with point-of-care technology. However, telehealth applications have continued to develop for almost every facet of health care, with a general understanding that increased transmission speed and capacity are always on the horizon.

Today, the use of telehealth has great potential for improving health care in traditionally underserved populations, particularly those who are located in geographies isolated from healthcare providers and those in areas where healthcare providers and facilities are limited in number. Healthcare access for all is consistent with the missions of the World Health Organization (WHO) and the U.S. Department of Health and Human Services (HHS, 2013)—via its *Healthy People 2020* initiative. The HRSA works to increase and improve the use of telehealth through the creation of new telehealth projects, the administration and evaluation of grant programs, and the promotion of a fluid exchange of knowledge about "best practices" in areas of telehealth.

▶ Domains of Telehealth Applications

Technological communication provides the opportunity for the optimal delivery of services without complications related to the physical transportation of messages or people. Being able to work outside the realm of familiar face-to-face interactions provides greater efficiency and increased frequency of communication. In the modern-day use of telehealth, four domains of applications are available: real-time applications, store and forward applications, remote patient monitoring, and mobile health. The availability of telecommunications technologies and the type of information to be transmitted plus concerns about urgency and budget influence which type of telehealth application is most appropriate.

Real-time applications (live video synchronous) are commonly transmitted in the form of live audio/video, telephone, or webcam with transmission occurring simultaneously with the capture of the information. Using Skype to visit with a colleague is an example of a real-time telehealth application. Video-chat platforms, such as Skype, were developed for marketing to the general consumer, and not for health care. The choice to use Skype would be optimal if the user has a computer with high-speed Internet access and anticipates a casual discussion without the need for strict privacy. Another example is the use of telepresence robotics. The robot is actually an iPad on a Segway (Double Robotics, n.d.).

The robot is able to view and hear the healthcare provider, and the healthcare provider is able to view what the robot is looking at. Connection to the robot can be made anywhere using a computer, tablet, or smartphone. The robot is able to maneuver throughout its remote location and can zoom in and/or view from a wide angle. Nursing programs across the country are using telepresence robots in their simulation laboratories to prepare their students for telehealth and interprofessional practice. For example, advance practice nursing students (nurse practitioners, clinical nurse specialists, nurse anesthetists, nurse midwives) can enter a simulation scenario with traditional nursing students through the telepresence robots and create an added dimension to the simulation scenario.

Store and forward applications (asynchronous) capture data, images, sound, and video, and store the information to be forwarded to healthcare providers at a later time. Examples of this application would be recording a visit or treatment to be consulted at a later date, or transmitting digital images such as X-rays and photographs. The Veterans Health Administration (VHA) has been using this type of application in the areas of radiology, dermatology, and ophthalmology. For example, veterans with diabetes are screened for retinopathy using retinal images that are stored and forwarded to healthcare providers for possible treatment (Veterans Health Administration, n.d.).

Remote patient monitoring (RPM) is the transmission of an individual's personal health and medical data to the healthcare provider in a different location for diagnosis and treatment. This application allows the monitoring of patients outside of the traditional clinical settings, such as the home. The delivery of care right to the home affords patients the comfort, freedom, and independence to live a quality life. Examples include glucometers, blood pressure cuffs, and pulse oximetry through the use of sensors. RPM is particularly useful in the monitoring of patients with chronic diseases. For example, continuous glucose monitors are minimally invasive devices that track interstitial glucose levels at intervals

through the day independently of patient actions. This method of glucose observation provides a much clearer look at patients' glucose dynamics, alleviates the need for patients to actively monitor their glucose, and is capable of being communicated directly to healthcare providers (Klonoff, 2005).

This type of application has been found to increase accessibility to care, reduce hospital readmissions, and decrease healthcare costs.

Mobile health (mHealth) is the transmission of health information and services via mobile technologies such as smartphones, tablets, and personal digital assistants (PDAs) (WHO, 2011). Information can range from texts focusing on health promotion and education to national alerts regarding disease outbreaks. Healthcare providers are able to use the mobile health application to communicate with patients, access critical health information, discuss care coordination with other healthcare team members, and provide remote monitoring. Patients can use this application for communicating with healthcare providers, tracking their personal health data, and accessing their clinical health records.

Laws and policies that pertain to the protection of patient healthcare information are important in the selection of telehealth applications and have implications regarding practice for nurses and advanced practice nurses (nurse practitioners). This is discussed later in the chapter.

▶ Privacy, Ethics, and Limitations in Telehealth

Patient Privacy

Privacy concerns are some of the most important issues healthcare providers face. Patients have the right to keep their healthcare information private and protected, and it is the responsibility of the provider to ensure this right is upheld and respected to the fullest. The use of telehealth services carries with it a host of specific privacy issues. Healthcare providers must ensure that any means of communication that is used, be it videoconferencing, direct messaging, or vital sign communication through biometric devices, is compliant with the Health Insurance Portability and Accountability Act (HIPAA). One of the most important caveats of HIPAA compliance relating to telehealth is the rule that providers use technology with the ability to produce audit trails, so that any potential security breaches can be tracked. Healthcare providers are ethically driven to use telehealth to offer healthcare services to those who might otherwise not receive those services, but in doing so they should strive to adhere to best practices and a code of ethics. According to Fleming, Edison, and Pak (2009), the ethical code for telehealth pledges commitment to benevolent action, fairness, integrity, respect for others, avoiding harm, pursuing sound scholarship, and ensuring appropriate oversight. In order to ensure quality care without harm, a standardized code for telehealth practice would be valuable as an ongoing guide and reference.

Telehealth Ethics

The use of telehealth should not adversely affect the relationship between the patient and the provider, which should be characterized by mutual trust and respect. In addition, telehealth should not impair the ability of the provider to engage in autonomous decision making for the best interests of the patient. Telehealth technology can be overwhelming for some older adults who are unfamiliar with communication using video and webcams; it is unethical to expect older adults to use a technology that creates stress. Healthcare providers question the ethics of delivering a terminal diagnosis or other bad news to patients using telehealth technology (Fleming et al., 2009). Because privacy is always a concern in the use of Internet-based services, the use of telehealth is no exception. The use of any video or other recording of patients must be handled in a secure and safe manner, in such a way that it cannot be used for exploitation.

System Limitations and Downtime

As with all technological systems, the use of telehealth can have drawbacks. Computerized networks are subject to network errors and unscheduled episodes of downtime that, in the event of a health emergency, could prove devastating. Healthcare providers who intend to implement telehealth services should make reasonable efforts to provide safeguards against the different threats to technological integrity, such as network downtime and hardware failure. In addition to the concerns associated with physical technology, there are inherent limitations associated with telehealth services. Despite advances in technology, at times there is simply no acceptable substitute for a face-to-face examination by a healthcare provider. Video and audio may not be clear enough to enable the provider to gather all the information from a patient that is needed, and a personal visit may be warranted. It is the role of the healthcare provider to be aware of the limitations of telehealth systems and be willing to admit those limitations, provide acceptable solutions, and, if necessary, assert the need for in-person examinations.

Licensure Issues in the United States

A regulatory aspect that has proven to be an obstacle to the delivery of telehealth services is medical and nursing licensure across state boundaries. In the United States, medical and nursing licenses are assigned at the level of the states; physicians, advanced practice nurses, and nurses may legally practice only within the boundaries of their respective state licenses. With the advent of telehealth services, there has been an increased movement to enhance licensure portability within the United States (see **TABLE 13-2**). However, at this time, the ability to practice telemedicine within a particular state resides within the jurisdiction of the medical board of that state. According to information from the Federation of State Medical Boards (2012), all states require that interested parties obtain a license to practice medicine within the

TABLE 13-2 Alternative Proposals for Licensure That Would Facilitate the Practice of Telehealth by Healthcare Providers

Model	Explanation
Consulting exceptions	With a consulting exception, a physician who is unlicensed in a particular state can practice medicine in that state at the request of and in consultation with a referring physician. The scope of these exceptions varies from state to state. Most consultation exceptions prohibit the out-of-state physician from opening an office or receiving calls in the state. In most states, these exceptions were enacted before the advent of telehealth and were not meant to apply to ongoing regular telehealth links. However, some states permit a specific number of consulting exceptions per year.
Endorsement	State boards can grant licenses to health professionals in other states with equivalent standards. Health professionals must apply for a license by endorsement from each state in which they seek to practice. States may require additional qualifications or documentation before endorsing a license issued by another state. Endorsement allows states to retain their traditional power to set and enforce standards that best meet the needs of the local population. However, complying with diverse state requirements and standards can be time consuming and expensive for a multistate practitioner.
Reciprocity	A licensure system based on reciprocity would require the authorities of each state to negotiate and enter agreements to recognize licenses issued by the other state without a further review of individual credentials. These negotiations could be bilateral or multilateral. A license valid in one state would give privileges to practice in all other states with which the home state has agreements.
Mutual recognition	Mutual recognition is a system in which the licensing authorities voluntarily enter into an agreement to legally accept the policies and processes (licensure) of a licensee's home state. Licensure based on mutual recognition is comprised of three components: a home state, a host state, and a harmonization of standards for licensure and professional conduct. The health professional secures a license in his or her own home state and is not required to obtain additional licenses to practice in other states. The nurse licensure compact is based on this model.
Registration	Under a registration system, a health professional licensed in one state would inform the authorities of other states that he or she wished to practice part-time there. By registering, the health professional would agree to operate under the legal authority and jurisdiction of the other state. Health professionals would not be required to meet entrance requirements imposed upon those licensed in the host state, but they would be held accountable for breaches in professional conduct in any state in which they are registered. California had the authority to draft this type of model but never did so.

Model	Explanation
Limited licensure	Under a limited licensure system, a health professional would have to obtain a license from each state in which he or she practiced but would have the option of obtaining a limited license for the delivery of specific health services under particular circumstances. Thus, the system would limit the scope rather than the time period of practice. The health professional would be required to maintain a full and unrestricted license in at least one state. The Federation of State Medical Boards has proposed a variation of this model. According to the Federation, 16 states have adopted a limited licensure model.
National licensure	A national licensure system could be adopted at the state or national level. A license would be issued based on a universal standard for the practice of health care in the United States. If administered at the national level, questions might be raised about state revenue loss, the legal authority of states, logistics about how data would be collected and processed, and how enforcement of licensure standards and discipline would be administered. If administered at the state level, these questions might be alleviated. States would have to agree on a common set of standards and criteria ranging from qualifications to discipline.
Federal licensure	Under a federal licensure system, health professionals would be issued one license, valid throughout the United States, by the federal government. Licensure would be based on federally established standards related to qualifications and discipline and would preempt state licensure laws. Federal agencies would administer the system. However, given the difficulties associated with central administration and enforcement, the states might play a role in implementation.

Reproduced from Wakefield, M. K., Puskin, D. S., & Tipping, K. (2010). *Telehealth licensure report*. U.S. Department of Health and Human Services Human Resources and Services Administration. Retrieved from https://web.archive.org/web/20161221072700/https://www.hrsa.gov/healthit/telehealth/licenserpt10.pdf

state in which the patient is located. However, if the physician desires to practice only telemedicine, 10 states will allow for the provision of special purpose licenses that provide only for the practice of telemedicine. In addition, not every state requires that telemedicine services be reimbursed by insurers.

▶ Utilization of Telehealth

Telehealth for Chronic Conditions

According to the Centers for Disease Control and Prevention (2016), chronic conditions such as heart disease, type 2 diabetes, stroke, cancer, obesity, and arthritis are among the most costly and preventable.

In 2012, 117 million Americans were living with at least one chronic condition. One out of four adult Americans have two or more chronic conditions (Ward, Schiller, & Goodman, 2014). In 2010, chronic conditions accounted for 86% of the country's total health spending (Gertis et al., 2014). These conditions require frequent, if not constant monitoring, to minimize the potential for exacerbation of acute disease. This makes them perfect for telehealth applications. The most common form of telehealth associated with chronic conditions is telepresence.

Telemonitoring enables healthcare providers to monitor the relevant signs and symptoms of chronic diseases even when patients are out of the clinic. Telemonitoring systems not only give providers patients' vital signs, but they also provide patients with a way to update their providers on the subjective experiences of the illness.

From 2003 to 2007, the VHA rolled out a national home telehealth program known as Care Coordination/Home Telehealth (CCHT). The goal of the program was defined as

> The use of health informatics, disease management, and home telehealth technologies to enhance and extend care and case management to facilitate access to care and improve the health of designated individuals and populations with the specific intent of providing the right care in the right place at the right time. (Darkins et al., 2008)

The program focused on caring for patients with diabetes mellitus, congestive heart failure, hypertension, posttraumatic stress disorder (PTSD), chronic obstructive pulmonary disease (COPD), and depression. The tools available for use in the system included biometric devices that measured vital signs, messaging devices for patient input, videophones, and telemonitoring devices. In 2003 there were 2,000 patients enrolled in CCHT. By 2007 that number had grown to 31,570 (Darkins et al., 2008).

The most common conditions treated in CCHT were diabetes mellitus and hypertension, accounting for 48.4% and 40.3% of patients, respectively. This was followed by congestive heart failure and COPD, accounting for 24.8% and 11.6% of patients, respectively. Depression, PTSD, and other mental disorders accounted for 2.3%, 1.1%, and 1.2% of patients, respectively. The efficacy of CCHT was measured by the decrease in utilization of hospital services, as measured by both hospital admissions and bed days of care (BDOC). Each of the conditions treated saw utilization of hospital services fall by 20% or more. The largest decreases in hospital services were

associated with conditions such as depression, PTSD, and other mental disorders, with declines of 56.4%, 45.1%, and 40.9%. Hypertension and chronic heart failure saw decreases of 30.3% and 25.9%; treatment for COPD and diabetes declined by 20.7% and 20.4%.

Patients and healthcare providers reported that the most beneficial aspect of home telehealth associated with the CCHT program was the messaging system. A direct line of communication from patient to provider greatly increased the efficacy of and capacity for self-management of chronic diseases (Darkins et al., 2008). Increased communication between patients and their providers also may have improved patient satisfaction. Quarterly patient satisfaction surveys assessed over the duration of the 4-year CCHT project revealed an average satisfaction rate of 86% (Darkins et al., 2008).

Telehealth in Underserved and Rural Communities

An important function of telehealth is the provision of healthcare services to underserved and rural communities. In the United States in 2012, although 20% of the country's total population resided in rural areas, only 11% of U.S. physicians reported practicing in a rural area (Cromartie, 2012), and there was an even greater shortage of nurses, healthcare technicians, and nonphysician providers in those areas (Shea & Effken, 2008). Unfortunately, the lack of healthcare services and providers in rural areas can contribute to a self-reinforcing cycle. As the healthcare providers and facilities serving rural areas find themselves overworked and understaffed, rural opportunities may be less appealing to graduating medical students, and the cycle of underservice continues (Shea & Effken, 2008).

Conger and Plager (2008) found the advanced practice nurses transitioning into rural practices were more successful if they had a sense of connectiveness versus disconnectiveness. Nurse practitioners found connectiveness through the development of networks with colleagues (other nurse practitioners), development of a relationship with an urban healthcare center, communication through electronic resources, and finally, connection with the rural community and become a part of that community.

Telehealth has been viewed as a method for transforming health care in rural communities. Through the use of telehealth, rural communities can participate in teleconsultation with specialists and remote in-home monitoring, The National Rural Health Association (NRHA) has identified four areas that need to be addressed in order to advance telehealth in rural communities. The NRHA advocates for (a) a review of reimbursement policies based on the geographical location of urban versus rural, (b) telehealth rural facilities to perform credentialing of telehealth providers by proxy, (c) greater investment in broadband among federal and state regulators and private industry, and (d) more research to be performed on services provided to rural communities (Morgan, 2012).

A primary purpose of the VHA's CCHT program was to address the geographical diversity of its patients (Darkins et al., 2008). Of the 31,570 total patients in the program, 31.2% lived in urban areas, 21% lived in rural areas, and 1% lived in highly rural areas. Patients who were located in highly rural areas saw the largest declines in hospital utilization, with an average reduction of 50.9%. Patients residing in urban areas utilized hospital services an average of 29.2% less, while patients living in rural areas utilized hospitals 17% less frequently over the course of the project. These declines are substantial and highlight the fact that telehealth may be most useful for those who are the most isolated.

The VHA CCHT program numbers also illustrate how telehealth programs may benefit urban communities as well as rural communities (Darkins et al., 2008). Though rural communities can suffer from a lack of healthcare providers in close proximity, the density of urban communities can make it more difficult to get timely appointments despite increased numbers of providers in these communities.

In addition, urban communities typically have more consistent access to Internet services. For these reasons, telehealth for underserved groups within urban communities should also be a high priority.

Telehealth for Rehabilitation Patients

Telerehabilitation, also known as telerehab, is defined by the American Telemedicine Association as the use of information and communication technology services to deliver rehabilitation services (Brennan et al., 2010). Speech-language pathology services, with their attention to auditory and visual communication, are ideally suited for telerehabilitation services. However, many sources suggest that the routine practice of telerehabilitation in the United States has been limited due to regulatory issues relating to licensure and reimbursement, and variations in state-to-state requirements regarding the use of telerehab services (Cherney & van Vuuren, 2012). Despite these difficulties, a review of the literature suggests telerehabilitation technologies can be used to assist patients with motor speech disorders.

In a review of the international literature, Cherney and van Vuuren (2012) compared results of face-to-face assessments of dysarthria due to traumatic or hypoxic brain injury, Parkinson's disease, or stroke, to those conducted in the telerehab environment. Though there were technical difficulties within the telerehab environment, for the majority of acoustic and perceptual parameters, clinical criteria for both face-to-face and videoconferencing were similar. Cherney and van Vuuren further noted that the use of the small 128 kbit/second bandwidth hindered the detection of fine motor movements during videoconferencing, and that these difficulties were more apparent for patients with severe dysarthria.

Telehealth in Public Schools

Telehealth can be used to improve school-based health services, particularly in rural areas.

School-based telehealth includes using telephones, teleconferences, store and forward transmissions, or web cameras in the school to connect to a distant healthcare provider (ATA, 2013). Pediatric equipment such as an otoscope or camera that transmits a static image, or a stethoscope that transmits respiratory and heart sounds are valuable assets that enhance decision making for treatment when school nurses teleconsult with specialists. School nurses can use telehealth for managing common ailments encountered in the school setting, such as the examination of skin conditions (rashes, wheals, eruptions, blisters, and petechiae) and ear, nose, and throat disorders (infections of ears, tonsils, adenoids, and sinuses).

For example, a school without a full-time school nurse may elect to employ a traveling nurse who comes to the school several times a week to see children with minor illnesses/ injuries. If the traveling nurse determines that the health problem requires a more detailed assessment, telehealth equipment will be used to transmit to a school-based health center where a nurse practitioner will be available to diagnose and treat the child. This mode of healthcare delivery eliminates missed school days, reduces transportation costs, and decreases the cost of care (Wicklund, 2016).

Telehealth and Connecting Patients with Specialists

A particularly difficult problem within health care is how to connect the most qualified healthcare providers with the patients who need their specific skill sets. Far too often patients have to travel hundreds or even thousands of miles to visit an appropriate specialist. Telehealth can give these patients a way to meet with the specialist they need, without having to endure the costly, troublesome process of long-distance travel. In many circumstances, telehealth enables a patient's primary healthcare provider to communicate directly with a specialist about the patient's illness and adapt treatment based on the specialist's recommendations.

Teletrauma, the remote treatment of trauma situations, is an example of a real-time application that can connect patients with specialists. In teletrauma, patients in rural areas or towns without access to a trauma center are able to receive the expertise of a trauma surgeon via telecommunications networks. Teletrauma services are initiated as soon as a trauma patient arrives at the rural hospital. Immediate consultation using real-time video allows the remote expert trauma surgeon to evaluate the patient's condition on arrival and work with the local emergency provider to stabilize and engage in a diagnostic workup. Early intervention from the Level I trauma expert can prevent painful, time-consuming, and unnecessary transfers. If air transfer to a Level I trauma center is required, the expert surgeon's familiarity with the case from the initiation of care can improve the quality of care that patients receive (Bjorn, 2012). One example of lifesaving teletrauma services is the case of an 18-month-old child who was the only surviving victim of an automobile accident in the remote desert near Douglas, Arizona. At the time of the accident, a trauma surgeon was able to provide direct supervision to an on-site physician via telecommunications networks. After endotracheal intubation, the delivery of blood products, and large amounts of intravenous fluids, the child was stabilized and transported to the University of Arizona Medical Center (Erps, 2008).

Licensure across state boundaries within the profession of nursing is slightly different. In 1994, the National Council of State Boards of Nursing (NCSBN) crafted a model of mutual recognition of licensure, entitled the Interstate Compact Agreement (Hutcherson & Williamson, 1999). For nurses who were licensed in states that agreed to participate in the Interstate Compact Agreement, physical or electronic practice in the participating states was allowed, unless a nurse was under discipline or in a monitoring agreement that restricted practice to a home state. Currently, 25 state boards of nursing are members of the NCSBN Nurse Licensure Compact. Because of the reciprocity agreements between

BOX 13-1 Case Study

Obstetrics is one of the most litigious specialties in health care. Healthcare professionals who work in Labor and Delivery (L&D) units are encouraged to maintain competency in fetal monitoring through continuing education and certification. Commonly, nurses in L&D units will provide bedside care for the laboring client, while the physician or midwife may attend to other tasks, such as in the office or operating room, until delivery is closer. This commonly used care delivery model for the laboring client necessitates clear and concise communication between the L&D nurses and the primary care provider to ensure quality and safe care for both mother and baby.

Jessica is the unit manager of an L&D unit in a small rural hospital. All obstetrical services are provided to this community by one obstetrician who has a very busy solo practice. It is common for the obstetrician to have a full day of scheduled primary care in the office while a client labors in the hospital. The L&D nurses have recently expressed concern to Jessica about the delay in physician response regarding analysis of fetal monitor strips. The L&D nurses would like to have a quicker response from the physician when there is a pattern of concern on the monitor strip. In cases of obvious fetal distress and other obstetrical emergencies, the nurses felt justified in asking for the obstetrician's rapid presence on the unit. In cases of fetal monitoring strips demonstrating equivocal patterns, the nurses needed to collaborate and communicate quickly with the obstetrician for review of the strip and planning for immediate patient care. The L&D nurses were seeking resolution to this concern.

After much review of the literature and discussions with a colleague in a large teaching hospital, Jessica learned about AirStrip One, an innovative technology that allows care providers to collaborate in near real-time analysis of the fetal monitor strip interpretations despite geographic boundaries. Other data points, such as elements of the electronic health record, labs, and hemodynamics may transmit in tandem with the fetal monitor strip. The obstetrician can use a smartphone or tablet remotely to access a laboring client's fetal monitor strip. In talking with AirStrip One's developers, Jessica found that the telehealth product could meet the needs of the L&D unit, easily integrating with the existing fetal monitoring system to provide a high-quality, HIPAA-protected platform for data sharing and professional engagement among healthcare providers. After much collaboration with the company in reviewing the product's white papers and specifications, Jessica approached the obstetrician and L&D nurses who were relieved to learn of this technology.

After purchase of the telehealth technology, a policy for its use was drafted, and L&D nurses were trained in use of the product. Now, when a pregnant woman presents to the L&D unit, the nurses confidently initiate the obstetrical telehealth algorithm. The client's menstrual, sexual, and pregnancy history and vital signs are collected, the fetal monitor is applied, and AirStrip One is utilized to transmit the near real-time fetal monitor strip and medical data to be analyzed by the primary care provider as needed. The obstetrician continues to respond to immediate calls of distress, and the nurses continue to communicate throughout the course of labor with the reassurance that all parties have access to the same client data.

Check Your Understanding

1. Besides the L&D unit manager, which other stakeholders should have been involved in the discussion of telehealth to create a solution for this unit's concerns? Why?
2. How could the use of telehealth, as outlined in this case study, enhance unit morale and client outcomes?
3. How could telehealth, as utilized in this case study, decrease the risk of liability for the healthcare providers?

the 26 state boards of nursing, nurses who hold unencumbered licenses within those 26 member states may practice, physically or electronically, without incurring additional applications or fees (NCSBN, n.d.).

▶ Summary

The future of telehealth is limited only by policy and the imagination, not by technology. Continued research is required to develop best practices for telehealth delivery. Telehealth should not be considered a replacement for face-to-face interventions, but another tool to be utilized alongside face-to-face interventions in the pursuit of the highest quality of care. As research and practice continue, the telehealth field will continue to grow and change. Healthcare providers should embrace this change, work to stay abreast of technological changes, and constantly be reassessing their methods and standards of care. The ability to reach patients who otherwise would not have access to care is a tremendous opportunity for improving the quality of health in the United States. Whether in an urban or rural community, a busy hospital or a small private practice, patients and healthcare providers across all spectrums of health care can and will continue to benefit from telehealth services.

References

American Telemedicine Association. (n.d.). Telemedicine glossary. Retrieved from http://thesource.american-telemed.org/resources/telemedicine-glossary

American Telemedicine Association. (2013). *State Medicaid best practice: School-based telehealth*. Retrieved from http://www.amdtelemedicine.com/telemedicine-resources/documents/ATAstate-medicaid-best-practice---school-based-telehealth.pdf

Bashshur, R. L. (2002). Telemedicine and health care. *Telemedicine Journal and E-Health, 8*(1), 5–9.

Bjorn, P. (2012). Rural teletrauma: Applications, opportunities, and challenges. *Advanced Emergency Nursing Journal, 34*(3), 232–237.

Brennan, D. M., Tindall, L., Theodoros, D., Brown, J.,

Campbell, M., Christiana, D., . . . Lee, A. (2010). A blueprint for telerehabilitation guidelines. *Telemedicine E-Health, 17*, 662–665.

Center for Connected Health Policy. (n.d.). What is telehealth? Retrieved from http://www.cchpca.org/what-is-telehealth

Centers for Disease Control and Prevention. (2016). Chronic disease overview. Retrieved from https://www.cdc.gov/chronicdisease/overview/index.htm

Cherney, L. R., & van Vuuren, S. (2012). Telerehabilitation, virtual therapists, and acquired neurologic speech and language disorders. *Seminars in Speech and Language, 33*(3), 243–257. doi: 10.1055/s-0032-1320044

Cohen, J. (December 22, 2016). The growth of telehealth: 20 things to know. Retrieved from http://www.beckershospitalreview.com/healthcare-information-technology/the-growth-of-telehealth-20-things-to-know.html

Conger, M., & Plager, K. (2008). Advanced nursing practice in rural areas: Connectedness versus disconnectedness. *Online Journal of Rural Nursing and Health Care, 8*(1), 24–38.

Cromartie, J. (May 26, 2012). Population and migration. U.S. Department of Agriculture, Economic Research Service. Retrieved from https://www.ers.usda.gov/topics/rural-economy-population/population-migration.aspx

Darkins, A., Ryan, P., Kobb, R., Foster, L., Edmonson, E., Wakefield, B., & Lancaster, A. E. (2008). Care coordination/home telehealth: The systematic implementation of health informatics, home telehealth, and disease management to support the care of veteran patients with chronic conditions. *Telemedicine and e-Health, 14*(10), 1118–1125. doi: 10.1089/tmj.2008.0021

Double Robotics. (n.d.). Double 2: Features. Retrieved from https://www.doublerobotics.com/double2.html

Erps, K. (2008). A life saved through new teletrauma service. The University of Arizona Telemedicine Program. Retrieved from http://www.telemedicine.arizona.edu/app/press-releases/A%20Life%20Saved%20through%20New%20Teletrauma%20Service

Federation of State Medical Boards. (2012). *Telemedicine overview: Board-by-board approach*. Retrieved from http://www.fsmb.org/pdf/grpol_telemedicine_licensure.pdf

Fleming, D. A., Edison, K. E., & Pak, H. (2009). Telehealth ethics. *Journal of Telemedicine and eHealth, 15*(8), 797–803. doi: 10.1089/tmj.2009.0035

Gertis, J., Izrael, D., Deitz, D., LeRoy, L., Ricciardi, R., Miller, T., & Basu, J. (2014). *Multiple chronic conditions chart book*. Rockville, MD: Agency for Healthcare Research and Quality U.S. Department of Health and Human Services.

Health Resources and Services Administration. (2012). Telehealth. Retrieved from http://www.hrsa.gov/ruralhealth/about/telehealth/

Hudson, H., & Ferguson, S. (2011). *Telemedicine in Alaska: From ATS-1 to AFHCAN*. Anchorage, AK: The University of Alaska at Anchorage's Institute of Social and Economic Research. Retrieved from http://www.iser.uaa.alaska .edu/Projects/akbroadbandproj/telecomsymposium /HudsonATS1toAFHCAN.pdf

Hutcherson, C., & Williamson, S. (1999). Nursing regulation for the new millenium: The mutual recognition model. *Online Journal of Issues in Nursing, 4*(1). Available: www .nursingworld.org/MainMenuCategories/ANAMarket place/ANAPeriodicals/OJIN/TableofContents/Volume 41999/No1May1999/MutualRecognitionModel.aspx

Iafolla, T. (2015, August 20). 36 Telemedicine statistics you should know. Retrieved from http://blog.evisit .com/36-telemedicine-statistics-know

Institute of Health Care Improvement. (n.d.). Telehealth and the triple aim. Retrieved from http://www.ihi.org /Engage/Initiatives/TripleAim/Pages/default.aspx

Institute of Medicine. (2001). *Crossing the quality chasm: A new health system for the 21st century.* Washington, DC: National Academies Press.

Klonoff, D. C. (2005). Continuous glucose monitoring. *Diabetes Care, 28*(5), 1231–1239. doi: 10.2337//diacare .28.5.1231

Mallisee, M. E., & von Rosenberg, R. H. (1965). Closed circuit television in the rehabilitation of the mentally ill (unpublished manuscript). Retrieved from http:// library.ncrtm.org/pdf/357.015.pdf

Morgan, A. (2012). *Stakeholder perspectives. In the Institute of Medicine, The role of telehealth in an evolving environment* (pp. 115–122). Washington, DC: National Academies Press.

National Council of State Boards of Nursing. (n.d.). Nurse licensure compact. Retrieved from https://www.ncsbn .org/nlc.htm

National Council of State Boards of Nursing. (2014). The National Council of State Boards of Nursing position paper on telehealth nursing practice. Retrieved from https://www.ncsbn.org/3847.htm

Shea, K., & Effken, J. A. (2008). Enhancing patients' trust in the virtual home healthcare nurse. *IN: Computers, Informatics & Nursing, 26*(3), 135–141.

U.S. Department of Health and Human Services. (2013). *Healthy people 2020.* Retrieved from http://www .healthypeople.gov/2020/default.aspx

Veterans Health Administration. (n.d.). VA telehealth services. Retrieved from https://www.telehealth.va.gov/

Wakefield, M. K., Puskin, D. S., & Tipping, K. (2010). *Telehealth licensure report.* U.S. Department of Health and Human Services Human Resources and Services Administration. Retrieved from https://web.archive.org /web/20161221072700/https://www.hrsa.gov/healthit /telehealth/licenserpt10.pdf

Ward, B., Schiller, J., & Goodman, R. (2014). Multiple chronic conditions among US adults: A 2012 update. *Preventing Chronic Disease, 11.* doi: 10.5888/pcd11.130389.

Wicklund, E. (January 6, 2016). Telemedicine offers new benefits for schools. mHealth Intelligence. Retrieved from http://mhealthintelligence.com/news /telemedicine-offers-new-benefits-for-schools

Winters, J. M., & Winters, J. M. P. (2007). Videoconferencing and telehealth technologies can provide a reliable approach to remote assessment and teaching without compromising quality. *Journal of Cardiovascular Nursing, 22*(1), 51–57.

World Health Organization. (2011). *mHealth: New horizons for health through mobile technologies.* Retrieved from http:// www.who.int/goe/publications/goe_mhealth_web.pdf

CHAPTER 14

Mobile Health Applications

Mladen Milosevic, PhD
Louise C. O'Keefe, PhD, CRNP, RN
Emil Jovanov, PhD
Aleksandar Milenkovic, PhD

LEARNING OBJECTIVES

1. Define mobile health (mHealth) and mHealth applications.
2. Describe mHealth systems architecture.
3. Identify the potential of mobile applications in health care.
4. Describe challenges to the adoption of mHealth applications.

KEY TERMS

mHealth	Mobile health monitoring	Wearable sensors
Mobile apps	Smartphones	

▶ Chapter Overview

This chapter discusses mobile health, or **mHealth**—an emerging practice of medicine, public health, and wellness enabled and supported by mobile communication devices such as **smartphones**, smart watches, and tablets. Continual advances and proliferation of

mobile computing and communication devices, wearable health monitors, cellular networks, satellites, and cloud computing services will likely make mHealth a mainstream healthcare service in the future. The mHealth technologies can be used by healthcare providers (HCPs) to improve healthcare delivery and by consumers to improve their own health. The use of mHealth has the potential to reduce healthcare costs and improve quality of life, but challenges with the technology still exist.

▶ Introduction

The National Institutes of Health (NIH) Consensus Group defined mHealth as "the use of mobile wireless communication devices to improve health outcomes, health care services, and health research" (Health Resources and Services Administration [HRSA], n.d.). mHealth holds the promise to radically modernize and change the way healthcare services are deployed and delivered. mHealth applications can enhance diagnosis, help prevent diseases, improve treatments, improve accessibility to health care, and advance health-related research. There is overlap of mHealth with telehealth, but mHealth tends to be more distributed and includes technology used by HCPs with patients and by consumers without the supervision of HCPs.

A typical mHealth system used by HCPs consists of devices used by patients, such as weight scales, glucometers, or **wearable sensors**, that transmit data by wireless technology to a patient's smartphone or other mobile communication device (Rajan, 2012). The communication device uses cellular technology to send data to a designated server, which in turn sends data to the HCP. In this way, patients use devices that allow monitoring of particular health parameters anywhere, called **mobile health monitoring**, and data from patients' medical devices populate HCPs' electronic health records (EHRs). The transactions are transparent to patients and HCPs, but sophisticated networks make mHealth possible (Rajan, 2012).

▶ mHealth Benefits

mHealth represents a new trend in healthcare management and delivery. Improved availability and immediate feedback facilitate a shift in care from reaction to symptoms to promotion of wellness and health. Mobile health monitoring

and integrated information system support provide distinct benefits to each segment of the healthcare system. Benefits for patients include increased access to healthcare information, increased quality of life by focusing on prevention and early detection of disease, better diagnostics, affordability, instantaneous feedback, improved confidence, and promotion and encouragement of healthy lifestyles. Benefits for HCPs include better diagnostics and treatment facilitated by collection and processing of records collected at home and during daily living activities, monitoring of reaction (including adverse) to drugs and treatment, and instantaneous suggestions and advice to patients. Benefits for informal caregivers include remote monitoring and access to real-time and long-term trends of healthcare parameters. This is particularly important in the case of care for chronically ill family members. Researchers will benefit from significantly larger and more relevant databases of patient records. Physiological records collected at home will better represent the state of users and dynamics of daily and monthly changes of relevant physiological parameters. Data mining of large databases will provide assessment of patient-specific responses and treatments and discovery of new approaches.

▶ Driving Forces for mHealth

The anticipated change and emerging new services are well timed to help cope with the imminent crisis in healthcare systems caused by current economic, social, and demographic trends. The overall healthcare expenditures in the United States reached $3.2 trillion, or $9,990 per person, in 2015 (Centers for Medicare & Medicaid Services, 2015); accompanying the expenditures are reduced numbers of uninsured Americans under age 65, from 28.2 million in 2011 to almost 49.9 million Americans in 2011 (DeNavas-Walt, Proctor, & Smith, 2011; Centers for Disease Control and Prevention, 2016). On the other hand, many companies have already been plagued by high and rising costs of health care. With current trends in healthcare costs, it is projected that the total healthcare expenditures will reach $4.5 trillion by 2020, or almost 20% of the gross domestic product (GDP), threatening the well-being of the entire economy (Centers for Medicare & Medicaid Services [CMS], 2010). The Brookings Institute estimates that nearly $200 billion could be saved in healthcare expenditures with the use of mHealth (West, 2012).

Current demographic trends suggest two significant phenomena: an aging population due to increased life expectancy, and the demographic peak of baby boomers in the over-65 age group. Life expectancy has increased from 49 years in 1901 to 77.6 years in 2003, and it is projected to reach 82.6 years by 2040 (National Institute on Aging, 2013). According to the U.S. Census Bureau (2011), the number of elderly over age 65 is expected to double from 39.6 million in 2009 (or 13% of the total population) to nearly 70 million by 2025, when the youngest baby boomers retire, and reach 88.5 million by 2050 (or 20% of the total population). This trend is global, and the worldwide population over age 65 is expected to almost triple from 545 million in 2011 to 1.55 billion in 2050 (National Institute on Aging, 2013). These statistics underscore the need for more scalable and more affordable healthcare solutions.

At the same time, advances in technology are occurring at a rapid pace, and technology is being adopted by millions of people in the United States and across the world. The Pew Internet and American Life Project reported that as of November 2016, 95% of adult Americans own cell phones, and 77% of adult Americans own smartphones (Pew Research Center—Internet & Technology, 2017). The ownership of all mobile technologies in the United States is on the rise, with 77% of Americans using smartphones (see **FIGURE 14-1**). New wearable technology—electrocardiography (ECG) sensors, electroencephalography (EEG) sensors, motion sensors, and many other types—is emerging rapidly (Wearable Technologies, 2013). Electronic sensors, power sources, and wearable materials are integrated in fabric, polymers, and metals, like recently introduced Levi's Commuter Trucker Jacket made in collaboration with Google (Levi's Commuter Jacket, 2017). The market for wearable technology is expected to exceed $6 billion by the year 2016 (Wearable Technologies, 2013). The company, Wearable Technologies, describes a new gadget each month on its website; however, not all technologies are for health and wellness.

The ubiquity of smartwatches has facilitated a new generation of health monitoring applications and improved the robustness of existing applications. New generations of smartwatches feature continuous measurement of physiological parameters, such as heart rate, galvanic skin resistance (GSR), and temperature. Typical applications include physical activity monitoring (Wright, Brown, Collier, & Sandberg, 2017), behavioral

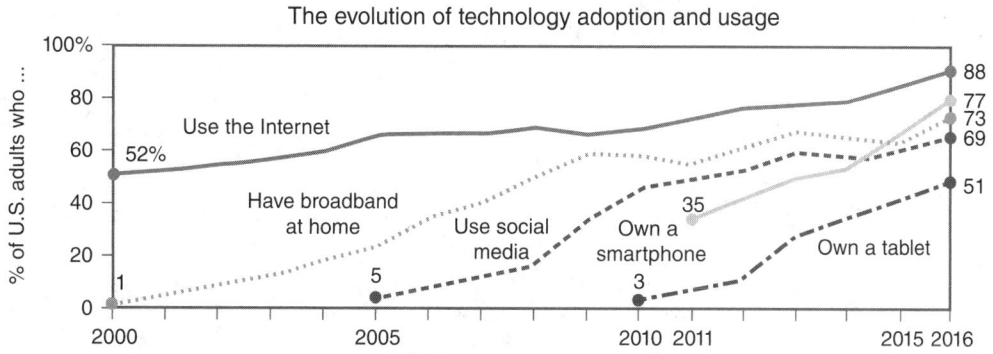

FIGURE 14-1 Record shares of Americans now own smartphones, have home broadband.

Reproduced from Smith, A., & Pew Research Center. (2017). Record shares of Americans now own smartphones, have home broadband. Retrieved from http://www.pewresearch.org/fact-tank/2017/01/12/evolution-of-technology/

monitoring (Amiri et al., 2017), and advanced notifications and reminders. Preliminary analysis demonstrates that the performance of existing smartwatches is sufficient to support longitudinal monitoring of health status and analysis of health and wellness trends (Jovanov, 2015). Integration of smartwatches with other wearable sensors and Internet of Things (IoT) environmental monitoring will enable new generation of applications and provide support for patients, caregivers, and physicians.

▶ mHealth Systems for HCPs and Researchers

Jovanov, Milenkovic, Otto, and De Groen (2005) developed an mHealth system incorporating

a number of components, ranging from personal health monitors worn by patients to medical services running on computer servers accessed over the Internet. **FIGURE 14-2** shows a three-tiered mHealth architecture, which is described in detail in the sections that follow (Jovanov et al., 2005; Milenkovic, Otto, & Jovanov, 2006). Tier 1 consists of one or more wearable monitors (mHealth monitors), Tier 2 includes an mHealth application (mHealth app) running on a personal communication device, and Tier 3 includes mHealth services accessed via the Internet.

Tier 1

A pivotal part of the mHealth system is Tier 1. It includes one or more wearable devices strategically placed on the human body that can

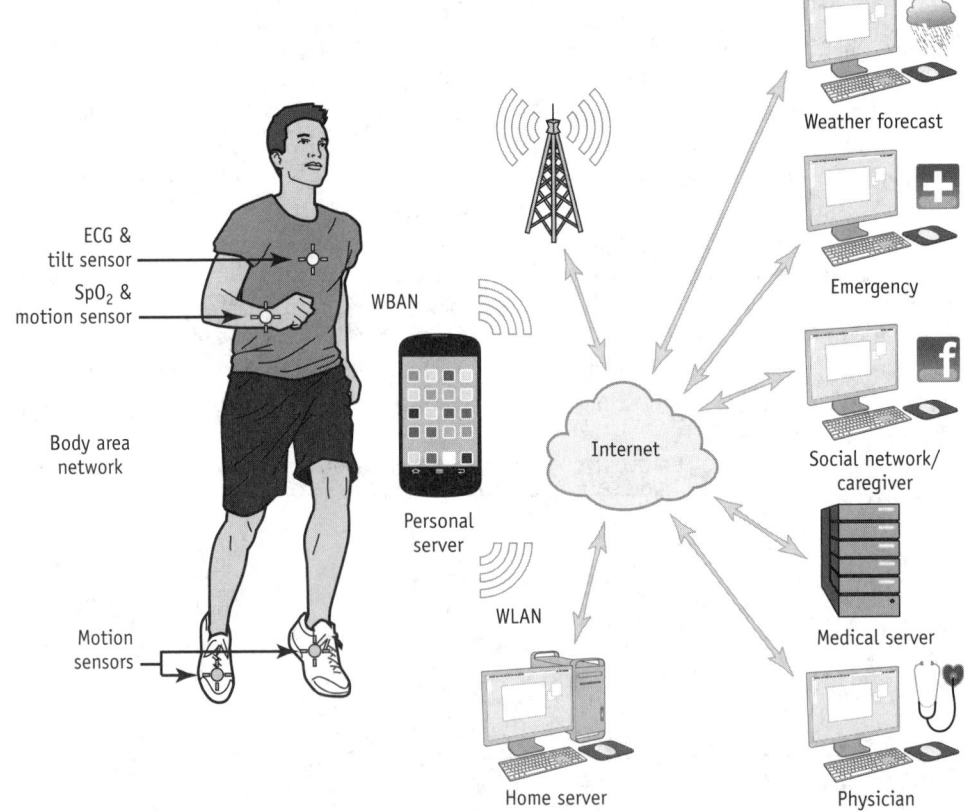

FIGURE 14-2 mHealth architecture.

monitor (a) physiological signals; (b) body posture, type, and level of physical activity; and (c) environmental conditions (Jovanov et al., 2005; Milenkovic et al., 2006). The exact number and type of physiological signals to be measured, processed, and reported depends on the mHealth application. Tier 1 may include any subset of the following physiological sensors:

- ECG sensor for monitoring heart activity
- EEG sensor for monitoring brain electrical activity
- Electromyography (EMG) sensor for monitoring muscle activity
- Photoplethysmography (PPG) sensor for monitoring of pulse and blood oxygen saturation
- Cuff-based pressure sensor for monitoring blood pressure
- Resistive or piezoelectric chest belt sensor for monitoring respiration (breathing rate)
- Galvanic skin response (GSR) sensor for monitoring a subject's autonomous nervous system arousal
- Blood glucose level sensor
- Thermistor for monitoring of body temperature

In addition to the physiological signals, mHealth wearable monitors may include sensors that can help determine user's location, discriminate between user's states (e.g., lying, sitting, walking, or running), or estimate the type and level of the user's physical activity (e.g., low-, moderate-, or high-intensity aerobic activity; Jovanov et al., 2005; Milenkovic et al., 2006). These monitors typically include the following:

- Localization sensor (e.g., global positioning system [GPS])
- Tilt sensor for monitoring of trunk position
- Gyroscope-based sensor for gait-phase detection
- Accelerometer-based motion sensors on extremities and trunk to estimate type and level of the user's activity
- Smart sock or an insole sensor to count steps and/or delineate phases and distribution of forces during individual steps

Environmental conditions may often influence the user's physiological state (e.g., it has been shown that blood pressure may depend on the subject's ambient temperature) or accuracy of the sensors (e.g., background light may influence the readings from PPG sensors). Consequently, mHealth monitors may benefit from integrating the third group of sensors that provide information about environmental conditions, such as humidity, light, ambient temperature, atmospheric pressure, and noise (Jovanov et al., 2005; Milenkovic et al., 2006).

A number of commercial wearable monitors have been introduced recently. **FIGURE 14-3** shows a subset of commercially available wearable monitors used at Tier 1. Other examples include the Zephyr Technologies BioHarness device placed in a chest belt or shirt with a conductive textile that can monitor a user's heart activity, including heart rate, R wave to R wave (RR) intervals, or even ECG signal; breathing rate; and body posture and level of activity by integrating inertial sensors (Zephyr BioHarness BT, n.d.). Several manufacturers introduced headphones with EEG sensors for monitoring brain electrical activity (Emotiv, 2013).

Tier 2

Tier 2 encompasses a mHealth application that runs on a personal device. A typical mHealth app provides interfaces to (a) the mHealth monitors to configure them and retrieve data

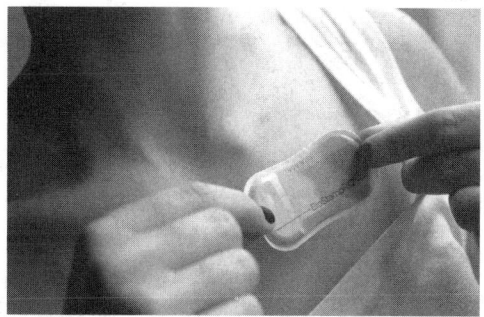

FIGURE 14-3 Example of a commercially available physiological sensor used at Tier 1.
Courtesy of MC10, Inc.

periodically from them; (b) the user to report the status, and provide feedback and guidance; and (c) the medical servers to upload the status information and receive feedback generated at the server (Jovanov et al., 2005; Milenkovic et al., 2006).

The proliferation of smartphones with standardized operating systems (OS) such as Apple's iOS or Google's Android makes smartphones an ideal platform for mHealth applications. A user's health data collected from mHealth monitors can be sent to the medical servers and then integrated into the user's medical record. **FIGURE 14-4** shows examples of several recent smartphones and tablets suitable for running mHealth applications.

Tier 3

Tier 3 includes mHealth servers accessed via the Internet. In addition to the medical server, the last tier may encompass other servers, such as informal caregivers, commercial healthcare services, and even emergency services (Jovanov et al., 2005; Milenkovic et al., 2006). The medical server keeps electronic medical records of registered users and provides various services to the users, medical personnel, and informal caregivers. It is the responsibility of the medical server to authenticate users, accept health-monitoring session uploads, format and insert the session data into corresponding medical records,

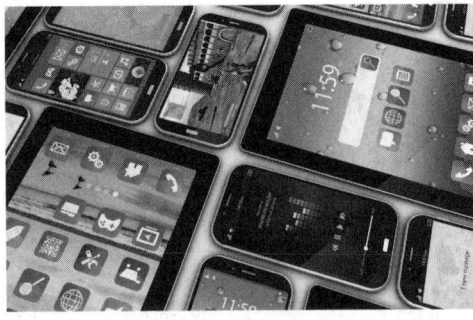

FIGURE 14-4 Examples of commercially available smartphones and tablets.

© Georgejmclittle/Shutterstock

analyze the data patterns, recognize serious health anomalies in order to contact emergency caregivers, and forward new instructions to the users, such as HCP-prescribed exercises (Jovanov et al., 2005; Milenkovic et al., 2006). The patient's HCP can access the data from his or her office via the Internet and examine them to ensure the patient is within expected health metrics (heart rate, blood pressure, activity), ensure that the patient is responding to a given treatment, or that a patient has been performing prescribed exercises. A server agent may inspect the uploaded data and create an alert in the case of a potential medical condition.

The large amount of data collected through these services can also be used for knowledge discovery through data mining. Integration of the collected data into research databases and quantitative analysis of conditions and patterns likely will prove invaluable to researchers trying to link symptoms and diagnoses with historical changes in health status, physiological data, or other parameters (e.g., gender, age, weight). In a similar way, mHealth systems could significantly contribute to monitoring and studying of drug therapy effects (Jovanov et al., 2005; Milenkovic et al., 2006).

An example of successful deployment of a telehealth system, that could also be considered an mHealth system, with a significant impact was recently shown by Banner Health and Philips (Banner Health and Philips eIAC Pilot, 2015). In this pilot program, the authors focused on patients with complex medical situations due to multiple chronic conditions, since these types of patients generate 50% of overall healthcare spending. Patients were part of an eIAC program that combines mobile and monitoring technologies (such as tablet, blood pressure cuff, weight scale), which monitor and educate, with a transformed clinical model that unites care team members and connects it with the patient. The pilot examined 128 patients who had at least one year pre-eIAC and one year post-eIAC follow-up to see the prolonged impact of the eIAC program on patient outcomes. The analysis of patient results over the first full year of the program revealed that the eIAC program helped reduce overall costs of care by 34.5%, reduce hospitalizations by 49.5%, reduce the number of days in hospital by 50%, and reduce the 30-day readmission rate by 75%.

▶ mHealth System in Action: A Case Study of Cardiac Rehabilitation

Peter is recovering from a heart attack. After his release from the hospital, Peter attends supervised cardiac rehabilitation for several weeks. His recovery process goes well, and Peter is to continue a prescribed exercise regimen at home. However, the unsupervised rehabilitation at home does not go well for Peter. He does not follow the exercise regimen as prescribed. He exercises but does not truthfully disclose to the treating HCP the minimal intensity and duration of his exercise. As a result, Peter's recovery is slower than expected, which raises concerns about his health status by his HCP. Is the damage to Peter's heart greater than initially suspected, or is he not adherent to the medical plan? The latter question is not answerable if his HCP has no way to verify his adherence to the exercise program.

An mHealth monitoring system offers a solution for Peter and all persons undergoing cardiac rehabilitation at home. Peter is equipped with an mHealth monitor that captures his heart activity and his physical activity. The time and duration of his normal and exercise activity are recorded, and the level of intensity of the exercise can be determined by calculating an estimate of energy expenditure from the motion sensors. The information is available on Peter's smartphone, which runs an mHealth app for cardiac rehabilitation. This app may also assist Peter in his exercise efforts: It may alert him that he has not initiated or is not reaching his intended goals, or generate warnings in case of excess exercise (e.g., heart rate is above the maximum threshold for a person of his age, weight, and condition).

Through the Internet, his HCP can collect and review all data, verify that Peter is exercising regularly, issue new prescribed exercises, adjust data threshold values, and schedule office visits. Peter's description of his progress continues to be important, but his HCP no longer needs to rely on only subjective descriptions. Instead the HCP has an objective and quantitative data set of his level and duration of exercise. In addition, Peter's parameters of heart rate variability provide a direct measure of his physiological response to the exercise, serving as an in-home stress test. Substituting these remote stress tests and data collection for in-office tests, Peter's HCP reduces the number of office visits. This decreases healthcare costs and makes better use of the HCP's time.

▶ mHealth Applications (Apps) for HCPs

With the recent explosion of the number of smartphone applications and the increase in smartphone performance, a number of **mobile apps** for HCPs have become available. Mobile apps for HCPs are built primarily for Apple iOS and Android OS. The iTunes store contains a large number of apps for HCPs, as does the Google Play store. Currently, there are about 8,000 mHealth apps in the Google Store application, and more than 20,000 in the Apple App store. Both app stores include medical references, patient education, and healthcare workflow management (Dolan, 2012).

Medical References

Medical reference applications help medical professionals and other users find information related to a broad spectrum of medical topics, such as anesthesiology, cardiology, and dermatology. Medical reference applications, such as Netter's Anatomy Atlas (Elsevier, 2012; Skyscape, 2012), Dorland's Illustrated Medical (Mobile Systems, Inc., 2013a, 2013b), Surgical Anatomy (Archibald Industries, 2011), and

BioDigital Human (BioDigital Systems, 2012), provide detailed information and graphical illustrations of the human anatomy. These applications can be used by students in many different health disciplines, HCPs, or other interested individuals. The Epocrates application (Epocrates, 2013) is designed to help HCPs, and it is particularly helpful to nurses as it includes a review of drug prescribing and safety information for thousands of drugs, checking for potentially harmful drug–drug interactions, black box warnings, off-label indications, national and regional healthcare insurance formularies for drug coverage information, and helps identify pills by imprint code and physical characteristics. Epocrates can also perform dozens of commonly used calculations, such as body mass index (BMI) and glomerular filtration rate (GFR). HCPs can access medical news and research information using Epocrates.

Mobile applications can facilitate evidence-based practice (EBP) and allow easy integration of clinical expertise and external scientific evidence with high-quality services delivered to the patient. A widely used EBP app is UpTo-Date (2013). It provides a synthesis of research evidence and recommendations for practice. Isabel (https://www.isabelhealthcare.com) is a diagnosis assistance app that provides HCPs with assistance in double-checking their diagnoses. Isabel has a database of more than 6,000 disease presentations, based on validated studies, which aid the practitioner by building a list of differential diagnoses. Read by QxMD (https://www.qxmd.com) centralizes personalized medical literature, allowing the practitioner to keep abreast of issues in their specialty. The user of Read by QxMD has the ability to search PubMed. Another application that facilitates EBP is the Evidence Based Treatment of Behavioral Symptoms of Dementia application (University of Illinois, 2013), which is used to assist HCPs to assess patients for dementia. Similarly, the BrainAttack application (PHI Consulting, 2012) facilitates determining tissue plasminogen activator (tPA) eligibility for acute stroke victims. Heart Failure Trials by Clinical AppStracts LLC (n.d.) is an app to help HCPs keep track of clinical trials for the treatment of heart failure.

Patient Education

Apps can be used to provide education for patients during interactions with HCPs. For example, the Cardiac Catheterization application (ArchieMD, Inc., 2013) uses visual animations for patient education about heart procedures. The Assist Me with Inhalers application (Saralsoft LLC, 2012) teaches patients how to use their inhalers. Another useful and highly rated patient education tool, drawMD, is available for iPads (drawMD, 2013). Using this app, HCPs in many different specialties can open anatomical images and draw directly on the image to explain procedures or surgery. The images can be saved to EHRs as documentation of patient education. MediBabble (http://medibabble.com) for Android and iOS, translates preset phrases into five different languages to help HCPs obtain an accurate history from non-English-speaking patients.

Healthcare Workflow Management

Healthcare workflow management applications assist HCPs in their everyday activities. HCPs can remotely access patients' historical health records and their current vitals or use them for pharmaceutical calculations. AirStrip Technologies (2010) has developed a hospital workflow management mobile application, AirStrip Patient Monitoring, for real-time and historical access of patients' physiological data. Healthcare workflow management applications can also help patients to communicate with their HCP's office to see their appointment summary, lab results, and other personal health data.

▶ mHealth Apps for Consumers

Consumers like gadgets! The Pew Research Center's Internet & American Life Project reported smartphone users engage in many different activities including checking news and weather forecasts, getting navigation directions, using social media, checking bank balances, getting coupons, and getting health information (Brenner, 2013). Around 40% of adults responding to the Pew survey download apps, and 30% report using smartphones for health and wellness monitoring and management. According to the IMS Institute for Healthcare Informatics, there are now more than 165,000 mobile health applications available for consumers (Constantino, 2015). There has been a 106% increase in the amount of health-related iOS apps since 2013 (Constantino, 2015). Nearly a quarter of consumer apps deal with chronic disease management and the other two-thirds target fitness and wellness (Constantino, 2015).

Most health-related smartphone apps are dedicated to health and wellness monitoring and management. Such applications include monitoring and management of cardio fitness, diet, medication adherence, stress, sleep, mental health, and chronic disease. In order to perform a specific task, the apps need some type of input information. This information can be manually entered by users or it can be automatically sensed by built-in sensors.

Calorie Counter by FatSecret (FatSecret, 2013) and MyPlate (LIVESTRONG.COM, 2011) are examples of applications that help users to keep track of their meals, exercise, and weight. These applications rely on user input as the source of the necessary information. Users can manually enter the name, type, and number of calories for each nutrient, or they can use a built-in barcode scanner through the smartphone's camera. Similarly, Fitness Buddy FREE (Azumio, Inc., 2013) is designed to help with training regimens. The application can help in learning new exercises, keeping track of all workouts, and potentially improving motivation, and enforcing commitment to fitness goals.

Applications that were previously described rely solely on user input as their source of information. Although this approach can be cheaper and easier to use because it does not require additional devices to be purchased and connected to a smartphone, user input often lacks sufficient accuracy, and in some cases is not suitable for use in health care. Tracking of physical activity is one example where manual user input through surveys can be used but may not be accurate because it relies on the user's subjective assessment. A better approach for obtaining accurate data is using sensors, such as those used for tracking physical activity. Accupedo Pedometer (Corusen LLC, 2013) is a smartphone app that uses the smartphone's built-in sensors to assess the number of steps the user makes during his or her daily activities. Other applications such as the Endomondo Sports Tracker (Endomondo Sports Tracker, n.d.) utilize external sensors such as external pedometers and bike speed and cadence sensors to assess a user's physical activity. Furthermore, the Endomondo Sports Tracker supports continuous tracking of cardio fitness using external heart rate monitors. Mobile apps can provide effective medical notifications/reminders, such as the Medisafe Pill Reminder & Medication Tracker (MediSafe, 2017). Mobile applications can also provide support for battling anxiety by sending gentle deep breathing reminders throughout the day (Breathe, 2017).

The effect of consumer mHealth apps on wellness or disease self-management is uncertain, and more research is needed (Anderson & Emmerton, 2016; Vodopivec-Jamsek, de Jongh, Gurol-Urganci, Atun, & Car, 2012). Healthcare systems and professionals are excited at the potential for chronic disease management with the use of mHealth apps. RPM1000, a mobile health application from Tactio Group Health, allows patients to monitor conditions such as obesity, hypertension, congestive heart failure, chronic obstructive pulmonary disease, and diabetes. This app not only monitors the disease condition, but can synch with health trackers to provide coaching and health education unique to the medical condition (Tactio Group Health, 2015). However, studies of particular chronic conditions have shown some promise. Studies of smoking cessation with medications and text messaging to support behavior change and tips for quitting have been shown to be effective (Whittaker et al., 2012). For people seeking weight loss, one study showed that mobile technology that delivered messages enhanced adherence and improved weight loss (Burke et al., 2012). Other studies show that people who use mHealth applications have consistent exercise patterns and improved self-efficacy (West, 2012). **BOX 14-1** provides a case study for consumer use of mHealth apps.

▶ mHealth Challenges

Health-monitoring systems have benefited from the fact that mHealth technologies are driven by consumer markets, particularly cell phone technology and portable communication platforms (e.g., smartphones, laptops, tablets). This is evident by a significant improvement of power efficiency of processors and microcontrollers since the 1990s. This trend will continue as basic technologies continue to mature. However, the full potential of mHealth-based systems can be achieved only if all users are aware of the remaining technological challenges. As wearable monitoring technology progresses from academic prototypes to commercial products, it is important to understand current challenges and interaction of humans with technology. Acceptance of mHealth systems is and will continue to be determined primarily by ease of use and reliability, meaningful feedback to users, price, and privacy and security of data (Bhuyan et al., 2016; Zapata, Fernandez-Aleman, Idri, & Toval, 2015).

Human factors, such as wearability, reliability, and interface design are crucial for any personal technology, particularly if it is to be used by older adults. It is necessary to employ user-centered design and quantify users' satisfaction of wearable health monitoring systems for everyday use (McCurdie et al., 2012). Research and clinical studies are needed to further evaluate new systems

---

BOX 14-1 Case Study

Amanda is a 42-year-old female diagnosed with type 2 diabetes. She feels that it was only a matter of time before she was diagnosed because her mother and sisters all have diabetes. Amanda is 40 pounds overweight and knows that she needs to control her weight to help with better control of her "sugar." A friend of hers suggested using a health app targeted to help those with diabetes. Amanda is skeptical but knows that she has to do something and not "end up on insulin shots." Amanda's friend shows her how to download the free app from the app store on her smartphone. Amanda is excited that the app can track her glucose levels by synching with her glucometer. She can even manually upload the glucose readings if she wishes. The app will display critical state messages if her glucose goes above a certain reading. The app uses the same criteria as the American Diabetes Association for glucose readings. The app can integrate data from her fitness tracker; blood pressure, hemoglobin A1c levels, and weight. This gives Amanda a clear picture of what is going on with her health and she can share this data with her nurse practitioner during her visits. To her surprise, Amanda also receives coaching messages from her app that encourage her to be more active and count the amount of fluid and vegetable intake for the day. Amanda is excited about the feedback she is receiving from her app and feels that this makes her accountable for actions related to her health. After a month of using the app, Amanda has lost 5 pounds and is more active.

Check Your Understanding

1. Does Amanda need to be supervised by an HCP to use mHealth apps?
2. Does Amanda need to be concerned about her health data on the smartphone?
3. Would the U.S. Food and Drug Administration (FDA) be interested in regulating the mHealth apps that Amanda used?

to test the willingness of users to adopt mHealth technologies. Wearability is mostly determined by the size and weight of sensors, ease of mounting and application, and seamless integration of sensors in the system. Size and weight of sensors are mostly determined by the size and weight of batteries selected to support certain sensor functionality for a predefined period of time. Some of the widely accepted technologies, such as WiFi and Bluetooth, do not provide the power efficiency necessary for ambulatory health monitoring systems. Therefore, sensor design must take into account user factors from the beginning of sensor design. New technologies, such as smart textiles, allow for integration of sensors into clothing and commonly used objects, and this will likely improve acceptance of such systems (McCurdie et al., 2012).

Reliability issues span all components in mHealth systems. Individual sensors and their communication networks (short-range communication in the wireless body area networks and/or long-range communication over a cell phone network) must provide continuous, high-quality service. Dropped data due to problems with sensors or communication technology remains an issue. Medical servers will need to have redundancy and backup. Servers will need to handle vast amounts of data generated from mobile health monitoring, and this means servers will need to be managed by network experts. The reliability and validity of feedback to HCPs and patients is particularly important if data analytical techniques are used. The techniques require advanced statistics and computer coding; data scientists who understand physiological data will be required.

Issues related to privacy, integrity, and confidentiality of protected health information were addressed by the Health Insurance Portability and Accountability Act of 1996 (HIPAA) and updated by the Health Information Technology for Economic and Clinical Health (HITECH) Act of 2009. mHealth systems must provide support for privacy and confidentiality on each level of the system. For covered entities (hospitals, medical practices, and other HCPs) and business associates of covered entities,

administrative and technological practices to safeguard protected health information must be planned, implemented, and regularly evaluated. Failure to comply with regulations will result in fines (Rinehart-Thompson, 2013).

The FDA (2013) announced its plans for regulation of a subset of mobile medical devices. According to industry estimates, by 2018, 50% of the more than 3.4 billion smartphone and tablet users will have downloaded mobile health apps (FDA Mobile Medical Applications, n.d.). The FDA regulations for mobile medical applications will

> focus on a subset of mobile apps that either have traditionally been considered medical devices or affect the performance or functionality of a currently regulated medical device. The FDA believes that this subset of mobile apps poses the same or similar potential risk to the public health as currently regulated devices if they fail to function as intended. (FDA, 2013)

In its final report, *Mobile Medical Applications: Guidance for Industry and Food and Drug Administration Staff,* the FDA limited the regulatory reach based on the *intended use* for mobile medical apps. Apps available for use by the general public on iTunes or Google Play are specifically not regulated by the FDA. The definition of a medical device and intended use are provided next.

Products that are built with or consist of computer and/or software components or applications are subject to regulation as devices when they meet the definition of a device in section 201(h) of the FD&C Act. That provision defines a device as "an instrument, apparatus, implement, machine, contrivance, implant, in vitro reagent, or other similar or related article, including any component, part, or accessory," that is " intended for use in the diagnosis of disease or other conditions, or in the cure, mitigation, treatment, or prevention of disease, in man, " or "intended to affect the structure or any function of the body of man or other animals . . ." Thus, software applications that run on a desktop computer, laptop computer, remotely on a website or "cloud," or on a handheld computer may be subject to device regulation if they are intended for use in the diagnosis or the cure, mitigation, treatment, or prevention of disease, or to affect the structure or any function of the body of man. The level of regulatory control necessary to assure safety and effectiveness varies based on the risk the device presents to public health. (FDA, 2013, pp. 7) An increasing number of mHealth apps are FDA approved. **TABLE 14-1** provides several examples of mHealth devices

and apps approved by the FDA. Other relevant mHealth resources and their Internet addresses are located in **TABLE 14-2** and at the companion website to this text.

▶ Summary

The proliferation of mobile computing and communication devices designed to improve health and wellness will continue to influence the care provided by nurses and all HCPs in the future. As the life expectancy and healthcare needs of U.S. citizens increase, the capabilities of mHealth

TABLE 14-1 mHealth Apps Approved by the FDA

mHealth App	Available from
AT&T mHealth DiabetesManager, FDA-approved mobile app designed to coach patients through positive behavior change and decision making.	https://www.corp.att.com/healthcare/wfm/docs/mhealth.pdf
AliveCor is an app and portable device that works as a portable ECG heart monitor.	https://store.alivecor.com/
The iExaminer turns the PanOptic Ophthalmoscope into a mobile digital imaging device allowing you to view and take pictures of the eye.	https://www.welchallyn.com/content/welchallyn/americas/en/products/categories/physical-exam/eye-exam/ophthalmoscopes--wide-view-direct/panoptic_ophthalmoscope.html
MobiUS portable ultrasound uses a specially designed ultrasound wand to allow physicians to view ultrasound images on their smartphones.	http://www.mobisante.com/products/product-overview/
BodyGuardian allows physicians to remotely monitor their patients' vital signs using a wireless monitor.	http://www.preventicesolutions.com/services/body-guardian-heart.html
MedWatcher, created in collaboration with the FDA and Center for Devices and Radiologic Health (CDRH), provides news and alerts for medical devices, drugs, and vaccines.	https:// play.google.com/store/apps/details?id=org.medwatcher&feature=search_result#?t=W251bGwsMSwyLDEsIm9yZy5tZWR3YXR-jaGVyll0.

TABLE 14-2 Internet Resources for mHealth	
Resource	**Website**
U.S. Department of Health and Human Services: Your Mobile Device and Health Information Privacy and Security	http://www.healthit.gov/providers-professionals/your-mobile-device-and-health-information-privacy-and-security
Wearable Technologies: Gadgets of the Month	http://www.wearable-technologies.com/gadgets-of-the-month/
Your Mobile Device and Health Information Privacy and Security: Videos	http://www.healthit.gov/providers-professionals/videos
Mobile Device Privacy and Security: Tips to Protect and Secure Health Information	http://www.healthit.gov/providers-professionals/how-can-you-protect-and-secure-health-information-when-using-mobile-device
U.S. Food and Drug Administration: Draft Guidance for Industry and Food and Drug Administration Staff—Mobile Medical Applications	http://www.fda.gov/downloads/Medical Devices/DeviceRegulationandGuidance/Guidance Documents/UCM263366.pdf

applications to collect physiological data and interface with smartphones and Internet-based medical servers will become critical in monitoring patients' responses and adherence to treatments. In addition, the aggregation of data generated from wearable physiologic sensors and their companion devices will continue to assist researchers and HCPs in answering clinical questions.

References

AirStrip Technologies LLC. (2010). AirStrip—Patient monitoring. Retrieved from https://itunes.apple.com/us/app/airstrip-patient-monitoring/id399665195?mt=8

Amiri, A. M., Peltier, N., Goldberg, C., Sun, Y., Nathan, A., Hiremath, S. V., & Mankodiya, K. (2017). WearSense: Detecting autism stereotypic behaviors through smartwatches. *Healthcare, 5*(1), 11. doi: 10.3390/healthcare5010011

Anderson, K., & Emmerton, L. M. (2016). Contribution of mobile health applications to self-management by consumers: Review of published evidence. *Australian Health Review, 40,* 591–597. doi: 10.107/AH15162

Archibald Industries. (2011). Surgical anatomy—Premium edition. Retrieved from https://itunes.apple.com/us/app/surgical-anatomy-premium-edition/id368728329?mt=8

ArchieMD, Inc. (2013). ICHealth: Cardiac catheterization. Retrieved from https://itunes.apple.com/us/app/archiemd-ichealth-cardiac/id592468810?mt=8

Azumio, Inc. (2013). Fitness buddy free. Retrieved from https://itunes.apple.com/us/app/fitness-buddy-free-300+-exercise/id514780106?mt=8

Banner Health and Philips eIAC Pilot. (2015). Banner Health reduces hospital admissions by nearly 50 percent managing high-cost patients by leveraging Philips' telehealth program. Retrieved from http://http://www.usa.philips.com/a-w/about/news/archive/standard/news/press/2017/20170123-Banner-Health-reduces-hospital-admissions-nearly-50-percent-managing-high-cost-patients-leveraging-Philips-telehealth-program.html

Bhuyan, S. S., Lu, N., Chandak, A., Kim, H., Wyant, D., Bhatt, J., Kedia, S., & Chang, C. F. (2016). Use of mobile health applications for health-seeking behavior among US adults. *Mobile Systems, 40*(153), 1–8. doi: 10.1007/s10916-0492-7

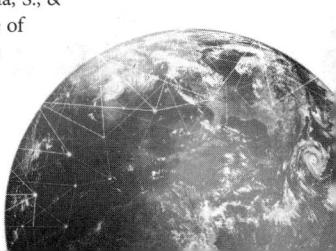

BioDigital Systems. (2012). BioDigital human. Retrieved from https://itunes.apple.com/us/app/bio-digital-human/id581713009?mt=8

Breathe. (2017). Calming reminders for mindful breathing. Retrieved from https://itunes.apple.com/us/app/breathe-calming-reminders-for-mindful-breathing/id976954751?mt=8

Brenner, J. (2013). Internet & American Life Project. *Pew Internet: Mobile*. Retrieved from http://pewinternet.org/Commentary/2012/February/Pew-Internet-Mobile.aspx

Burke, L. E., Styn, M. A., Sereika, S. M., Conroy, M. B., Ye, L., Glanz, K., ... Ewing, L. J. (2012). Using mHealth technology to enhance self-monitoring for weight loss: A randomized trial. *American Journal of Preventive Medicine, 43*(1), 20–26. doi: 10.1016/j.amepre.2012.03.016

Centers for Disease Control and Prevention. National Center for Health Statistics (2016). Health insurance coverage. Retrieved from https://www.cdc.gov/nchs/fastats/health-insurance.htm

Centers for Medicare & Medicaid Services. (2010). *National health expenditure projections 2010–2020*. Retrieved from https://www.cms.gov/Research-Statistics-Data-and-Systems/Statistics-Trends-and-Reports/NationalHealthExpendData/downloads/proj2010.pdf

Centers for Medicare and Medicaid Services. (2015). Historical: National health expenditure data. Retrieved from https://www.cms.gov/Research-Statistics-Data-and-Systems/Statistics-Trends-and-Reports/_NationalHealthExpendData/NationalHealthAccountsHistorical.html

Clinical AppStracts LLC. (n.d.). Heart failure trials. Retrieved from https://play.google.com/store/apps/developer?id=Clinical+AppStracts+LLC&hl=en

Constantino, T. (2015). Patient options expand as mobile healthcare apps address wellness and chronic disease treatment needs. *IMS Institute for Healthcare Informatics*. Retrieved from: http://www.imshealth.com/en/thought-leadership/quintilesims-institute/reports/patient-options-expand-as-mobile-healthcare-apps-address-wellness-and-chronic-disease-treatment-needs

Corusen LLC. (2013). Accupedo pedometer. Retrieved from https://play.google.com/store/apps/details?id=com.corusen.accupedo.te&feature=search_result

DeNavas-Walt, C., Proctor, B., & Smith, J. (2011). *Income, poverty, and health insurance coverage in the United States: 2010*. Retrieved from http://www.census.gov/prod/2011pubs/p60-239.pdf

Dolan, B. (2012). An analysis of consumer health apps for Apple's iPhone 2012. *Mobi Health News*. Retrieved from http://mobihealthnews.com/17925/just-launched-our-2012-consumer-health-apps-report/

drawMD. (2013). Retrieved from http://www.drawmd.com/

Elsevier. (2012). Netter's anatomy atlas. Retrieved from https://itunes.apple.com/us/app/netters-anatomy-atlas/id461841381?mt=8

Emotiv. (2013). EEG features. Retrieved from http://www.emotiv.com/eeg/

Endomondo Sports Tracker. (n.d.). Retrieved from https://play.google.com/store/apps/details?id=com.endomondo.android&hl=en

Epocrates. (2013). Epocrates. Retrieved from https://itunes.apple.com/us/app/epocrates/id281935788?mt=8&ign-mpt=uo%3D6

FatSecret. (2013). Calorie counter by FatSecret. Retrieved from https://itunes.apple.com/us/app/calorie-counter-by-fatsecret/id347184248?mt=8

FDA, Mobile medical applications. (n.d.) Retrieved from https://www.fda.gov/medicaldevices/digitalhealth/mobilemedicalapplications/ucm255978.htm

Health Resources and Services Administration (HRSA). (n.d.). mHealth. *Health Information Technology and Quality Improvement*. Retrieved from http://www.hrsa.gov/healthit/mhealth.html

Jovanov, E. (2015, August). *Preliminary analysis of the use of smartwatches for longitudinal health monitoring*. Paper presented at the 37th Annual International Conference of the IEEE Engineering in Medicine and Biology Society, Milan, Italy.

Jovanov, E., Milenkovic, A., Otto, C., & De Groen, P. C. (2005). A wireless body area network of intelligent motion sensors for computer assisted physical rehabilitation. *Journal of Neuroengineering and Rehabilitation, 2*(1), 6. doi: 10.1186/1743-0003-2-6

Levi's Commuter Jacket. (2017). Retrieved from http://www.levi.com/US/en_US/features/levi-commuter-xgoogle-jacquard/

LIVESTRONG.COM. (2011). MyPlate calorie tracker. Retrieved from https://itunes.apple.com/us/app/calorie-tracker-livestrong.com/id295305241?mt=8

McCurdie, T., Taneva, S., Casselman, M., Yeung, M., McDaniel, C., Ho, W., & Cafazzo, J. (2012). mHealth consumer apps: The case for user-centered design. *Biomedical Instrumentation & Technology*, 49–56.

MediSafe. (2017). Retrieved from https://itunes.apple.com/us/app/medisafe-pill-reminder-medication-tracker/id573916946?mt=8.

Milenkovic, A., Otto, C., & Jovanov, E. (2006). Wireless sensor networks for personal health monitoring: Issues and an implementation. *Computer Communications, 29*(13–14), 2521–2533. doi: 10.1016/j.comcom.2006.02.011

Mobile Systems, Inc. (2013a). Dorland's illustrated medical dictionary. Retrieved from https://play.google.com/store/apps/details?id5com.mobisystems.msdict.embedded.wireless.elsevier.dorlandsillustrated&feature5search_result#?t5W251bGwsMSwxLDEsImNvbS5tb2Jpc3lzd GVtcy5tc2RpY3QuZW1iZWRkZWQud2lyZWxlc3Mu ZWxzZXZpZXIuZG9ybGFuZHNpbGx1c3RyYXRlZCJd

Mobile Systems, Inc. (2013b). Dorland's illustrated medical dictionary (32nd ed.). Retrieved from https://itunes.apple.com/us/app/dorlands-illustrated-medical/id447024921?mt=8

National Institute on Aging. (2013). *Unprecedented global aging examined in new Census Bureau report commissioned by the National Institute on Aging.* Retrieved from http://www.nia.nih.gov/news-room/2009/07/unprecedented-global-aging-examined-new-census-bureau-report-commissioned-national

Pew Research Center—Internet & Technology. (2017). Mobile fact sheet. Retrieved from http://www.pewinternet.org/fact-sheet/mobile/

PHI Consulting. (2012). BrainAttack. Retrieved from https://itunes.apple.com/app/brainattack/id581546430?mt=83D2

Rajan, R. (2012). The promise of wireless: An overview of a device-to-cloud mHealth solution. *Biomedical Instrumentation & Technology,* 26–32.

Rinehart-Thompson, L. A. (2013). *Introduction to health information privacy and security.* Chicago, IL: American Health Information Management Association Press.

Saralsoft LLC. (2012). Assist me with inhalers. Retrieved from https://itunes.apple.com/us/app/assist-me-with-inhalers/id590417707?mt=8

Skyscape. (2012). Netter's atlas: Human anatomy. Retrieved from https://play.google.com/store/apps/details?id=com.skyscape.packagenetteranfivektwokgdata.android.voucher.ui&hl=en

Tactio Health Group (2015). Tactio Health Apps. Retrieved from: https://www.tactiohealth.com/about-us/

University of Illinois. (2013). Evidence based treatment of behavioral symptoms of dementia. Retrieved from https://itunes.apple.com/us/app/evidence-based-treatment-behavioral/id598716627?mt=8

UpToDate. (2013). Product. Retrieved from http://www.uptodate.com/home/product

U.S. Census Bureau. (2011). Newsroom: Profile American facts for features: Older Americans. Retrieved from http://www.census.gov/newsroom/releases/archives/facts_for_features_special_editions/cb11-ff08.html

U.S. Food and Drug Administration. (2013). *Mobile medical applications: Guidance for industry and Food and Drug Administration staff.* Retrieved from http://www.fda.gov/downloads/MedicalDevices/DeviceRegulationandGuidance/GuidanceDocuments/UCM263366.pdf

Vodopivec-Jamsek, V., de Jongh, T., Gurol-Urganci, I., Atun, R., & Car, J. (2012). Mobile phone messaging for preventive health care. *Cochrane Database of Systematic Reviews, 12*(CD007457). doi: 10.1002/14651858.CD007457.pub2

Wearable Technologies. (2013). Wearable technologies. Retrieved from http://www.wearable-technologies.com/

West, D. (2012). How mobile devices are transforming healthcare. *Issues in Technology Innovation, 18,* 1–14.

Whittaker, R., McRobbie, H., Bullen, C., Borland, R., Rodgers, A., & Gu, Y. (2012). Mobile phone-based interventions for smoking cessation. *Cochrane Database of Systematic Reviews, 11*(CD006611). doi: 10.1002/14651858.CD006611.pub3

Wright, S. P., Brown, T., Collier, S. R., & Sandberg, K. (2017). How consumer physical activity monitors could transform human physiology research. *American Journal of Physiology—Regulatory, Integrative and Comparative Physiology.* doi: 10.1152/ajpregu.00349.2016

Zapata, B. C., Fernandez-Aleman, J. L., Idri, A., & Toval, A. (2015). Empirical studies on usability of mHealth apps: A systematic literature review. *Journal of Medical Systems, 39,* 1–19.

Zephyr BioHarness BT. (n.d.). Components. Retrieved from http://www.zephyranywhere.com/products/bioharness-3

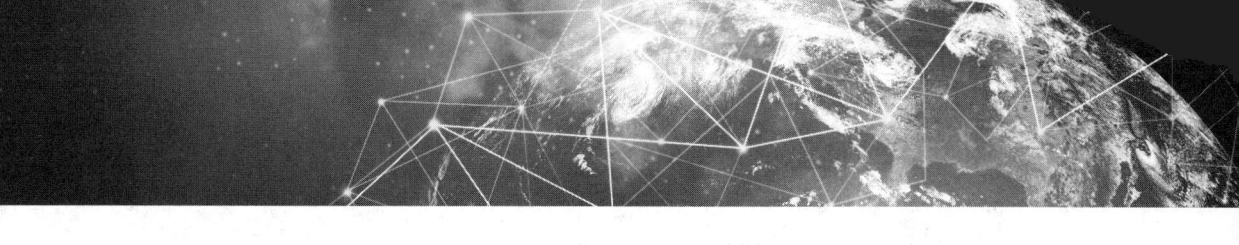

CHAPTER 15

Informatics and Public Health

Pamela V. O'Neal, PhD, RN
Brenda Talley, PhD, RN, NEA-BC
Susan Alexander, DNP, ANP-BC, ADM-BC
Ellise Adams, PhD, CNM

LEARNING OBJECTIVES

1. Review concepts used in the study of public health.
2. Describe methods used to assess the health of populations and communities.
3. Examine informatics tools used in the surveillance and management of acute and chronic diseases.

KEY TERMS

Census Data Mapper
Community
Epidemiology

Population
Public health informatics
Public health nursing

Reference maps
Thematic maps
Vital statistics

▶ Chapter Overview

Innovative applications for health information technology (health IT) continue to emerge, as in the challenging field of public health, where tools can be used in disaster planning, management of outbreaks of communicable disease, and addressing of disparities in health among communities and populations. In this chapter, the reader is introduced to concepts needed to understand the study of public health, such as communities and populations. Tools that are widely used to assess the health of communities and populations are reviewed, along with innovative informatics approaches that can be applied to the study of public health. Finally, future directions in the study of public health informatics are reviewed.

▶ Concepts in Public Health

There are many ways in which communities and populations are examined, and informatics tools are used to assess various aspects of health and disease in both communities and populations. To grasp the potential benefits of the tools, an understanding of concepts that are commonly used in the field of public health is necessary.

A Population

The term **population** has a specific meaning to healthcare professionals in the field of public health. The American Nurses Association (2007, p. 5) defines population as "those living in a specific geographic area or those in a particular group who experience a disproportionate burden of poor health outcomes." Analysis of health data demonstrates that some population subtypes may have a greater propensity toward disease and accidents. Targeted information about the health risks of populations can assist public health professionals in drafting programs to address these risks. For example, *Healthy People* is an ongoing project containing goals and objectives designed to improve the health of U.S. citizens (U.S. Department of Health and Human Services [HHS], 2013) (**TABLE 15-1**). An updated version of *Healthy People* is released every 10 years, and *Healthy People 2020* is the fourth generation of the document. Although the entire *Healthy People 2020* document may be downloaded, it is quite lengthy. Specific topics are easier to access and review online. Searches can be conducted

---

TABLE 15-1 Mission of *Healthy People 2020*

- Identify nationwide health improvement priorities.

- Increase public awareness and understanding of the determinants of health, disease, and disability, and the opportunities for progress.

- Provide measureable objectives and goals that are applicable at the national, state, and local levels.

- Engage multiple sectors to take actions to strengthen and improve practices that are driven by the best available evidence and knowledge.

- Identify critical research, evaluation, and data-collection needs.

Reproduced from U.S. Department of Health and Human Services. Office of Disease Prevention and Health Promotion. (2017). *Healthy People 2020*. Washington, DC. Retrieved from http://healthypeople.gov/2020/about/default.aspx

by topic, which include health conditions or specific populations or by objectives that are contained in the document. *Healthy People 2020* can be used both as a foundation for health and wellness activities and as a guide for measurement of activities by local groups.

The Community

Groups of people may be designated a "**community**" on the basis of many parameters. Each community has its own unique characteristics and dynamics. Those who reside in the community have similarities as they share a common greater environment and experience similar social interactions. Community residents may have shared history, values, and concerns. However, some communities are more homogeneous than others. Understanding the similarities and differences among those who live in a given community is critical in defining and prioritizing the health risks specific to that community, as well as assessing the resources and motivations required to reduce risks. Priorities may differ within the community; the priorities of the community may well differ from those on the "outside" who find themselves engaged in trying to work with the community to improve health outcomes and the well-being (however that is defined!) of the community.

A community may be defined broadly as "a collection of people who interact with one another and whose common interest or characteristics is the basis of unity" (Allender, Rector, & Warner, 2009, p. 6), or slightly more specific as "a group of people who share something in common and interact with one another, who may exhibit commitment with one another and may share a geographic boundary" (Lundy & Janes, 2009, p. 16).

As with communities, tools are available for the systematic assessment of defined populations. Some, such as the Population Health Assessment and Surveillance (PHAS), offer a general framework to gather and analyze information as well as provide guidance to implement and evaluate strategies (Government of Nova Scotia, 2011).

The Vulnerable Populations Assessment Tool for assessing the risk to vulnerable populations especially during special conditions such as evacuation due to extreme weather conditions or disease outbreaks (which can occur in rapid succession) is used by the Florida Department of Health (n.d.) and is accessible online.

Epidemiology

Epidemiology is a field of science that studies health and disease in defined populations or communities. The statistical analysis of data that is collected in epidemiological research studies can assist public health professionals with tasks such as creating and revising public health programs or identifying risk factors for disease (Porta, 2008). Principles of epidemiological research can be used in many ways. Field epidemiologists are often called on to review the outbreaks of epidemics; hospital epidemiologists use similar techniques to identify patterns of disease occurrence, such as nosocomial infections, in hospitals (Porta, 2008). The techniques of epidemiological research can be applied to any community or population of interest, and used to assess relationships between characteristics or behaviors of the community and health. In a sample of 173 nurses employed in North Carolina and West Virginia, Bae (2013) identified a significant association between mandatory overtime and verbal abuse after controlling for other variables such as work setting, workload, and the educational level of the nurse.

Public Health Nursing

Public health nursing is a specialty field in nursing that combines populations, community, health, epidemiology, and informatics. Public health nursing is the "practice of promoting and protecting the health of populations using knowledge from nursing, social, and public health sciences" as defined by the American Public Health Association's Public Health Nursing Section (American Public Health

Association, 2013). Public health nurses are involved in policy development, health promotion, and disease prevention in public and private and local and global health areas. Examples of common population health issues are immunizations, infection prevention, environmental health, and emergency management. Community participatory health promotion and prevention is an evolving strategy used in working with populations (Kulbok, Thatcher, Park, & Meszaros, 2012). Several professional organizations support public health nursing, such as the Association of Community Health Nurse Educators (ACHNE), Association of Public Health Nurses (APHN), American Public Health Association Public Health Nursing Section (APHA and PHN Section), and National Association of School Nurses (NASN). Public health nurses use data to treat, manage, and improve the health of populations.

Public Health Informatics

As public health professionals address issues within their field, knowledge of informatics tools and applications, in addition to training in concepts and practices specific to public health, is necessary for all disciplines within the specialty. In a recent survey of 56 public health workers, Hsu et al. (2012) identified the most important competency as leadership and system thinking skills. Respondents identified the need to integrate health IT tools into the systems-level thinking necessary to construct and execute public health policy decisions. There is a global need for workforce development in the field of **public health informatics**, to train a workforce familiar with concepts inherent in public health, health promotion, health services research, and information and communications technologies (Gebbie, Rosenstock, & Hernandez, 2003). A review of educational programs in the field of public health informatics by Joshi and Perin (2012) identified only 15 programs across 13 institutions, mainly in the United States. None of the programs offered a doctoral degree in public health

informatics, and only seven could be taken in an online format.

Informatics and communications technology tools to support the work of the nurse in public health are widely available, particularly in the field of chronic disease management. However, barriers to the adoption of these technologies have been reported including themes such as capacity building, confidence and trust in the technology, and competence (Courtney-Pratt et al., 2012). Without question, the adoption of tools, even as they are intended to reduce workload, can initially increase it. Strategies to increase ease of adoption, such as consideration of physical office setup, adequate resources, and initial and ongoing training, are needed (Courtney-Pratt et al., 2012). It is important to involve public health nurses in the design of informatics tools that can increase efficiency in daily work activities, but also support them during times of public health crises.

▶ Methods of Describing the Health of Communities and Populations

Similar to the manner in which an individual is assessed, a community or population can be assessed in a manner using selected criteria. Statistics that describe the health of a population or a community cannot be fully understood without demographic information. For example, understanding the impact and significance of 100 cases of a disease may differ if the occurrence is in a city with a population of 1 million, rather than a smaller city with a population of 1,000. Making connections to demographic factors, such as socioeconomic status, age, gender, occupation, geographic location, and other parameters provides context for the interpretation of the effects of a disease or disorder. By utilizing this approach to the analysis of information, a better estimate of the burden of disease, the vulnerabilities, and the disparities in health outcomes for a specific population can be acquired. Several models based in nursing and public health offer a framework for appraisal of communities and populations and are available in an online format.

An example of a resource that local communities can use to improve the health of their members is the Mobilizing for Action through Planning and Partnerships (MAPP) framework. The framework offers both resources and tools to enhance community involvement in decision making, the setting of priorities, the appraisal of needed resources, and community engagement in effecting change. Targeted assessments, such as the Community Themes and Strengths Assessment, Local Public Health Systems Assessment, Forces of Change Assessment, and the Community Health Status Assessment are available in the MAPP Clearinghouse. Specifically, the Community Health Status Assessment is used to analyze "data about health status, quality of life, and risk factors in the community" (National Association of County and City Health Officials, 2013). MAPP also gives annual Model Practices Awards to those partnerships that best demonstrate ways in which health departments and local communities work together to address local health issues.

Facilitating change in a community or a population can be a difficult and overwhelming task. The initial step in facilitating change is often the assessment of readiness to change. Other online tools are available for communities and populations who wish to begin the change process. The Community Health aNd Group Evaluation (CHANGE) tool provides resources for building community teams, gathering and analyzing information, and developing plans to improve a community's health (CHANGE, n.d.). The CHANGE tool can be used by community planners for focused assessments and to target change efforts in five sectors: community-at-large, community institutions/organizations, health care, schools, and work sites. Successful change efforts include the substitution of healthy food items in school vending machines, the establishment of community gardens and farmers' markets in low-income areas to increase access to fresh

fruits and vegetables, and enhancing the ability of pedestrians and bicyclists to use public streets (CHANGE, n.d.).

Populations and communities are multidimensional. Thorough assessment of these entities often includes collection of many different data points, such as personal income, gender, ethnicity, age, and home ownership, requiring the collection of data from discrete members. Historically, data has been collected telephonically, through in-person examinations or interviews, or by mailouts, all of which require entry into a database by someone other than the person who obtained the data point. Health-related data is frequently included in these assessments, typically by self-reports from patients. The proliferation of electronic records has allowed for healthcare facilities to export health-related data to larger, federally maintained databases, removing the step of indirect entry that is required with some surveys.

Assessments with Indirect Entry to Databases

The most inclusive and comprehensive source of demographic data is maintained by the U.S. Department of Commerce in the Census Bureau. According to constitutional law, a census of the population of the United States is conducted every 10 years, and census records date back to 1790. According to U.S. Census 2010 Fast Facts, the largest city in the United States is New York, New York, with a population of 8.1 million, and the U.S. population experienced a 9.7% increase from 2000 figures. Many data visualization tools, including mapping tools and other statistical analysis tools, are available on the Census Bureau website. Census data is collected through a mail canvass of state government offices that are involved with the administration of state-level taxes. If necessary, phone calls, repeat mailings, and emails can be used until a sufficient sample of the population is achieved. Data that are collected are aggregated and are accessible to the public on the Census Bureau website.

Census Bureau Maps

A variety of interactive maps enable the retrieval of census data in graphic form, which can be used for illustration and education. For example, **reference maps** are designed to show geographic locations and features, such as rivers, but do not contain demographic data. **Thematic maps** display socioeconomic, demographic, or business-related data about an area, and may build on reference maps. The **Census Data Mapper** is an application that allows users to create custom maps containing county-level demographic data (**FIGURE 15-1**).

The America's Economy app, designed to deliver updates on 19 key economic indicators, is no longer supported by its agency developers

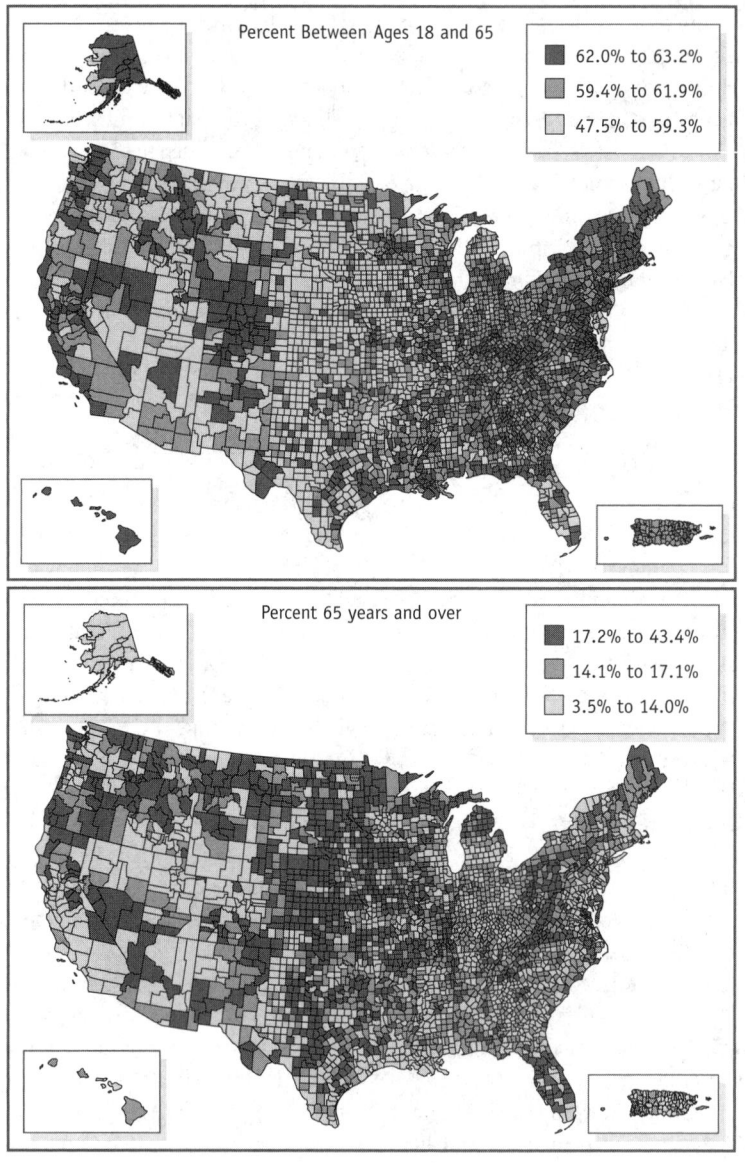

FIGURE 15-1 Percent of U.S. population aged 65 years and older.

Courtesy of U.S. Census Bureau. Available at https://www.census.gov/quickfacts/map/IPE120213/00

from the U.S. Census Bureau, the U.S. Bureau of Labor Statistics, and the Bureau of Economic Analysis. These agencies now offer regular updates on economic indicators using a web-based approach of regularly updated economic indicators (https://www.census.gov/economic-indicators/). Content from the webpage, maintained by the U.S. Census Bureau, is freely available to developers who wish to create their own mobile applications using topics such as employment, manufacturing, and retail sales. Data from sources such as the American Community Survey, also supported by the U.S. Census Bureau, offer detailed information about the American people and our workforce. Data from the Survey can be extracted to address queries such as numbers of U.S. civilians with disabilities (**FIGURE 15-2**).

American Community Survey

The American Community Survey (ACS) is an ongoing statistical survey, used by the U.S. Census Bureau that samples a small percentage of the population every year, to gather information needed by communities to plan investments and services (U.S Department of Commerce, U.S. Census Bureau, 2010). Data from the ACS helps to determine priorities in allocating an additional $400 billion in federal and state funds annually, and data analysis is used to make decisions on topics ranging from school lunch programs to the need for new hospitals. Though the ACS samples a smaller percentage of the population, it contains more questions on topics in addition to demographics, such as family information, employment, veteran status, health insurance, and disabilities. The results are obtained by estimating from fewer individuals than the 10-year census, but the report provides a deeper set of information than the census.

One-, three-, and five-year estimates of data from the ACS can be retrieved from the website using interactive searches based on topics such as age, gender, geography, ethnicity, employment, and housing. Results of the searches can then be displayed visually by using embedded tools for generation of charts and maps. The website also contains a selection of pre-constructed charts that can be edited according to user preference (**TABLE 15-2**).

Federal Surveillance Programs

Data is to be used to inform consumers and health professionals and drive decisions in health care. The Centers for Disease Control and Prevention (CDC) has developed an interactive database system that provides information on many health-related topics.

Various topics include birth defects and developmental disabilities, child and adolescent health, chronic disease, diabetes, environmental health, global health, infectious disease, injury, maternal and child health, occupational safety and health, oral health, population, and vaccination coverage. These databases are continuously updated, easily accessible, and provide information that can be easily applied to a variety of populations. Innovation in health care requires healthcare professionals to be familiar with current data sources, analyze data related to practice, and incorporate the information to change policies, promote healthy behaviors, and prevent disease. Knowing where to find resources and how to use these resources can have a direct impact on patient outcomes. Healthcare professionals need to know the latest information related to health diseases and trends in populations. The CDC provides many resources that are beneficial to healthcare professionals, and the data can lead to advances in healthcare management strategies (**FIGURE 15-3**).

Behavioral Risk Factor Surveillance System

The CDC initiated the Behavioral Risk Factor Surveillance System (BRFSS) in 1984 in an effort to systematically collect data on the health behaviors of Americans. Data collection expanded to all 50 states in 1993. The BRFSS is a phone-based survey tool designed to collect a person's self-reported responses to questions on health behaviors, covering items such as the use of alcohol, tobacco, and seat belts, or history of medical conditions. Responses are then entered

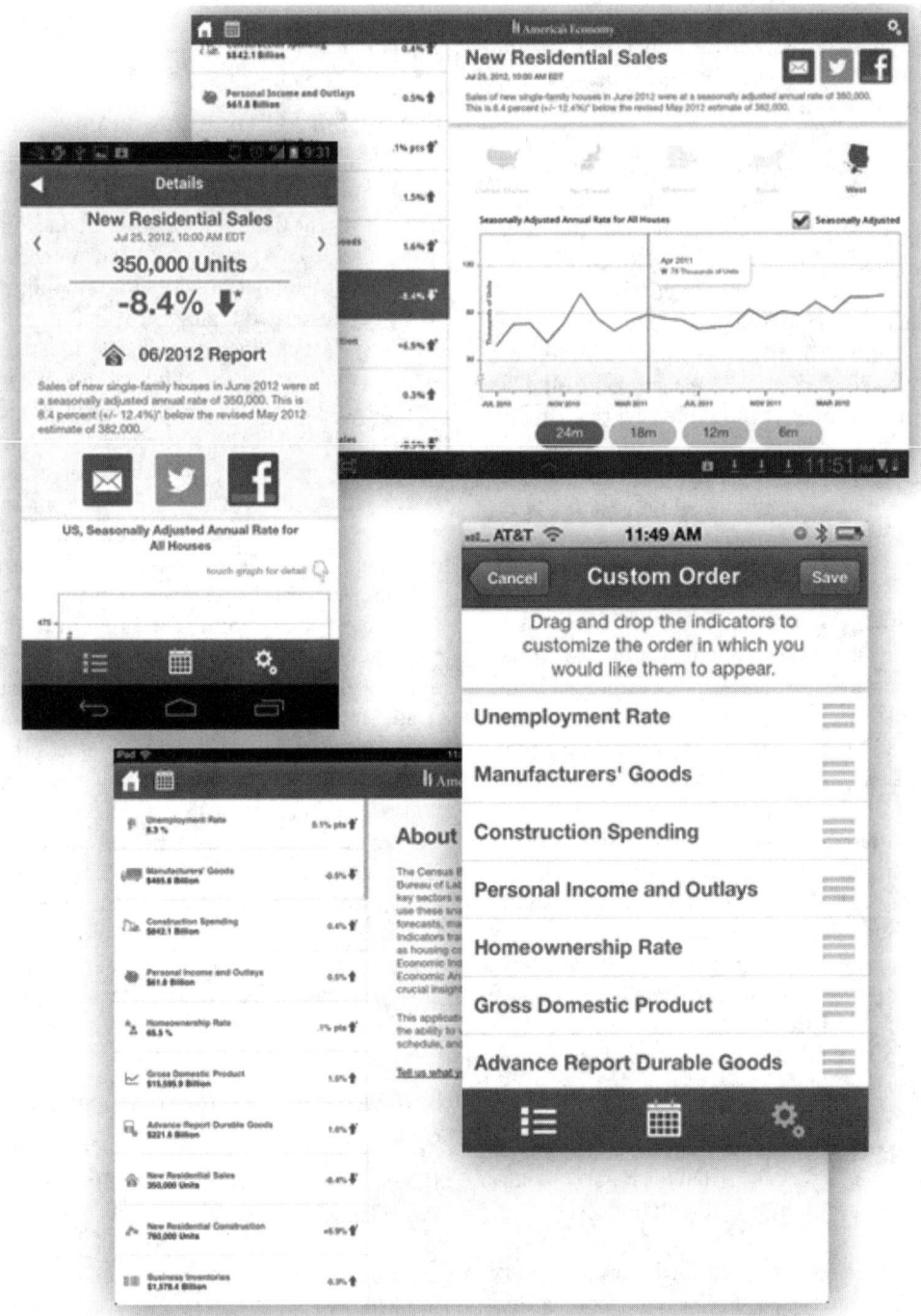

FIGURE 15-2 Screen capture of America's Economy app.

Courtesy of U.S. Census Bureau. Available at http://www.census.gov/mobile/

TABLE 15-2 U.S. Department of Commerce, U.S. Census Bureau: 2009–2011 American Community Survey, 3-Year Estimates

Disability Status of the Civilian Noninstitutionalized Population	Estimate	Margin of Error	Percentages and Total Numbers
Total civilian noninstitutionalized population	304,085,860	± 8,917	304,085,860
With a disability	36,499,048	± 58,831	12.0%
Under 18 years	73,901,825	± 11,968	73,901,825
With a disability	2,942,519	± 16,660	4.0%
18 to 64 years	190,999,705	± 12,599	190,999,705
With a disability	19,141,182	± 44,271	10.0%
65 years and over	39,184,330	± 8,251	39,184,330
With a disability	14,415,347	± 26,918	36.8%

Data from U.S. Department of Commerce, Census Bureau, American Community Survey. (2010). About the American Community Survey. Retrieved from http://www.census.gov/acs/www/about_the_survey/american_community_survey/

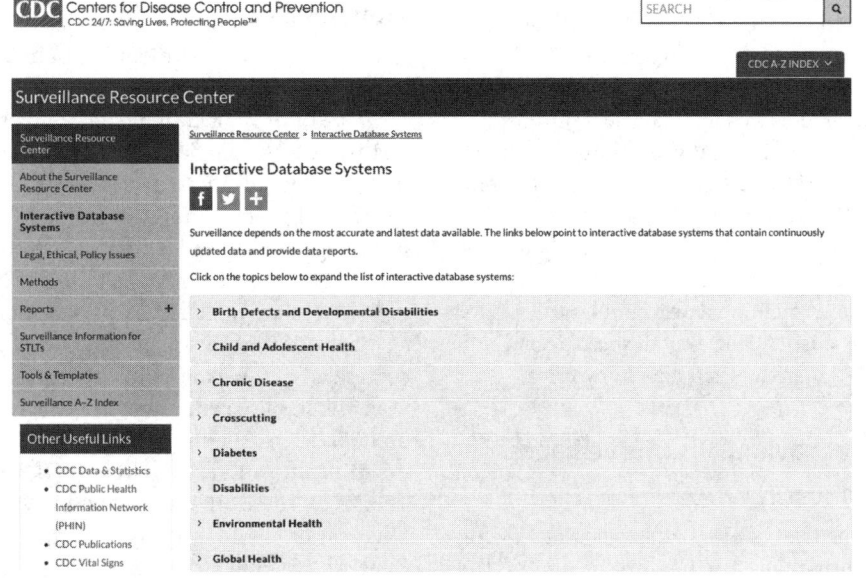

FIGURE 15-3 Screen capture of CDC Surveillance Resource Center.

Courtesy of Centers for Disease Control and Prevention.

in databases, and interested users can query the databases with a simple web-based tool (BRFSS, n.d.). Because survey items remain largely consistent from year to year, users can construct queries to compare responses between states and regions of the country by year of survey.

The BRFSS databases are maintained by the CDC and are available for use by investigators in assessing the health of specific populations and communities and health-related trends. Interested users must apply to the CDC in order to obtain needed datasets. Information is available in data sets that can be queried by state, year, and category.

National Health and Nutrition Examination Survey

Using the National Health and Nutrition Examination Survey (NHANES), information is collected both from physical examinations as well as by interview. NHANES collects and analyzes health and nutritional information on adults and children. NHANES is a major program of the CDC's National Center for Health Statistics (NCHS). Additional information gathered include dental and eye health, information related to diabetes, kidney, heart disease, and osteoarthritis, as well as other topics. NHANES is one of the earliest collections available, beginning in the 1960s. Numerous surveys and physical examinations have created searchable data sets on multiple populations and in many locations. Due to the complexity of the resources available, it is recommended that the brief, easily available tutorials be used before seeking information. Though the NHANES is intended to be representative of all Americans, intentional oversampling allows for reliable statistics. However, the health condition of older Americans is a stated objective.

Youth Behavioral Risk Surveillance System

While the CDC's BRFSS focuses on assessing the health-related behaviors of adults, the Youth Behavioral Risk Surveillance System (YBRSS) collects data on six categories of health-risk behaviors that are leading causes of death and disability in America's youth (YBRSS, n.d.). The YBRSS is administered annually in paper form to selected populations of middle- and high-school students across the United States. Survey items include questions about alcohol, drug, and tobacco use; sexual health; diet and physical activity; and violence and unintentional injuries. The prevalence of medical conditions such as obesity and asthma are also assessed. Much of this information is available in report form, with numerous publications available; responses are entered into databases that can be searched by data points such as sites of participation and survey topics. Searches may be further refined, with the selection of gender, age, race, and grade in school as additional data points. Results from the YBRSS are used by investigators to create projects designed to address high-risk health behaviors in adolescents.

Assessments with Direct Entry into Databases

Vital Statistics

Local and state departments of public health are charged with the responsibility of collecting **vital statistics**, including data points such as births, deaths, marriages, divorces, and fetal death. Although these data may be retrieved electronically from individual departments, it is aggregated by the National Vital Statistics System (NVSS). Users can get direct access to individual state and territory information, such as a copy of a birth or marriage certificate or aggregated national mortality data for a specified year. The site also contains prespecified datasets on items such as multiple births, maternal and infant health, and family growth (**TABLE 15-3**). The NVSS site is maintained by the CDC, the Division of Vital Statistics, and the National Center for Health Statistics.

TABLE 15-3 Programs Related to National Vital Statistics System	
Programs	**Internet Address**
Linked Birth and Infant Death Data	http://www.cdc.gov/nchs/linked.htm
National Survey of Family Growth	http://www.cdc.gov/nchs/nsfg.htm
Match Multiple Birth Data Set	http://www.cdc.gov/nchs/nvss/mmb.htm
National Death Index	http://www.cdc.gov/nchs/ndi.htm
National Maternal and Infant Health Survey	http://www.cdc.gov/nchs/nvss/nmihs.htm
National Mortality Followback Survey	http://www.cdc.gov/nchs/nvss/nmfs.htm
Vital Statistics of the United States	http://www.cdc.gov/nchs/products/vsus.htm
National Vital Statistics Reports	http://www.cdc.gov/nchs/products/nvsr.htm
Other selected reports	http://www.cdc.gov/nchs/products.htm

Data from Centers for Disease Control and Prevention. (2013). National Vital Statistics System. Retrieved from http://www.cdc.gov/nchs/nvss.htm

Though a vast array of data is collected by Departments of Health in each state, its use in research can be limited by difficulties in access. Not every state has the tools necessary to access the data so that it can be used for research purposes. Investigators at the University of Utah have developed an alternative method of querying the Utah Population Health Database (UPDB) (Hurdle et al., 2013). The query tool, called Utah Population Database Limited, rapidly determines the availability of specified cohorts for researchers. Users can select a cohort from UPDB datasets, gain access to limited family or pedigree information, and gather preliminary results that are used to refine a query tool used to generate data for research (Hurdle et al., 2013). To date, the tool has been used to create cohorts used to study conditions including spondyloarthritis, breast cancer, and pregnancy complications co-occurring with cardiovascular disease.

Healthcare Cost and Utilization Project

Many states collect health-related information on hospital admissions, discharges, ambulatory surgeries, and emergency department visits. The Healthcare Cost and Utilization Project (HCUP) is a collection of databases maintained by the Agency for Healthcare Research and Quality (AHRQ). States may choose to participate in submitting deidentified data to the HCUP databases. Databases may then be queried to identify, track, or analyze national trends in healthcare utilization, access, charges, quality, and outcomes (HCUP Databases, 2013). Use of state-level data can yield similar information for a specific state or group of states. Investigators who are interested in using the data for research purposes can submit an application to obtain copies of necessary files, with fees ranging from $20–$800 (HCUP Databases, 2013).

▶ Applying Informatics Tools to Improve Public Health

Public Health Informatics Surveillance and Support

Converting data to information and then to knowledge is challenging when electronic medical records are complex, contain silos of multiple layers of data, and are not easily accessible. Retrieving data can be aided by organizations and informaticians. The Task Force for Global Health, a 502(c)(3) nonprofit organization affiliated with Emory University, developed a program called Public Health Informatics Institute (PHII). This institute promotes informatics in "improving health worldwide by transforming health practitioners' ability to use information effectively" (PHII, 2016). This institute worked with the CDC to develop a framework to electronically report cases of sexually transmitted diseases (**FIGURE 15-4**). Various organizations are available to assist with data access, retrieval, and interpretation. Support from an informatician can be helpful to understand data and improve public health outcomes.

Prevention and Surveillance of Communicable Disease

Some communities experience exceptional conditions that can have an adverse effect on the well-being of citizens. Two of these conditions

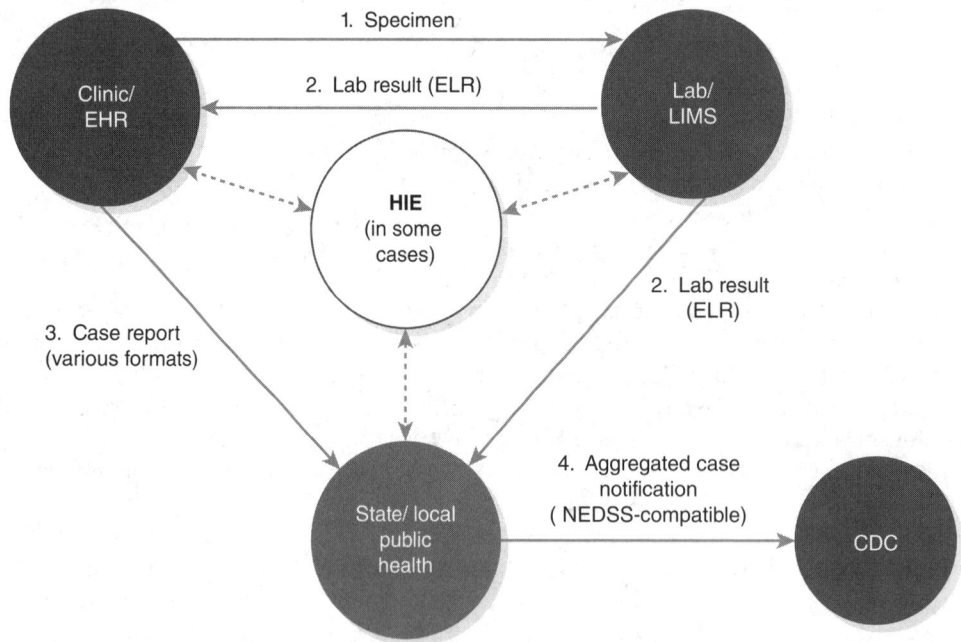

FIGURE 15-4 The context of electronic case reporting.

Reproduced from Public Health Informatics Institute. (2016). Advancing electronic case reporting of sexually transmitted infections: Technical guidance for Public Health Departments, Version 2. Public Health Informatics Institute. Supported by cooperative agreement number U38OT000216-2 from the Centers for Disease Control and Prevention, Division of STD Prevention.

are disasters, both natural and man-made, and occurrences of communicable disease outbreaks. Online resources can be helpful in assessing the state of the community. In addition to examining real-time information, examination of the experiences of other communities in similar experiences may aid a community in preparing or responding to adverse events.

Prevention of Disease Outbreaks

According to the World Health Organization, more than 900 million international journeys are undertaken annually (WHO, 2012). Global travel exposes people to many varieties of health risks. Immunizations for diseases such as yellow fever or typhoid, and empowering patients for self-treatment of conditions such as traveler's diarrhea, are often necessary when people travel to less-developed areas of the world. A surveillance network known as Global TravEpiNet was created by the CDC, in conjunction with Massachusetts General Hospital, in 2009. It consists of member organizations scattered across the United States who contribute data on the demographic characteristics, travel patterns, and pretravel health care of people traveling internationally from the United States. Analyses of the data on traveler population subtypes is ongoing, including pediatrics, immunocompromised individuals, frequent business travelers, those who travel to zones where yellow fever is endemic, and use of vaccines for rabies and Japanese encephalitis (Global TravEpiNet, 2012). In an analysis of data contributed to the Global TravEpiNet database by member sites, LaRocque et al. (2012) found that more than 90% of travelers to areas of West Africa, where malaria is endemic, were prescribed malaria chemoprophylaxis. These results are important, as they may reduce the risk of importing cases of malaria to the United States. Further analysis of data from Global TravEpiNet revealed reasons for missed vaccinations in international travelers, such as patient refusal, time constraints, or lack of vaccine availability (LaRocque et al., 2012). Targeted identification of the causes for missed

vaccinations is the initial step in crafting strategies to improve vaccination rates, and eventual reduction in the risk of communicable diseases.

Surveillance of Communicable Diseases

In the United States, the responsibility for surveillance of disease and wellness lies with the CDC. The CDC is the collector of information, functions as the repository, and prepares the information for consumption on several levels. Originally called the Communicable Disease Center, the CDC was established in 1946 in Atlanta, Georgia, to deal with the serious issue of malaria in the southern United States. Probably the most traditional of the responsibilities expected of the CDC is surveillance of communicable diseases. The surveillance of reportable diseases actually involves many systems that report to the CDC. The CDC has the responsibility of aggregating, compiling, and communicating the information. The list of reportable conditions is revised as new trends emerge (CDC, 2010) **(FIGURE 15-5)**.

Disease-specific data. Also accessible through the CDC data and statistics portal are links to collections of disease-specific resources. The CDC produced numerous collections of data and statistics on health and disease conditions. Especially useful in the assessment of community needs would be information on incidence, prevalence, risk factors, and disparities in outcomes, including differences in racial and ethnic groups. Factors such as cost and level of disability aid in describing the impact of the condition on the community, as well as the individual. Full-text articles relating current information are also available. Information specific and unique to the disease or condition is included with each topic. Relevant webinars and podcasts are included as resources on the site.

CDC Epi Info 7

Epi Info 7 is a resource of software and rapid assessment tools that can be deployed by

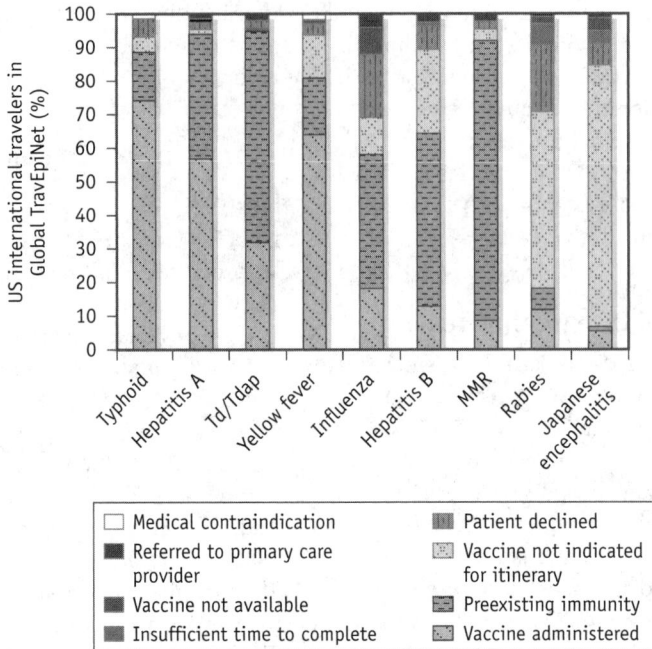

FIGURE 15-5 Selected immunization status and vaccine use among U.S. international travelers in Global TravEpiNet.

Reproduced from LaRocque, R.C., Rao, S.R., Lee, J., Ansdell, V., Yates, J.A., Schwartz, B.S.,...Global TravEpiNet Consortium. (2012). Global TravEpiNet: A national consortium of clinics providing care to international travelers - Analysis of cemographic characteristics, travel destinations, and pretravel healthcare of high-risk US international travelers, 2009-2011. *Clinical Infectious Diseases, 54*(4), 455-462. p. 7 (Figure 2). Reprinted by permission of Oxford University Press.

public health professionals, including nurses, physicians, and field epidemiologists, in areas lacking in technological resources and/or by those who do not have an extensive background in the use of technology. It can be used when there are disease outbreaks or to develop small surveillance systems in rural areas. It is an Internet-based software package, available in the public domain, that can be used to quickly construct questionnaires and databases, perform rapid data entry, and perform analysis with epidemiologic statistics. Analytical visualization, by use of graphs and maps, is also included. At this time, the application is limited to Windows-based operating systems. The website contains a variety of training resources and free downloads.

Management of Chronic Diseases

According to estimates from the National Center for Health Statistics (2013) cardiovascular disease (CVD) is the most common cause of death in the United States, occurring at a rate of 193.6 per 100,000 of the population. Myocardial infarction, commonly called a "heart attack," is one example of an acute manifestation of CVD that can result in sudden death. The insertion of a stent through an occluded coronary artery and the restoration of perfusion to the cardiac muscle may reduce the morbidity and mortality associated with CVD. Once inserted, the stent is left in place, and the risk of reocclusion of the stent is a great concern for both the cardiologist and patient. Efforts to reduce the risk of stent reocclusion led to the development of drug-eluting stents (DES). These types of stents are designed to slowly release drugs that block the proliferation of cells leading to restenosis. When a patient's CVD warrants the use of a stent to restore myocardial circulation, cardiologists can choose between use of the DES or a traditional bare metal stent (BMS).

In 2006, the results of a randomized clinical trial on outcomes for patients who used DES were released, suggesting that patients who received this type of stent were at increased risk for restenosis within the first 6 months post stent deployment, and further recommending that this group of patients use dual antiplatelet therapy for longer periods of time than originally recommended (Pfisterer et al., 2006). This incident is an example of a need for the rapid translation of research findings into practice. Major medical societies in the United States jointly issued a Clinical Alert and Science Advisory to stress the importance of compliance with dual antiplatelet therapy. Staff at the Duke University Heart Center supplemented this education campaign by sending letters to each of their patients who had a history of DES insertion, using records from their in-house registry, instructing the patients to speak with their HCPs about the need for continued dual antiplatelet therapy to prevent restenosis of the stents. Results of their targeted patient campaign revealed increased patient self-reports of clopidogrel (an antiplatelet therapy recommended to be used along with aspirin) at 6 and 12 months following initiation of the campaign (Eisenstein et al., 2012). There was no reported increase in the use of clopidogrel for patients who received BMSs (Eisenstein et al., 2012).

When combined with geospatial data mapping, clinical information mined from EHR systems can offer rich insight into which patients with chronic diseases exist in communities. Califf, Sanderson, and Miranda (2012) combined clinical data from Duke Medical Center with geospatial mapping data on points such as housing, social stressors, neighborhoods, and culture, hoping to gain more detail about the environmental factors that influence the lives and health of patients. A second project, focusing on adults with type 2 diabetes mellitus, extends the dual approach to other counties in North Carolina, Mississippi, and West Virginia. The projects are ongoing, and results are expected to better demonstrate the effects of community-based interventions on patients with chronic diseases. Studies such as these using geospatial mapping are expected to add to the knowledge base about long-term clinical outcomes for patients with chronic diseases, such as diabetes (Califf et al., 2012).

Disaster Planning—National and International

Planning for disasters requires the collaboration of multiple disciplines to achieve preparedness goals. In training exercises, staff can practice using technological devices, such as handheld GPS devices to produce specific coordinates that can be used for search-and-rescue efforts. Outbreaks of disease, that can quickly become global health threats, can occur in any country. In 2005, WHO issued revised International Health Regulations (IHR). The revised IHR addressed the need for strengthening global alerting and response systems, and it required participating countries to "develop and strengthen field systems, tools, methodologies, and capacity for risk assessment, communication and information management, outbreak logistics, and field deployment" (WHO, 2007, p. 24).

In developed countries, such as the United States, computerized disease biosurveillance systems are based on data reported from electronic health records (EHRs) or electronic medical records (EMRs), such as claims data from office or hospital visits, prescription drug sales, or nurse hotline data, and reported to local and regional public health departments (Campbell et al., 2012). In countries without stable Internet access, extensive use of EMR or EHR systems, and other electronic resources, disease surveillance is more difficult, and outbreaks can be more difficult to detect until the disease has become widespread.

Two low-cost biosurveillance systems, designed for use in areas with unreliable access to the Internet and data feeds from electronic records, have been developed by the U.S. Department of Defense, the Veterans Administration, and the Johns Hopkins University Applied Physics Laboratory: the Electronic Surveillance System for Early Notification of Community-based Epidemics (ESSENCE) Desktop Edition (EDE) and an Open source version of ESSENCE (OE). Both of the systems utilize freely available open source software and are low cost. EDE can run on a stand-alone desktop computer, with data entered by personnel or by simple short message service (SMS) text messages via smartphones. OE can be used as a stand-alone system or connected to the Internet, with data being entered directly into the OE server or via the Internet. A pilot study of EDE use began in 2009, in the Philippines, where healthcare personnel used SMS messaging to send daily patient data to a receiver phone connected to a computer at a city health office. Prior to implementation of the SMS messaging system, a 2-week delay between case presentation of diseases and reporting to the city office was common. After implementation of the messaging system and the EDE surveillance, 90% of local health clinics were using SMS messaging to send daily reports of fever to local health offices (Campbell et al., 2012).

Federal Agencies Responsible for Public Health Efforts

U.S. Department of Labor, Occupational Safety and Health Administration (OSHA).
OSHA offers educational programs for emergency workers and community leaders and planners. Modules range from natural disasters, chemical and biological hazards, radiation release, and oil spills, to acts of terrorism. They provide guidelines for communities. In conducting a community assessment, evaluation of the community's disaster plan is a critical component. These resources could be used as a benchmark for local communities in developing disaster planning.

U.S. Department of Homeland Security, Federal Emergency Management Agency (FEMA).
The Federal Emergency Management Agency (FEMA) is probably the best-known resource for community planning. In addition to the vast resources and support for disaster preparedness, FEMA also provides a framework for the establishment of a community's emergency preparation plan. FEMA's *Comprehensive Preparedness Guide* is available online as well as a tool for evaluation.

▶ Future Directions

This chapter contains numerous examples of the many ways data can be used to inform models of public health care and research, along with tools that are both in development and present use. However, the need to further adapt and transform present surveillance systems to more fully meet the needs of public health practice is ongoing and has been identified by the CDC as an important future direction to meet healthcare needs of the 21st century (Savel, Foldy, & CDC, 2012). At present, the most pressing need is the further development of health IT tools in order to link to data that have not traditionally been available to public health professionals, such as data contained in the EHRs of medical practices and hospitals (**FIGURE 15-6**). Regularly sharing these data would improve the timeliness of public health surveillance, but is a source of controversy due to concerns of confidentiality violations and data ownership (Savel & Foldy, 2012). Strategies to improve data sharing include (Savel & Foldy, 2012, p. 32):

- Deidentification of data
- Use of a subset of restricted data that complies with regulations concerning release
- Development of agreements in which data can be released only for public health surveillance purposes

Savel and Foldy (2012) further suggest that the offer of feedback or incentives to the agency who owns the data may also be successful in promoting the sharing of data for public health purposes.

The personally controlled health record (PCHR) has been investigated by other authors

Activities:
ongoing, systematic

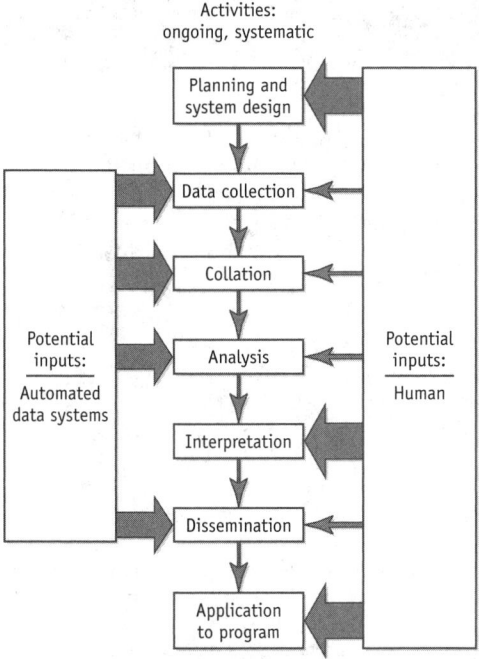

* The size of the arrow indicates the relative human and automated inputs into each activity

FIGURE 15-6 Optimal balance of humans and automated inputs into ongoing systematic public health surveillance system activities.

Data from Savel, T. G., Foldy, S., & Centers for Disease Control and Prevention. (2012). The role of public health informatics in enhancing public health surveillance. *MMWR, 61*(Suppl. 03)., 20–24.

as a mechanism for increasing the sharing of personal health data for public health surveillance efforts. In a PCHR, participants have control over a web-based, digital collection of their personal medical history, including elements such as medical illnesses and medications, age, weight, vital signs, immunization history, and other elements. Participants have the option to decide if they would like data from the PCHR released, and to whom the information would be released. In this model, patients could consent to sharing of their PCHR to a public health agency, without the intervention or consultation of their HCP. Weitzman, Kelemen, Kaci, and Mandl (2012) conducted a web-based survey of 261 users on their willingness to share data maintained in a PCHR, via a hospital patient portal system. In the survey, respondents reported greater willingness to share all categories of health information with a state or local public health authority than with an outside health provider (63.3% v. 54.1%) (Weitzman et al., 2012). The authors suggest that further efforts are needed in order to increase public knowledge of the need to share comprehensive information, to support better understanding of the health of populations and communities.

BOX 15-1　Case Study

Andrea is an area coordinator for a public health office in a southeastern state. As Andrea visits the county health departments in her area, she is confronted with a seeming increase in sexually transmitted infections (STI) in 15- to 19-year-old females. By consulting two resources, Andrea is able to determine whether the state and county statistics for STIs substantiate the clinic findings.

First, Andrea consults the National Center for HIV/AIDS, Viral Hepatitis, STD and TB Prevention Atlas (http://www.cdc.gov/nchhstp/Default.htm) to determine state rates of the STIs (per 100,000). By choosing the parameters of disease, year, race, gender, and age, this tool provides rates for diseases, which can then be compared with other states. Many state health departments provide these same rates by county or region. For example, the Georgia Health Department uses a system called the Online Analytical Statistical Information System (OASIS) to provide information about STIs (https://oasis.state.ga.us/PageDirect.aspx?referer=STD)

Once Andrea frames the scope of the problem, she prepares to address the clinical issue. Using the CHANGE method to address issues of health care, Andrea begins to assemble a team of leaders. Key

(continues)

BOX 15-1 Case Study (*Continued*)

partners, such as the city councils of all affected areas, school boards, providers of health insurance, girls and boys clubs, city sports leagues and YMCAs, and area hospitals and clinics, can combine efforts to make a stronger impact on this issue by developing common objectives. The CHANGE method advocates for a thorough community assessment to reflect the needs, wants, and desires of the people most directly affected by a rising STI rate among teenage girls. After the team is assembled and the community assessment is complete, the key partners can begin to design changes in policy, systems, and environments to address this healthcare need.

Check Your Understanding

1. How would the team assess the impact of their intervention?
2. What tools could be used to assess the impact of the team's efforts?
3. What other public health informatics resources are available to use in describing the at-risk behaviors for young adults?

▶ Summary

Health information and tools are rich in variety, reliability, and quality. This chapter explores selected online, easily accessible resources for information and tools needed to assess communities and populations. Included are data sets, interactive tools, and frameworks useful to communities, though this is not an exhaustive presentation. The volume of resources could be overwhelming; individuals will find that employing an assessment framework will help focus the selection of resources. At the same time, new and updated resources are constantly being made accessible.

References

Allender, I. J., Rector, C., & Warner, K. (2009). *Community health nursing: Promoting and protecting the public's health* (7th ed.). Philadelphia: Lippincott, Williams, and Wilkins.

American Nurses Association. (2007). *Public health nursing: Scope and standards of practice.* Silver Springs, MD: American Nurses Association.

American Public Health Association, Public Health Nursing Section. (2013). *The definition and practice of public health nursing: A statement of the public health nursing section.* Washington, DC: American Public Health Association.

Bae, S. H. (2013). Presence of nurse mandatory overtime regulations and nurse and patient outcomes. *Nursing Economic$, 31*(2), 59–89.

Califf, R. M., Sanderson, I., & Miranda, M. L. (2012). The future of cardiovascular clinical research: Informatics, clinical investigators, and community engagement. *Journal of the American Medical Association, 308*(17), 1747–1748.

Campbell, T. C., Hodanics, C. J., Babin, S. M., Poku, A. M., Wojcik, R. A., Skora, J. F., . . . Lewis, S. H. (2012). Developing open source, self-contained disease surveillance software applications for use in resource-limited settings. *BMC Medical Informatics and Decision Making, 12,* 99. doi: 10.1186/1472-6947-12-99

Centers for Disease Control and Prevention. (n.d.). Adolescent and school health: Youth Risk Behavior Surveillance System. Retrieved from http://www.cdc.gov/healthy youth/yrbs/index.htm

Centers for Disease Control and Prevention. (2010). EpiInfo. Retrieved from http://wwwn.cdc.gov/epiinfo/

Centers for Disease Control and Prevention. (2010). MMWR weekly: Summary of notifiable diseases. Retrieved from http://www.cdc.gov/mmwr/preview/mmwrhtml /mm5953a1.htm

Centers for Disease Control and Prevention. (2013). National Vital Statistics System. Retrieved from http://www.cdc .gov/nchs/nvss.htm

Courtney-Pratt, H., Cummings, E., Turner, P., Cameron-Tucker, H., Wood-Baker, R., Walters, E. H., & Robinson, A. L. (2012). Entering a world of uncertainty: Community nurses' engagement with information and communication technology. *CIN: Computers, Informatics, Nursing, 30*(11), 612–619. doi: 10.1097/NXN .0b013e318266caab

Eisenstein, E. L., Wojdyla, D., Anstrom, K. J., Brennan, J. M., Califf, R. M., Peterson, E. D., & Douglas, P. S. (2012). Evaluating the impact of public health notification: Duke clopidogrel experience. *Circulation: Cardiovascular Quality and Outcomes, 5*(6), 767–774. doi: 10.1161 /CIRCOUTCOMES.111.963330

Florida Department of Health. (n.d.) Vulnerable Populations Assessment Tool. Retrieved from http://www.doh.state. fl.us/demo/BPR/PDFs/VPAssessmentTool.doc

Gebbie, K., Rosenstock, L., & Hernandez, L. M. (Eds.) (2003). *Who will keep the public healthy? Educating public health professionals for the 21st century.* Washington, DC: National Academies Press.

Global TravEpiNet. (2012). Materials, updates, and postings. Retrieved from http://www2.massgeneral.org/id /globaltravepinet/materials/

Government of Nova Scotia. (2011). Population health assessment and surveillance. Retrieved from http:// www.gov.ns.ca/hpp/populationhealth/

HCUP Databases. (2013). Healthcare Cost and Utilization Project (HCUP). Rockville, MD: Agency for Healthcare Research and Quality. Retrieved from http://www .hcup-us.ahrq.gov/databases.jsp

Healthy People 2020. (2013). Healthy people topics and objectives. Retrieved from http://www.healthypeople. gov/2020/topicsobjectives2020/default.aspx

Hsu, C. E., Dunn, K., Juo, H. H., Danko, R., Johnson, D., Mas, F. S., & Sheu, J. J. (2012). Understanding public health informatics competencies for mid-tier public health practitioners: A web-based survey. *Health Informatics Journal, 18*(1), 66–76. doi: 10.1177 /1460458211424000

Hurdle, J. F., Haroldsen, S. C., Hammer, A., Spigle, C., Fraser, A. M., Mineau, G. P., & Courdy, S. J. (2013). Identifying clinical/translational research cohorts: Ascertainment via querying an integrated multi-source database. *Journal of the American Medical Informatics Association, 20*(1), 164–171. doi: 10.1136/amiajnl-2012-001050

Joshi, A., & Perin, D. M. (2012). Gaps in the existing public health informatics training programs: A challenge to the development of a skilled global workforce. *Perspectives in Health Information Management, 9,* 1–13.

Kulbok, P. A., Thatcher, E., Park, E., & Meszaros, P. S. (2012). Evolving public health nursing roles: Focus on community participatory health promotion and prevention. *OJIN: The Online Journal of Issues in Nursing, 17*(2), Manuscript 1. doi: 10.3912/OJIN.Vol17No02Man01

LaRocque, R. C., Rao, S. R., Lee, J., Ansdell, V., Yates, J. A., Schwartz, B. S., . . . Global TravEpiNet. (2012). Global TravEpiNet: A national consortium of clinics providing care to international travelers—Analysis of demographic characteristics, travel destinations, and pretravel healthcare of high-risk US international travelers, 2009–2011. *Clinical Infectious Diseases, 54*(4), 455–462. doi: 10.1093/cid/cir839

Lundy, K. S., & Janes, S. (2009). *Community health nursing: Caring for the public's health* (3rd ed.). Burlington, MA: Jones and Bartlett Learning.

National Association of County and City Health Officials. (2013). The National Connection for Public Health. Mobilizing for Action through Planning and Partnerships (MAPP). Retrieved from http://www.naccho.org /topics/infrastructure/mapp/

National Center for Health Statistics. (2014). *Health, United States, 2013: With special feature on prescription drugs.* Hyattsville, MD.

Pfisterer, M., Brunner-La Rocca, H. P., Buster, P. T., Rickenbacher, P., Hunziker, P., Mueller, C., . . . Basket-Late Investigators. (2006). Late clinical events after clopidogrel discontinuation may limit the benefit of drug-eluting stents. *Journal of the American College of Cardiology, 48*(12), 2584–2591.

Porta, M. (2008). *A dictionary of epidemiology* (5th ed.). New York, NY: Oxford University Press.

Public Health Informatics Institute. (2016). Overview. Retrieved from https://www.phii.org/overview

Savel, T. G., Foldy, S., & CDC. (2012). The role of public health informatics in enhancing public health surveillance. *MMWR Surveill Summ, 61*(Suppl), 20–24.

U.S. Department of Commerce, U.S. Census Bureau. (n.d.). What is the census? Retrieved from http://www.census .gov/2010census/about/

U.S. Department of Commerce, U.S. Census Bureau. (n.d.). Explore the 2010 Census. Retrieved from http://www .census.gov/2010census/about/interactive-form.php

U.S. Department of Commerce, U.S. Census Bureau. (n.d.). Mobile apps. Retrieved from http://www.census.gov /mobile/

U.S. Department of Commerce, U.S. Census Bureau. (n.d.). About the form. Retrieved from http://www.census .gov/2010census/about/interactive-form.php

U.S. Department of Commerce, U.S. Census Bureau. (n.d.) Mobile apps: America's economy. Retrieved from http:// www.census.gov/mobile/

U.S. Department of Commerce, U.S. Census Bureau, American Community Survey. (2010). About the American Community Survey. Retrieved from http://www.census.gov/acs /www/about_the_survey/american_community_survey/

U.S. Department of Health and Human Services. (2013, July 13). About Healthy People. Retrieved from http:// healthypeople.gov/2020/about/default.aspx

U.S. Department of Health and Human Services. Centers for Disease Control and Prevention. (n.d.). Community Health Assessment aNd Group Evaluation (CHANGE) action guide: Building a foundation of knowledge to prioritize community needs. Retrieved from http:// www.cdc.gov/healthycommunitiesprogram/tools /change.htm

U.S. Department of Health and Human Services. Centers for Disease Control and Prevention. Office of Surveillance,

Epidemiology, and Laboratory Services. (n.d.). BRFSS: Prevalence and trends data. Retrieved from http://apps.nccd.cdc.gov/brfss/

U.S. Department of Labor, Occupational Health and Safety Administration. (n.d.). Emergency preparedness and response. Retrieved from http://www.osha.gov/SLTC/emergencypreparedness/index.html

Weitzman, E. R., Kelemen, S., Kaci, L., & Mandl, K. D. (2012). Willingness to share personal health record data for care improvement and public health: A survey of experienced personal health record users. *BMC Medical Informatics and Decision Making, 12*, 39. doi: 10.1186/1472-6947-12-39

World Health Organization. (2007). *International health regulations (2005). Areas of work for implementation.* Retrieved from http://www.who.int/ihr/finalversion9Nov07.pdf

World Health Organization. (2012). International travel and health. Retrieved from http://www.who.int/ith/en/

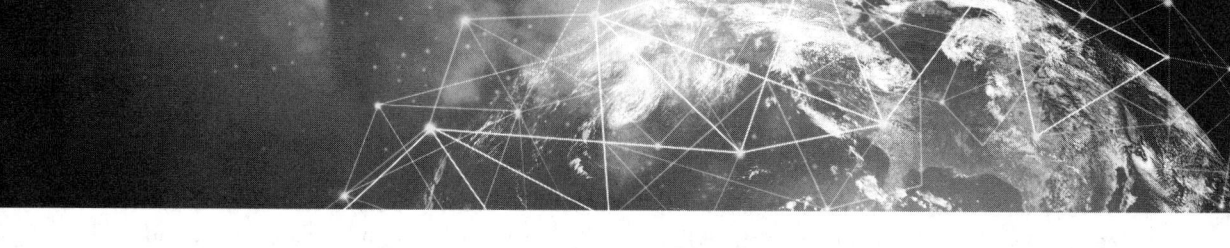

CHAPTER 16

Digital Patient Engagement and Empowerment

Heather Carter-Templeton, PhD, RN-BC
Xiaohua Sarah Wu, MSN, RN, FNP-BC
Ellise D. Adams, PhD, RN, CNM

LEARNING OBJECTIVES

1. Understand patient engagement and empowerment and the role of digital tools and the Internet.
2. Explore current perspectives on digital patient engagement and empowerment.
3. Discuss the challenges and issues related to the use of the Internet in patient engagement and empowerment.
4. Describe the revolutionary digital changes in healthcare delivery systems.
5. Recognize future trends in patient engagement and empowerment in the digital era.

KEY TERMS

Digital divide
Health literacy
Internet

Patient empowerment
Patient engagement
Personal health record (PHR)

Shared decision making
Social media
Telehealth

▶ Chapter Overview

This chapter reviews the healthcare information technology revolution and the innovations that influence interactions between healthcare providers (HCPs) and patients. Its specific focus is on the ways in which patients engage and are empowered by the use of information technology. Tools used to facilitate patient engagement, such as the Internet, social media, and personal health records, are discussed in this chapter. While advancements in technology promise an endless number of possibilities for accessing healthcare information, there are challenges that should not be overlooked. Recognizing and addressing challenges can make these technologies more useful in providing patient-centered health care and improving patient engagement and empowerment (**FIGURE 16-1**).

▶ Introduction

The onset of the information age has led to revolutionary changes in the delivery of health care. The capacities of the information age and the needs of patients have led HCPs to alter traditional methods of patient engagement and develop new methods of assisting with patient

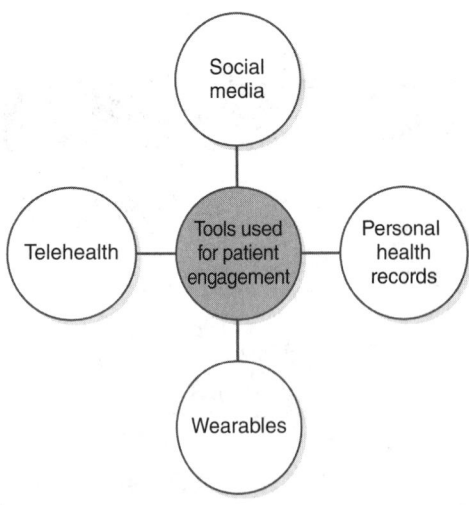

FIGURE 16-1 Patient engagement tools.

engagement, promotion, and empowerment. As public health promotion becomes an increasingly significant priority, methods that lead to improved collaboration between patients and HCPs will continue to be an important trend in the evolution of health care.

▶ Engagement and Empowerment

Patient engagement is a set of reciprocal tasks performed by patients and HCPs in a collaborative effort to promote and support active patient involvement in their own health care (Coulter, 2011). Essentially, patient engagement refers to patients and HCPs working together to improve patient care and patients' health. Historically, patient engagement included the use of educational materials such as brochures or pamphlets along with face-to-face encounters. With advancements in technology, patient engagement can also occur through the use of social media, secured messaging systems, online communities, wearable technology, and mobile devices, augmenting the face-to-face encounters. Tools used to engage patients are further explained in this chapter.

Patient engagement can occur at any point along the healthcare continuum. When more than one viable treatment or screening option exists, patient engagement can raise the patient's awareness and understanding of treatment options and possible outcomes. Many want to be engaged in their care and health-related decisions, and may experience better outcomes when this happens.

Patient empowerment is the practice of maximizing the number of opportunities made available to patients to endow them with a better sense of control over their own health care, which can only lead to well-informed decisions and an improved collaborative dynamic with HCPs (Coulter, Safran, & Wasson, 2012). Empowerment encourages patients to share their preferences and values with HCPs to form plans of care that are based on the best available evidence and that also reflect patients' best interests. For example, the anterior cruciate ligament (ACL) is a commonly injured ligament of the knee. With the same severity of injury, the treatment plans for ACL injury can vary from altered activity level with conservative management to surgical intervention to repair or even replace the injured ligament. The different approaches for treatment are dependent on a patient's goal of activity level. An 18-year-old football player who wants to play ball in college may choose to have his torn ACL reconstructed surgically, but a 30-year-old working mother may opt for an alteration of her level of activity rather than having surgery. Allowing patients to make these types of decisions about their care is one of the primary means of empowering patients with regard to their own health care.

The integration of the Internet into day-to-day life and the access to vast amounts of healthcare information has transformed patients into more active healthcare consumers, particularly in terms of how they seek and accept medical advice. The Internet has afforded opportunities to bridge the information gap between patients and providers. Many patients have begun to transition from being passive recipients of the healthcare plans or decisions made by their HCP to being more actively engaged in the decisions surrounding their own health care (White & Herzlinger, 2004). Today's patients can acquire access to their personal health data and then join appropriate groups, using avenues such as social media, to share experiences and coping mechanisms. It is common to see patients arrive for a visit with a stack of printouts from online resources already in hand, as well as a list of questions on which they wish to consult with their HCPs.

When the visit with the HCP becomes more collaborative, it is the perfect time to encourage patients to engage in decisions about their health. **Shared decision making** is most effective whenever patients are fully aware of the risks, benefits, and their own preferences (or values). HCPs can use technology and digital tools to integrate patients' values with scientific evidence in an effort to provide treatment alternatives that are amenable with the patients' goals. However, HCPs must always be sure to impress upon patients the objective risks and benefits of each alternative (Eysenbach, 2000). When patients make more responsible choices, they will in turn experience positive results, which help to further reinforce those healthy choices (Juengst, Flatt, & Settersten, 2012). Shared decision making is becoming more and more valuable in management of chronic diseases, such as diabetes. A patient's increased involvement in decision making about his or her own health management, which may include lifestyle changes, diet modification, medication regimens, and regularly scheduled appointments with the HCP, may maximize the likelihood of the patient's compliance with the plan of care (Muhlbacher, Stoll, Mahlich, & Nubling, 2013). Furthermore, contemporary health care tries to focus on the value or efficacy of decisions from the perspective of the patients, another way to encourage patient engagement and self-care. Patients are truly empowered by efforts that help them engage in the planning of their care, as well as by tools that help improve their ability to understand, cope, and manage health in their lives (Mittler, Martsolf, Telenko, & Scanlon, 2013). In order to have patient engagement, empowerment, and shared decision making, patients must be able to understand information about their own health. The term **health literacy** is used to describe "the degree to which individuals can obtain, process, and understand the basic health information and services they need to make appropriate health decisions" (Institute of Medicine [IOM], 2004, p. 1). Just as one's level of education plays a role in health literacy, many other skills, such as communicating, having adequate background information, and advocating for one's self, are also critical components of health literacy. In the United States, 36% of adults have low levels of health literacy, meaning they have difficulty in locating, comprehending, and applying health information (Sheridan et al., 2011).

Health literacy, which includes numeracy skills and knowledge of health topics, is dependent on individual and environmental elements. The following may influence a person's health literacy levels: communication skills of the patient and healthcare provider, knowledge of health matter of patient and healthcare provider, culture, healthcare system burden, pressures/concerns of the situation. One's health literacy level may have an effect on a person's ability to navigate the healthcare system, share personal health information, engage in care management, and understand probability and risk associated with their conditions (U.S. Department of Health and Human Services [HHS], n.d.).

In the digital era, patients with low levels of health literacy may be at a serious disadvantage. Without the ability to interpret health-related information, the increased use of information technology in health care means little to these patients. A patient who is without health literacy skills can make few or no well-informed decisions, which directly impairs patient empowerment. In 2010, the HHS released a national action plan to improve health literacy in which it hopes to bridge the chasm of knowledge between what professionals know and what patients know. The plan includes (1) simplifying and standardizing the health information available to patients; (2) providing clinicians with formal training in communicating with lower level literacy patients; (3) expanding community services in terms of providing culturally and linguistically appropriate health information; and (4) increasing the use of evidence-based health literacy research, practices, and interventions (HHS, 2010). These efforts to improve communication between HCPs and low health-literacy patients can greatly foster patient engagement and empowerment.

Communication about health and health literacy are related. The Office of Disease Prevention and Health Promotion (n.d.) defines health communication as referring to "human and digital interactions that occur during the process of improving health and health care." Public health requires effective health communication among patients and providers.

Healthcare Information Revolution

There is little doubt that the Internet has taken over the global communication landscape. The revolutionary impact of the Internet, sometimes called the "third industrial revolution," has changed the way HCPs share data and communicate (Rifkin, 2011). The use of personal computers, laptops, and mobile Internet devices, such as smartphones and tablets, has dramatically changed the means by which patients seek access to healthcare information. Widespread use of the Internet has led developers of healthcare information systems to shift their focus toward developing products for patients (Eysenbach, 2000). In the late 1990s, Eysenbach (2000) foresaw an "information age healthcare system" in which patients would use technology to gain access to information and assume more responsibility for their own health care (p. 1715). It is believed that patient empowerment will result in more efficient use of healthcare resources, with an emphasis on preventive care (Eysenbach, 2000). Legislation designed to promote the implementation of patient-centered healthcare information technologies, such as the Health Information Technology for Economic and Clinical Health (HITECH) Act of 2009, ensures that healthcare delivery systems will continue to address patients' needs, values, and preferences (Eysenbach, 2000).

Internet

The **Internet** has "world-wide broadcasting capability, a mechanism for information dissemination, and a medium for collaboration and interaction between individuals and their computers without regard for geographic location" (Leiner et al., 1997). The Internet is proving to be a major source of health information for patients (Moretti, de Oliveira, & Koga da Silva, 2012). In 2010, a survey showed that three-quarters of adults in the United States use the Internet, and 59% of all adults have looked online for healthcare information, such as specific disease information or treatment options (Fox, 2011). The range of available healthcare information has expanded through the use of Internet-based tools such as email, websites, search tools, discussion forums, blogs, and videos, with websites being the tool that people choose to browse most frequently (Pew Internet & American Life Project, 2013).

There are two general categories of healthcare-related websites: government-sponsored and nongovernmental, which can be either commercial or nonprofit. HCPs should understand the need for a thorough evaluation of healthcare information that is present on the Internet. In general, websites sponsored by schools of medicine, nursing, or allied health professions, medical centers, or the U.S. government are more likely to provide accurate and thorough information. Trustworthy websites are available for consumers to seek health information (**TABLE 16-1**).

Websites that seek to provide healthcare information should also be evaluated in terms of effectiveness from the perspective of the patient. Research suggests that the effectiveness can be assessed in four dimensions: accessibility, content, marketing, and technology (**TABLE 16-2**; Ford, Huerta, Schilhavy, & Menachemi, 2012).

Today, websites often represent the initial point of contact that patients establish with healthcare organizations such as hospitals, government agencies, and insurance companies

TABLE 16-1 Trustworthy Websites for Consumer Health Information

Title of Agency or Organization	Website
American Association of Retired Persons	http://www.aarp.org/health/
Agency for Healthcare Research and Quality	http://www.ahrq.gov/patients-consumers/
Centers for Medicare & Medicaid Services	http://www.cms.gov
Leapfrog Group	http://www.leapfroggroup.org
Mayo Clinic	http://www.mayoclinic.com
Medline Plus	http://www.medlineplus.gov
National Institute on Aging	http://www.nia.nih.gov
NIH Senior Health.gov	http://www.nihseniorhealth.gov
PubMed	http://www.ncbi.nlm.nih.gov/pubmed
U.S. Centers for Medicare & Medicaid Services	http://www.healthcare.gov/
U.S. Department of Health and Human Services	http://www.hhs.gov/ocr/privacy/hipaa/understanding/consumers/
U.S. Department of Labor	http://www.dol.gov/ebsa/consumer_info_health.html

TABLE 16-2 Website Effectiveness Assessment

Website Assessment Dimension	Definition	Utilization	Contributory Elements
Accessibility	A website's ease of use for healthcare patients with lower computer literacy levels	To reach as many users (patients) as possible	1. Spiderability: To ensure interoperability with search engines. This enables patients to easily find the healthcare information they need without navigating a complex site hierarchy. 2. Flash reliance: To avoid features relying on Flash that systematically limit some users' access levels, especially for Apple mobile products users. 3. Use of link states: To help patients move across the site with effective visual cues, such as use of color, to identify potential new links. 4. Use of alternative text: To convert images to text-only healthcare information that enables sight-impaired patients to navigate web pages through screen readers.
Content	A website's overall content quality without taking into consideration the technical limitations of the site	Promote and maintain effective consumer engagement	1. Quality: Well-chosen titles and descriptions can encourage consumer engagement. Ensure grammatically correct text and the right number of words on the web page. 2. Freshness: Up-to-date content is a positive indicator to patients that the organization is engaged in state-of-the-art activities. 3. Readability and visual interests: Healthcare web pages should use words and grammar consistent with 8th- to 11th-grade reading levels. Striving to increase the interest of websites leads to consumer engagement.
Marketing	How readily and reliably information is accessed using search engines	Become more accessible to search engines to increase a website's popularity	1. The amount of content: Content within a page becomes more accessible to search engines, which results in more consumer visits. 2. Popularity: More site traffic indicates higher popularity.
Technology	How well a website is designed, built, and maintained	Provide user-friendly website	1. Website download speed: The ideal loading time for a web page is 0.5 second or less. 2. Site structure and code quality: To build and maintain a well-performing website. 3. Content organization: Adding healthcare education video and graphics as web page content is a trend in healthcare consumer empowerment.

Reproduced from Ford, E.W., Huerta, T.R., Schilhavy, R.A., & Menachemi, N. (2012). Effective US health system websites: Establishing benchmarks and standards for effective consumer engagement. *Journal of Healthcare Management, 57*(1), 47–64.

(Ford et al., 2012). Websites that are designed to engage and empower patients send a clear message that patients' interests and needs are now the focus of the healthcare system.

Quality Control of Information Available to Patients

The rapid growth of health-related information available on the Internet could be overwhelming to patients. Research suggests that less than one-third of Internet users who follow medical advice or seek health information online describe the data as helpful (Fox, 2011). Approximately 3% of adults say they or others they know have been harmed in some way by online healthcare-related information (Fox, 2011). Finding useful and valid information on the Internet can be challenging and time consuming for patients, because it is difficult to filter out applicable and credible information from other less trustworthy information (Jadad, 1999).

One strategy to help patients judge the quality of a website's information is website certification (Moretti et al., 2012). Five "Cs" can be used to assess the quality of information on any website containing health-related information—credibility, currency, content, construction, and clarity (Roberts, 2010). The 5C evaluation tool, as described by Roberts, contains numerous questions in the five categories to guide an extensive assessment of any website.

When patients come to HCPs with health-related information obtained from online sources, they should be advised that although the Internet offers many tools to promote healthcare information exchange, the quality of the information is not standardized. Patients should be directed only to websites that have been thoroughly evaluated and deemed trustworthy by HCPs (Table 16-1). Direct instructions from a patient's HCP remain the most reliable information in forming a healthcare plan.

As wireless technologies grow and electronic medical information expands, mobile medical and health applications (apps) continue to impact the cyber infrastructure of health care (Abernethy, Wheeler, & Bull, 2011). As of May 2012, there were 10,000 apps available in the "medical section" of Apple's "App Store" and more than 3,000 on the Google Play store (Buijink, Visser, & Marshall, 2013). Although there is a promising future in apps for public health, challenges remain. Wireless medical device and software regulations to ensure the quality of health apps are set by different governmental agencies, such as the Federal Communications Commission (FCC) and the U.S. Food and Drug Administration (FDA).

▶ Tools Used to Facilitate Patient Engagement

Social Media

Social media is increasingly becoming the mechanism that patients use to seek and share healthcare information (Pho, 2013). **Social media** is defined as "the use of web-based and mobile technologies to turn communication into interactive dialogues" (Bradley, 2011). In an online environment, social media creates a powerful platform for the mass collaboration of people, who may or may not have had preexisting connections to exchange user-generated content (Kaplan & Haenlein, 2010). While social media is similar to television, radio, and newspaper in that it is a format that delivers a message, it is unique in its capability to create a platform for two-way communication, a dynamic known as "social networking" (French, 2010).

The most popular social media tools may be those that allow us to make and maintain social connections with others. These programs offer user-friendly ways to keep up with family and/or friends. Many relationships have been strengthened or maintained as a result, and some simply may not have ever been able to advance without these platforms. These sites and tools are truly social.

Social media are free, web-based platforms that facilitate interaction and networking among their communities. Social media offers a form of communication that allows users to create diverse content for the purposes of sharing with others via online environments. Different types of social media platforms exist including networking, media sharing, blogs, wikis, and microblogs. These tools facilitate interaction, community building, dissemination, and collaboration among users. Social media offers an alternative to long-established methods of sharing information by print, television, or radio, and offers new opportunities for an efficient means of sharing information (Verhoef, Van de Belt, Engelen, Schoonhoven, & Kool, 2014).

By using a social media platform, the concept of crowdsourcing and the potential for increased participation offers avenues to expand knowledge among patients and healthcare providers (Okun & Caligtan, 2014). In some cases, the research consumer may be connected with the authors/researchers due to the ability to connect and network easily with hashtags and individual contact information available on social media platforms (Leung, Tirlapur, Siassakos, & Khan, 2013).

The world of social media is not free of challenges and opposition. While social media connections are facilitated through technology, the technology should not necessarily be the focal point, but it should serve as the medium used to connect with others. Many may be apprehensive about using social media platforms to communicate with others, offering reasons such as "it takes too much time to learn," "it can't help healthcare providers," "it's likely to be prohibited in healthcare organizations," and "it will compromise patient confidentiality." Many have recognized that eliminating social media does not mitigate the hazards associated with it. Managing the stakes associated with communication channels demands leaders that work to create knowledge, engage stakeholders, and fine-tune based on reaction and responses. Social media has quickly developed and become an acceptable form of mass communication (Thielst, 2014).

Use of Social Networks by Patients

When social networking enables conversations with patients, rather than lectures, it becomes an act of engagement. Facebook and Twitter, well-known social networking media, have become venues of information exchange for patients. According to the Pew Research Center, a nonpartisan source of data analysis, 72% of adult Internet users report use of a social network for procuring health-related information about drugs or other treatments and for following healthcare organizations for information updates or procedure videos (Pew Internet & American Life Project, 2013). The percentage of adult Internet users who use a social network for health-related information has increased 11-fold, when compared to Pew Research Center's report in 2011 (Fox, 2011).

While a large number of people report using social media tools, it is important to be sensitive to trends with regard to age, gender, socioeconomic status, and race when thinking about patient engagement. Interesting trends were noted in a more recent report from the Pew Research Center (Perrin, 2015): while young adults (ages 18–29) are often the most likely users of social media, 35% of those 65 and older reported using social media. This was a greater than triple increase since 2010, when those in that age group reported using social media. Another interesting trend was the differences in men and women in regard to using social media. Sixty-eight percent of women use social media today, while 62% of men report using it. The use of social media also differs by race. Sixty-five percent of whites, 65% of Hispanics, and 56% of African Americans reported using social media.

As a teaching tool that increases patient awareness, information from social networking was found to be useful in facilitating self-care in terms of supporting diagnoses, managing conditions, and monitoring treatments and preventing disease (Griffiths et al., 2012). Latino and African American men who voluntarily used Facebook to post and discuss human immunodeficiency virus (HIV)–related topics were more likely to request an HIV testing kit (Young & Jaganath, 2013). Facebook was found to have a positive impact on allowing patients to shift from being mere passengers to responsible drivers of their health for a wide variety of issues, including maternal and infant care, depression, general wellness, and weight management (Prasad, 2013).

More than simply educating patients with medical knowledge, social media can provide an online environment for patients to discuss their health in virtual support groups. Some patients share their personal stories, including side effects of treatments and the psychological aspects of their illness. Patients with chronic illness, cancer, and rare diseases have found social media useful as a means for sharing stories, learning from others, and instilling hope to other members of the virtual group (Fox & Purcell, 2010).

Use of Social Networks by Nurses

Social media can be a tool for professional connections among nurses and can enrich nurses' knowledge when it is used mindfully and in accordance with professional standards. However, nurses must understand that posting information on social media outlets can be widely and rapidly disseminated to individuals other than those for whom the post was intended. In the social media environment, privacy is typically only an illusion. The most common concerns related to the use of social media by healthcare providers include patient confidentiality, privacy, and patient–provider relationships.

In October 2011, the American Nurses Association (ANA) (2011a, 2011b) released two guiding documents on social networking for nurses: *Social Networking Principles for Nurses* and *Fact Sheet—Navigating the World of Social Media* that can be found on the ANA website. Strategies that nurses can use to avoid breaches of patient privacy and confidentiality with social media have also been identified by the National Council of State Boards of Nursing (NCSBN). These strategies address the maintenance of professional boundaries and employer policies,

professional behavior in the online environment, and specifically recommend that nurses refrain from posting patient-related images or information that could lead to the identification of a patient (NCSBN, 2011). In addition, the NCSBN also recommends that nurses avoid posting disparaging remarks about patients, employers, or coworkers.

Use of Social Networks by Healthcare Organizations

The increasingly popular practice of patients using social networking for health-related information has resulted in the widespread adoption of social networking by healthcare organizations. A recent survey conducted by the Mayo Clinic found that 1,264 hospitals actively used and maintained officially sponsored accounts on Facebook, while 976 hospitals mentioned the exchange of healthcare information with their patients on Twitter (Bennett, 2013).

Many organizations have adopted Facebook to increase awareness and promote the healthcare system. The United Network for Organ Sharing (UNOS), which manages the U.S. organ transplant and organ procurement system, advocates for organ donation awareness on Facebook. They see Facebook as a key opportunity for broadening public awareness of the organ shortage and promoting the decision to become an organ donor. As of May 2012, Facebook users can share their organ status by accessing "Life event," selecting "Health and Wellness," and adding "choose Organ Donor" to be a registered donor. On the first day of the change, about 13,000 people in the United States registered to become organ donors. That is 20 times more than the average number of daily registrations (Stobbe, 2012).

Concerns and Future of Social Media

Although social networking is becoming more accepted as a vehicle for exchanging healthcare information, there are concerns associated with the use of large social networks as platforms for healthcare delivery. Confidentiality has been cited as the most troubling factor (Tang, Ash,

Bates, Overhage, & Sands, 2006). Because the networks are social in nature, certain groups, such as patient support groups and fund-raising groups, may prompt users to "surrender" their confidentiality by exchanging names, locations, symptoms, or lab results (Farmer, Burckner Holt, Cook, & Hearing, 2009). In light of this concern, patients and their caregivers must be made aware of the security risks involved in the disclosure of personal details on public networking sites.

Just as there are obvious benefits to patients who now have access to others with similar medical conditions, the practice of comparing treatment plans, procedure processes, and practice protocols may also create anxiety. Much of the information found on social networks, even the so-called "scientific" content, is often unauthorized, leaving many to question its accuracy and applicability (Farmer et al., 2009). With these concerns in mind, healthcare-focused networking, which is akin to Facebook but exclusive to HCPs and patients, seems to be an ideal solution. In 2013, Dabo Health, partnering with the Mayo Clinic, launched a full version of a healthcare-focused networking site (https://www.dabohealth.com /welcome) that is limited to use by HCPs. Though the site remains in development, Dabo Health is striving to reach the goal of providing relevant and accurate healthcare-related content to users. Another healthcare-focused networking site is called Sharecare, which is found at http://www. sharecare.com. At Sharecare, experts in particular healthcare topics answer questions posed by consumers. Nurses who are members of the Sigma Theta Tau International Honor Society of Nursing can apply to become experts for Sharecare.

▶ Examples of Patient-Digital Interactions

Wearables

Wearable fitness trackers and smartphone companion applications (apps) have become very popular and have great potential for improving

diet and exercise monitoring and adherence. These tools can be used with devices to collect information on activity, sleep, or to log dietary intake. In theory, the use of these devices should improve dietary intake and physical activity behaviors, however, they may have greater appeal for niche audiences who are concerned about monitoring these physical parameters. Because of the capacity of the wearables to collect a wide range of data from the user, including movement, sleep, number of steps taken, further increase in the use of the devices and expansion to previously untapped markets is predicted.

Personal Health Records

In 2005, President George W. Bush and Secretary Mike Leavitt set a specific goal for health care. By 2014, the U.S. Government would implement a program to "create a personal health record that patients, doctors, and other health care providers could securely access through the Internet no matter where a patient is seeking medical care" (HHS, 2006). Since then, there has been a remarkable adoption of **personal health records (PHRs)** at all levels of government and health care.

Despite the increased attention, there is no uniform definition of PHR, but there are several characteristics used to classify PHR (**TABLE 16-3**). One of the most often cited definitions comes from the Markle Foundation (2003), a private foundation that promotes the use of information technology in health and national security. Its definition of PHR is "an electronic application through which individuals can access, manage and share their health information, and that of others for whom they are authorized, in a private, secure, and confidential environment" (p. 3). The American Health Information Management Association (AHIMA e-HIM Personal Health Record Work Group, 2005) adds the following:

> The personal health record is an electronic, universally available, lifelong resource of health information needed by individuals to make health decisions. Individuals own and manage the information in the PHR, which comes from

TABLE 16-3 Characteristics of Personal Health Records

Comprehensive, Longitudinal Data Storage

Data ownership, control, and privacy
Portability
Data sharing
Technology independence
Access
Unique and desired services
Customization

Types of Personal Health Records

Stand-alone personal health records
Untethered personal health records
Tethered personal health records

Data from Gibson, B., & Charters, K. G. (2012). Personal health records. In Nelson, R., & Staggers, N., *Health informatics-e book: An interprofessional approach,* (2nd ed., pp. 241–254). St. Louis, MO: Elsevier.

health care providers and the individual. The PHR is maintained in a secure and private environment, with the individual determining rights of access. The PHR is separate from and does not replace the legal record of any provider. (p. 64)

Data Entry and Management

A PHR is an individualized, web-based, decision-support tool that patients can access from home computers or other mobile devices. A PHR is different from an electronic health record (EHR), which is often used by HCPs for entering healthcare documentation and data on patients. Unlike with an EHR, the patient plays a pivotal role in the collaborative process of PHR data entry and retrieval. Although HCPs may import healthcare data to PHRs, patients should be the only individuals who have the access to maintain information, manage, and make decisions based on their own health information. A PHR provides patients with healthcare information that is truly customized and accurate, such as patients' allergies, lab results, pathology reports, prescribed medication lists, diagnoses, health insurance, and scheduled appointments.

Advantages of Adapting PHRs

The unique PHR data-entry method shared online by patients and providers has direct benefits, such as automated services, up-to-date consumer information, and improved consumer satisfaction (Klein-Fedyshin, 2002). Patients can request routine appointments, outpatient procedures, medicine refills, and referrals to specialists through PHR automated services. Automated services can provide efficient medical attention to patients and ease HCPs' workload by shortening communication time between patients and providers.

PHRs have the capacity to facilitate record-keeping processes between patients and HCPs. Traditionally, patient demographics and insurance information are often not current in medical records, which can result in miscommunication and patient dissatisfaction. Patients who have access to PHRs tend to check and update the data regularly (Ash, Berg, & Coiera, 2004). Effective communication and efficient medical services can improve overall consumer satisfaction.

The goal of PHR implementation is to offer patients the opportunity to leverage their own health information and have ongoing communication with their providers in order to engage in health-promoting behaviors and to develop continuity among HCPs (Tang et al., 2006). Although PHRs benefit patients the most, they are certainly advantageous to individuals involved in the process at all levels. Benefits for patients, HCPs, payers, employers, and public health are associated with the use of PHR (HHS, 2006; see **TABLE 16-4**).

Challenges and Concerns

Although the PHR offers great potential in empowering patients, those who need it most may find it challenging to enter and maintain their data. Groups who have experienced disparities in health care, such as the poor, uneducated, elderly, unemployed, and disabled, often lack access to information resources on the Internet (O'Grady et al., 2012). The **digital divide** includes a technical divide based on the availability of infrastructure and a social divide resulting from the skills required to manipulate and utilize healthcare resources. These skills are often referred to as health information literacy.

Crossing the Digital Divide

Bridging the digital divide and lessening disparity will require action from various government (federal, state, and local) agencies and stakeholders. In 2000, President Bill Clinton argued, "We must close the digital divide between those who've got the tools and those who don't." Hence, he proposed $2.25 billion of initiatives to bridge the digital divide (U.S. White House, 2000). In 2009, the stimulus package allocated $4.7 billion to the Broadband Technology Opportunities Program, of which a sum of no less than $2 billion was made available for competitive grants in an effort to expand public computer center capacity (U.S. Department of Commerce, 2009). These efforts clearly indicate that the development of a national information infrastructure has and continues to be a key priority for the federal government. As time progresses, the government should be able to utilize that infrastructure to reduce the costs of health care.

Though still early in development and use, PHRs appear to have positive effects on patient care experiences, health outcomes, and healthcare use. In summary, PHRs are an evolving concept with great potential to facilitate improvement in the health of individuals and the efficiency of healthcare. While current trends are encouraging and substantial progress has been made in recent years, significant work remains to be done if PHRs are to reach their full potential (Gibson, 2012).

Delivering Health Care Digitally

Telehealth makes it possible to deliver healthcare services to patients in rural, remote, and/or geographically isolated areas. Telehealth can equip patients to assist in taking control of their health. Telehealth offers patients more opportunities to connect with their providers, but issues of privacy and security continue to be a challenge. In addition, people with low health literacy or a lack of access to technology can be excluded from these avenues, such as telehealth, which may be used to connect with HCPs.

Often, patients who are geographically isolated or living in rural areas find it challenging to receive timely and consistent treatment. In addition, it may be hard to get feedback related to their health to their providers. Those dealing with chronic health conditions such as diabetes, cancer, heart disease, and acute diseases that require frequent and intense follow-ups, reminders, and support for patients may find access to care problematic. Telehealth, which dates back to 1897, can often offer solutions to those who face challenges to accessing health care. Patient engagement, patient empowerment, and shared decision making can be used together to design options that encourage the patient. Further, modern methods of communication, such as telehealth, can help bridge this gap between isolated patients and HCPs. (Schlachta-Fairchild, 2017).

Telehealth includes the use of telecommunications and information technology–enabled tools to deliver healthcare services. The term *telehealth* is often used synonymously with *telemedicine*, *e-health*, or *mhealth*. The Health Resources and Services (2012) administration

TABLE 16-4 Key Potential Benefits of PHRs and PHR Systems

Roles	Benefits
Patients and their caregivers	<ul><li>Support wellness activities</li><li>Improve understanding of health issues</li><li>Increase sense of control over health</li><li>Increase control over access to personal health information</li><li>Support timely, appropriate preventive services</li><li>Support healthcare decisions and responsibility for care</li><li>Strengthen communication with providers</li><li>Verify accuracy of information in provider records</li><li>Support home monitoring for chronic diseases</li><li>Support understanding and appropriate use of medications</li><li>Support continuity of care across time and providers</li><li>Manage insurance benefits and claims</li><li>Avoid duplicate tests</li><li>Reduce adverse drug interactions and allergic reactions</li><li>Reduce hassle through online appointment scheduling and prescription refills</li><li>Increase access to providers via e-visits</li><li>Improve documentation of communication with patients</li></ul>
Healthcare providers	<ul><li>Improve access to data from other providers and the patients themselves</li><li>Increase knowledge of potential drug interactions and allergies</li><li>Avoid duplicate tests</li><li>Improve medication compliance</li><li>Provide information to patients for healthcare and patient services purposes</li><li>Provide patients with convenient access to specific information or services (e.g., lab results, Rx refills, e-visits)</li><li>Improve documentation of communication with patients</li></ul>
Payers	<ul><li>Improve customer service (transactions and information)</li><li>Promote portability of patient information across plan</li><li>Support wellness and preventive care</li><li>Provide information and education to beneficiaries</li></ul>
Employers	<ul><li>Support wellness and preventive care</li><li>Provide convenient service</li><li>Improve workforce productivity</li><li>Promote empowered healthcare patients</li><li>Use aggregate data to manage employee health</li></ul>
Public health benefits	<ul><li>Strengthen health promotion and disease prevention</li><li>Improve the health of populations</li><li>Expand health education opportunities</li></ul>

Reproduced from U.S. Department of Health and Human Services, National Committee on Vital and Health Statistics.

define telehealth as "the use of electronic information and telecommunications technologies to support long-distance clinical health care, patient and professional health-related education, public health, and administration." Meanwhile, telenursing is the use of telehealth technology to specifically deliver nursing care.

Telehealth affords patients and providers a connection to deliver health care despite their geographic locations. Telehealth services can provide access to assessment, diagnosis, intervention, or consultation that may otherwise be impossible. Telehealth may also assist in conquering obstacles, such as healthcare provider shortages, physical limitations of patients, as well as financial and geographic barriers to accessing care. Telehealth technologies may include but are not limited to telephones, fax machines, emails, mobile phones, videoconferencing, remote patient-monitoring systems, remote vital sign monitoring, or online physician consultations (Schlachta-Fairchild, 2017).

Notwithstanding technological advances, telehealth holds great potential for decreasing care costs and increasing and improving timely and suitable treatments. However, legal and regulatory challenges exist. Provider licensure and the credentialing and privileging processes in facilities are obstacles to the widespread adoption of telehealth in the United States. Challenges surrounding provider reimbursement and integration with other health-related information technology and EHRs exist as well.

▶ The Future of E-Health Applications

Inherently, a healthcare system is labor intensive, and HCPs play important roles in the provision of effective and high-quality health care. Imbalances in the geographic distribution of skilled HCPs have a huge impact on the provision of high-quality health care for all patients (Nouhi, Fayaz-Bakhsh, Mohamadi, & Shafii, 2012). Today, healthcare technology is used widely to improve patient access to HCPs and promote patient empowerment. Along with technology innovation, more and more virtual healthcare teams are used to bridge the gaps in time, distance, and quality of health care. Virtual health care provides Internet-based, advanced care that monitors and manages patient care remotely. Trauma surgeons at the University of Arizona have developed a Voice-over-Internet-Protocol (VoIP) to provide real-time guidance in remote airway intubation by using video-laryngoscope and Skype over 3G wireless networks (Mosier, Joseph, & Sakles, 2013). Remote operators perform (or facilitate the performance of) procedures that can help ensure patient safety and improve outcomes (see **FIGURE 16-2**).

Based on the virtual healthcare concept, the virtual intensive care unit (vICU) is a model of future care that uses state-of-the-art technology to leverage the expertise and knowledge of experienced ICU HCPs to perform virtual rounds and critically ill patient management. The vICU was the idea of two intensivists from Johns Hopkins Hospital, Brian Rosenfeld, MD, and Michael Breslow, MD (Breslow et al., 2004; Nowlin, 2004). Imagine an extremely ill patient is connected to tubes and monitors that calculate every change in vital signs. In the meantime, ICU physicians and nurses who may be hundreds of miles away from the patients monitor these changes. Live audio and video are used

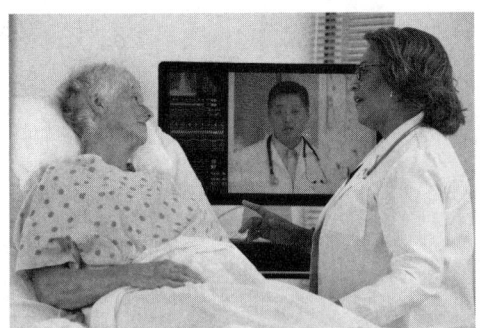

FIGURE 16-2 With the use of virtual health technologies, remote operators can offer assistance with procedures while improving patient safety and outcomes.

© Ariel Skelley/DigitalVision/Getty

to assess a patient. When something triggers an alarm, the vICU nurse can direct a camera in the patient's room to zoom in and visually examine the patient. The vICU nurse can then alert and coach the actual bedside nurse to provide appropriate nursing intervention. vICUs will not only bring the resources and expert care of experienced specialists to rural facilities but also provide an extra layer of safety to patient care.

Remote monitoring and management can be used for those who need chronic disease and/or post-acute care management at home. Patients or caregivers can use devices to upload blood pressure, heart rate, body temperature, weight, blood glucose levels, postsurgery drain output, and other relevant, measurable data. When multiple comorbidities compound the challenges in self-reporting and patient data

collection, invasive or noninvasive devices that automatically record data and detect changes are utilized to ensure patient safety (Bui & Fonarow, 2012). Noninvasive, wearable sensors have been widely used to collect and forward patient information to one or multiple recipients who can then provide appropriate feedback and/or responses (see **FIGURE 16-3**).

European pain management groups have put forth major efforts to develop wearable motion sensors within interactive garments to provide an engaging way to perform home-based therapeutic exercises in back pain management. The system allows patients to increase the amount of motor exercise they perform independently with real-time feedback based on data collected via wearable sensors embedded in the garment across the upper limb and trunk. A patient's activity-associated data are then stored in a

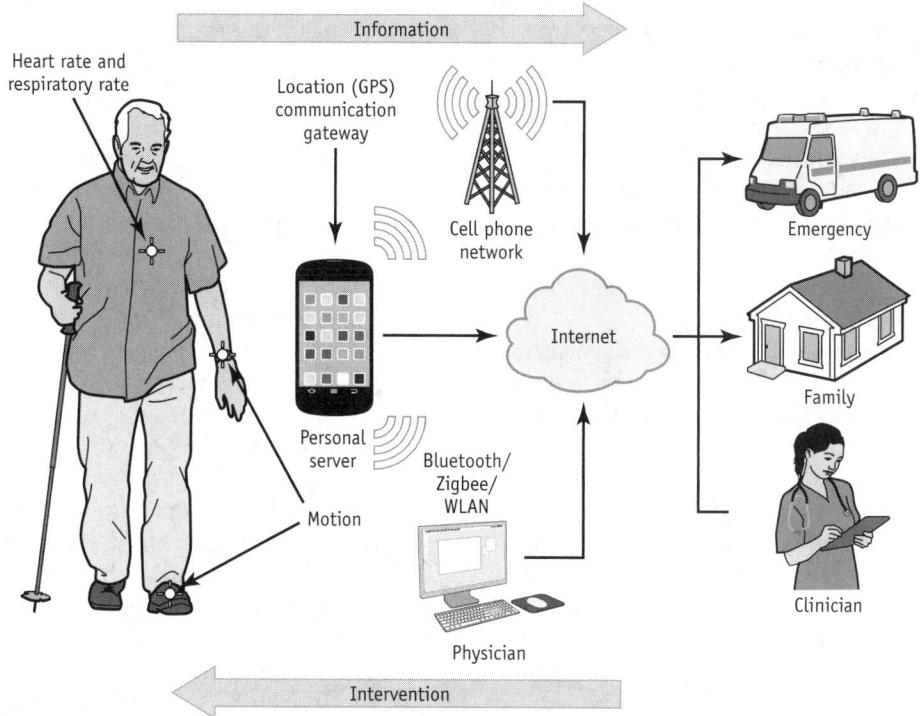

FIGURE 16-3 Illustration of a remote health-monitoring system based on wearable sensors.

Reproduced from Patel, S., Park, H., Bonato, P., Chan, L., & Rodgers, M. (2012, April 20). A review of wearable sensors and systems with application in rehabilitation. *Journal of NeuroEngineering and Rehabilitation, 9*(21). doi:10.1186/1743-0003-9-21. Creative Commons license available at https://creativecommons.org/licenses/by/2.0/

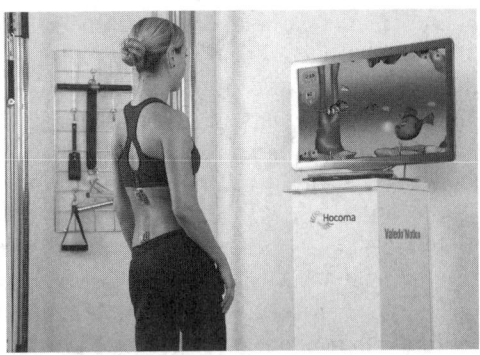

FIGURE 16-4 Low back pain therapy system with wireless wearable motion sensors and interactive games to perform therapeutic exercises.

Courtesy of Hocoma AG

central location where clinicians can access and review statistics (Patel, Park, Bonate, Chan, & Rodgers, 2012; **FIGURE 16-4**).

One such noninvasive, wearable garment system was implemented for remote fetal monitoring during a pregnancy to allow pregnant women to remain at home as much as possible. A group of experts received the recorded signals and then provided prompt feedback about the fetal condition. The system allowed a reduction in the costs inherent in fetal monitoring, improved the assessment of fetal conditions, and, most importantly, guaranteed a continuous and deep screening of the fetal health state whenever a particular pregnant woman was at home (Fanelli et al., 2010).

Patients with heart failure can benefit from implanting a hemodynamic monitoring device via right heart catheterization, which monitors intracardiac and pulmonary artery pressure when patients are at home. This monitoring device provides an early warning of potential decompensation and facilitates the day-to-day management by titrating medications on the basis of reliable physiological data (Bui & Fonarow, 2012; see **FIGURE 16-5**). Digital technology improvements, such as advanced cellular networks and wireless devices, have made prompt clinician feedback possible for

© nednapa/Shutterstock

those patients who choose to manage their health at home.

▶ Summary

The burgeoning use of digital tools in health care has resulted in novel methods of interprofessional communication and dissemination of information. We now face over 100,000 options when it comes to healthcare-related applications. Mobile patient portals are now available, and we have access to sophisticated wearable technologies and applications that facilitate connections with peripheral health devices used to monitor labs and vital signs.

Over the last 15 years we have seen tremendous growth and development of online sharing platforms. In addition, popular user-friendly tools and platforms such as Facebook, Twitter, LinkedIn, and Instagram have developed platforms that many use to share information with others. Many of these tools are ungoverned or unmonitored. To complicate matters, many institutions or organizations don't have policies used to guide employees or professionals within their discipline on how to use these tools. Furthermore, our federal government is encouraging patients to use their personal health records to work with their healthcare providers to improve their health. The merging of technology and promotion of patient empowerment has resulted in many consumers gaining access to an abundance of information about their conditions, providers, and choices.

Health information technology is changing the ways in which patients access and manage their own health care. Technologies such as the Internet, PHRs, and social media, promote patient engagement and empowerment. As we look to the future, our patients will have more opportunities to engage and connect with their healthcare providers via online or electronic applications. Further, digital natives, those born after 1993, are very skilled at using the Internet and electronic tools. In fact, their desire for immediate responses to questions and online tools drive many developers in their innovations. The notion of e-patients will be considered less of a novelty in the future.

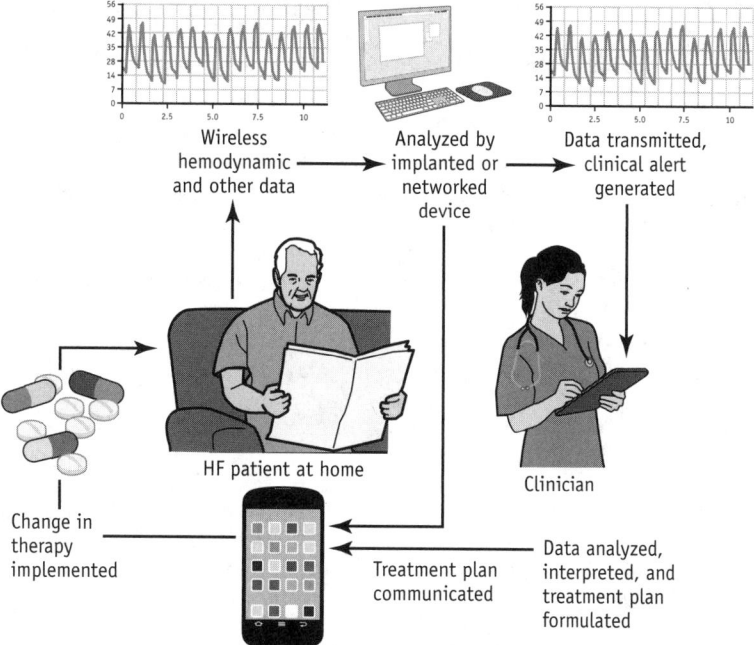

FIGURE 16-5 Home hemodynamic monitoring of chronic heart failure.

BOX 16-1 Case Study

Charlotte is a certified nurse-midwife (CNM) who is opening a freestanding birth center within 5 miles of a major community hospital. The birth center is accredited by the American Association of Birth Centers and has a collaborative agreement, including a transfer agreement with the community hospital and an obstetric practice consisting of three physicians and a women's health nurse practitioner.

In order to promote patient engagement and to provide a PHR, Charlotte installs iPad stations in her waiting rooms and antepartum assessment rooms. Using these electronic stations, pregnant women provide their health history and update their health status throughout pregnancy. The PHR is also accessible online and can be viewed by patients and HCPs at the birth center, obstetrician's office, and the hospital. This allows for a seamless, continuity of care should risks develop and the patient needs to transfer to an obstetrician's care.

Although intrapartum transfers from birth center to hospital comprised less than 12% of the population of women using a birth center, it is important for Charlotte to develop policies in conjunction with the obstetric practice and hospital to promote maternal and newborn safety. One reason for emergent transfer in the immediate postpartum period is postpartum hemorrhage (PPH). By using the protocols outlined in the *Obstetric Hemorrhage Toolkit* (California Maternal Quality Care Collaborative, 2007), Charlotte is able to provide the women and families the best care (see http://www.cmqcc.org/). This clinical information document provides antepartum, admission, and ongoing

(*continues*)

BOX 16-1 Case Study (*Continued*)

risk assessment procedures to identify patients at highest risk for PPH, parameters to diagnose PPH, and a protocol for management. For example, patients are screened for antepartum risks including severe anemia, history of labor uterine fibroids, body mass index greater than 35, estimated fetal weight greater than 4 kg, more than four previous vaginal births, history of bleeding disorders, and a lack of consent to receive blood products in an emergency. The protocols for management of PPH include active management of the third stage of labor by the CNM. Active management procedures are administration of 10 units Pitocin (oxytocin) intramuscularly and vigorous fundal massage following delivery of the placenta. Also, all birth center staff are educated in accurately estimating blood loss and implementing appropriate transfer protocols. Not only does this toolkit promote standardized, quality care between the healthcare professionals, but, when shared with the birth center patients, it promotes shared decision making and patient empowerment.

References

Abernethy, A. P., Wheeler, J. L., & Bull, J. (2011). Development of a health information technology-based data system in community-based hospice and palliative care. *American Journal of Preventive Medicine, 40*(5S2), S162–S172.

AHIMA e-HIM Personal Health Record Work Group. (2005). The role of the personal health record in the EHR. *Journal of AHIMA, 76*(7), 64A–64D.

American Nurses Association. (2011a). *Fact sheet: Navigating the world of social media.* Retrieved from http://www.nursingworld.org/FunctionalMenuCategories/AboutANA/Social-Media/Social-Networking-Principles-Toolkit/Fact-Sheet-Navigating-the-World-of-Social-Media.pdf

American Nurses Association. (2011b). *Social networking principles for nurses.* Retrieved from http://www.nursingworld.org/FunctionalMenuCategories/AboutANA/Social-Media/Social-Networking-Principles-Toolkit

Ash, J. S., Berg, M., & Coiera, E. (2004). Some unintended consequences of information technology in health care: The nature of patient care information system-related errors. *Journal of the American Medical Informatics Association, 11*(2), 104–112.

Bennett, E. (2013). Health care social media list. Retrieved from http://network.socialmedia.mayo-clinic.org/hcsml-grid/

Bradley, A. (2011, March 8). Defining social media: Mass collaboration is its unique value. *Gartner Blog Network.* Retrieved from http://blogs.gartner.com/anthony_bradley/2011/03/08/defining-social-media-mass-collaboration-is-its-unique-value/

Breslow, M. J., Rosenfeld, B. A., Doerfler, M., Burke, G., Yates, G., Stone, D. J., . . . Plocher, D. W. (2004). Effect of a multiple-site intensive care unit telemedicine program on clinical and economic outcomes: An alternative paradigm for intensivist staffing. *Critical Care Medicine, 32*(7), 1632.

Bui, A. L., & Fonarow, G. C. (2012). Home monitoring for heart failure management. *Journal of the American College of Cardiology, 59*(2), 97–104. doi: 10.1016/j.jacc.2011.09.044

Buijink, A. W., Visser, B. J., & Marshall, L. (2013). Medical apps for smartphones: Lack of evidence undermines quality and safety. *Evidence-Based Medicine, 18*(3), 90–92. doi: 10.1136/eb-2012-100885

California Maternal Quality Care Collaborative. (2007). Obstetric hemorrhage toolkit. Retrieved from https://www.cmqcc.org/ob_hemorrhage

Coulter, A. (2011). *Engaging patients in healthcare.* Maidenhead, England: Open University Press.

Coulter, A., Safran, D., & Wasson, J. H. (2012). On the language and content of patient engagement. *Journal of Ambulatory Care Management, 35*(2), 78–79. doi: 10.1097/JAC.0b013e31824a5676

Eysenbach, G. (2000). Consumer health informatics. *British Medical Journal, 320*(7251), 1713–1716.

Fanelli, A., Ferrario, M., Piccini, L., Andreoni, G., Matrone, G., Magenes, G., & Signorini, M. G. (2010). Prototype of a wearable system for remote fetal monitoring during pregnancy. *Conference Proceeding IEEE Engineering Medicine and Biology,* 5815–5818. doi: 10.1109/IEMBS.2010.5627470

Farmer, A. D., Burckner Holt, C. E. M., Cook, M. J., & Hearing, S. D. (2009). Social networking sites: A novel portal for communication. *Postgraduate Medical Journal, 85*(1007), 455–459.

Ford, E. W., Huerta, T. R., Schilhavy, R. A., & Menachemi, N. (2012). Effective US health system websites: Establishing benchmarks and standards for effective consumer engagement. *Journal of Healthcare Management, 57*(1), 47–64.

Fox, S. (2011). *The social life of health information, 2011.* Washington, DC: Pew Research Center's Internet & American Life Project. Retrieved from http://pewinternet. org/Reports/2011/Social-Life-of-Health-info.aspx

Fox, S., & Purcell, K. (2010). *Chronic disease and the Internet.* Pew Internet and American Life Project. Retrieved from http://pewinternet.org/~/media/Files/Reports/2010/PIP _Chronic_Disease_with_topline.pdf

French, D. (2010). The social media mindset: A narrative view of public relations and marketing in the Web 2.0 environment. *Media Psychology Review, 3*(1).

Gibson, B., & Charters, K. G. (2012). Personal health records. In Nelson, R., & Staggers, N., *Health informatics-e book: An interprofessional approach*, (2nd ed., pp. 241–254). St. Louis, MO: Elsevier.

Griffiths, F., Cave, J., Boardman, F., Ren, J., Pawlikowska, T., Ball, R., . . . Cohen, A. (2012). Social networks—the future for health care delivery. *Social Science & Medicine, 75*(12), 2233–2241.

Institute of Medicine. (2004). *Health literacy: A prescription to end confusion.* Retrieved from http://www.iom.edu/~ /media/Files/Report%20Files/2004/Health-Literacy-A -Prescription-to-End-Confusion/healthliteracyfinal.pdf

Jadad, A. R. (1999). Promoting partnership: Challenges for the Internet age. *British Medical Journal, 319,* 761–764.

Juengst, E. T., Flatt, M. A., & Settersten, R. A. (2012). Personalized genomic medicine and the rhetoric of empowerment. *The Hastings Center Report, 42*(5), 34–40.

Kaplan, A., & Haenlein, M. (2010). Users of the world, unite! The challenges and opportunities of social media. *Business Horizons, 53*(1), 61.

Klein-Fedyshin, M. S. (2002). Consumer health informatics: Integrating patients, providers and professionals online. *Medical References Services Quarterly, 21*(3), 35–50.

Leiner, B. M., Cerf, V. G., Clark, D. D., Kahn, R. E., Kleinrock, L., Lynch, D. C., . . . Wolff, S. (1997). A brief history of the Internet. *e-OTI: OnTheInternet. An International Electronic Publication of the Internet Society.* Retrieved from http://www.isoc.org/oti/printversions/0797prleiner .html

Leung, E., Tirlapur, S., Siassakos, D., & Khan, K. (2013). #BlueJC: BJOG and Katherine Twining Network collaborate to facilitate post-publication peer review and enhance research literacy via a Twitter journal club. *BJOG, 120*(6), 657–660.

Markle Foundation. (2003). *Final report, Personal Health Working Group.* Retrieved from http://www.markle.org /downloadable_assets/final_phwg_report1.pdf

Mittler, J. N., Martsolf, G. R., Telenko, S. J., & Scanlon, D. P. (2013). Making sense of "consumer engagement" initiatives to improve health and health care: A conceptual framework to guide policy and practice. *Milbank Memorial Fund, 91*(1), 37–77. doi: 10.1111/milq.12002

Moretti, F. A., de Oliveira, V. E., & Koga da Silva, E. M. (2012). Access to health information on the Internet:

A public health issue? *Journal of the Brazilian Medical Association, 58*(6), 650–658.

Mosier, J., Joseph, B., & Sakles, J. C. (2013). Telebation: Next-generation telemedicine in remote airway management using current wireless technologies. *Telemedicine and e-Health, 19*(2), 95–98. doi: 10.1089/tmj.2012.0093

Muhlbacher, A. C., Stoll, M., Mahlich, J., & Nubling, M. (2013). Patient preference for HIV/AIDS therapy—a discrete choice experiment. *Health Economics Review, 3*(1), 14. doi: 10.1186/2191-1991-3-14

National Council of State Boards of Nursing. (2011). *White paper: A nurse's guide to the use of social media.* Retrieved from https://www.ncsbn.org/Social_Media.pdf

Nouhi, M., Fayaz-Bakhsh, A., Mohamadi, E., & Shafii, M. (2012). Telemedicine and its potential impacts on reducing inequalities in access to health manpower. *Telemedicine and e-Health, 18*(8), 648–653. doi: 10.1089/tmj.2011.0242

Nowlin, A. (2004). Get ready for the virtual ICU. *Registered Nurse, 67,* 52.

Office of Disease Prevention and Health Promotion. (n.d.). *Health literacy and communication.* Retrieved from https://health.gov/communication/about.asp

O'Grady, L., Wathen, C. N., Charnaw-Burger, J., Betel, L., Shachak, A., Luke, R., . . . Jadad, A. R. (2012, January). The use of tags and tag clouds to discern credible content in online health message forums. *International Journal of Medical Informatics, 81*(1), 36–44.

Okun, S., & Caligtan, C.A. (2014). The evolving ePatient. In *Health informatics: An interprofessional approach.* (1st ed., pp. s212–221). St. Louis, MO: Elsevier Mosby.

Patel, S., Park, H., Bonato, P., Chan, L., & Rodgers, M. (2012). A review of wearable sensors and systems with application in rehabilitation. *Journal of NeuroEngineering and Rehabilitation, 9*(21). doi: 10.1186/1743-0003-9-21

Perrin, Andrew. (2015). Social media usage: 2005–2015. Retrieved from http://www.pewinternet.org/Commentary/2011/November/Pew-Internet-Health.aspx

Pew Internet & American Life Project. (2013). Pew Internet: Health. Retrieved from http://www.pewinternet.org /Commentary/2011/November/Pew-Internet-Health.aspx

Pho, K. (2013, February 3). 3 reasons why patients should use social media. Retrieved from http://www.kevinmd .com/blog/

Prasad, B. (2013). Social media, health care, and social networking. *Gastrointestinal Endoscopy, 77*(3), 492–495.

Rifkin, J. (2011). *The third industrial revolution: How lateral power is transforming energy, the economy, and the world.* New York, NY: Palgrave Macmillan.

Roberts, L. (2010). Health information and the Internet: The 5 Cs website evaluation tool. *British Journal of Nursing, 19*(5), 322–325.

Schlachta-Fairchild, L. R.-P. (2017). Telehealth and applications for delivering care at a distance. In R. Nelson (Ed), *Health informatics: An interprofessional approach* (pp. 131–152). St. Louis: Elsevier.

Sheridan, S. L., Halpern, D. J., Viera, A. J., Berkman, N. D., Donahue, K. E., & Crotty, K. (2011). Interventions for individuals with low health literacy: A systematic review. *Journal of Health Communication, 16*(3), 30–54.

Stobbe, M. (2012). 100,000 Facebook users use new organ donor option. *USA Today News.* Retrieved from http://usatoday30.usatoday.com/news/health/story/2012-05-02/facebook-organ-donation-option/54690366/1

Tang, P. C., Ash, J. S., Bates, D. W., Overhage, J. M., & Sands, D. Z. (2006). Personal health records: Definitions, benefits, and strategies for overcoming barriers to adoption. *Journal of the American Medical Informatics Association, 13,* 121–126.

Thielst, C. B. (2014). *Applying social media technologies in healthcare environments.* Chicago, IL: HIMSS.

U.S. Department of Commerce, National Telecommunications & Information Administration. (2009). American Recovery and Reinvestment Act of 2009. Retrieved from http://www.ntia.doc.gov/page/2011/american-recovery-and-reinvestment-act-2009

U.S. Department of Health and Human Services. (n.d.). Quick guide to health literacy: Fact sheet. Retrieved from https://health.gov/communication/literacy/quickguide/factsbasic.htm

U.S. Department of Health and Human Services. (2010). *National action plan to improve health literacy.* Retrieved from http://www.health.gov/communication/hlactionplan/pdf/Health_Literacy_Action_Plan.pdf

U.S. Department of Health and Human Services, Health Resources & Services Administration. (2012). Telehealth programs. Retrieved from https://www.hrsa.gov/ruralhealth/telehealth/

U.S. Department of Health and Human Services, National Committee on Vital and Health Statistics. (2006). *Report recommendation: Personal health records and personal health record systems.* Retrieved from http://www.ncvhs.hhs.gov/0602nhiirpt.pdf

U.S. White House. (2000). *The Clinton-Gore administration: From digital divide to digital opportunity.* Retrieved from http://clinton4.nara.gov/WH/New/digitaldivide/digital1.html

Verhoef, L. M., Van de Belt, T. H., Engelen, L. J., Schoonhoven, L., & Kool, R. B. (2014). Social media and rating sites as tools to understanding quality of care: A scoping review. *Journal of Medical Internet Research, 16*(2), e56.

White, T., & Herzlinger, R. E. (2004). *Consumer-driven health care: Implications for providers, payers, and policymakers.* San Francisco, CA: Jossey-Bass.

Young, S. D., & Jaganath, D. (2013). Online social networking for HIV education and prevention: A mix-methods analysis. *Sexually Transmitted Diseases, 40*(2), 162–167. doi: 10.1097/OLQ.0b013e318278bd12

Glossary

A

access control tools Safety measures to protect information built into electronic health record (EHR) systems, such as user-specific passwords and personal identification numbers.

Agency for Healthcare Research and Quality (AHRQ) U.S. government agency within the U.S. Department of Health and Human Services whose mission is to improve the quality, safety, efficiency, and effectiveness of health care for all Americans.

alert fatigue When false alerts occur frequently, staff members experience a lack of responsiveness to them, or a "cry wolf" bias.

algorithms A set of mathematical steps used for calculation, data processing, and automated reasoning.

anthropometry Workplace design principle that plays an important role in the design of the workplace in that it allows the worker to assume a comfortable working posture and promotes safety and efficiency as tasks are carried out.

artificial intelligence The ability of a computer to perform human-like behavior and/or analysis.

artificial neural network An information-processing system that is based on biological neural networks such as are present in the human nervous system.

association rules Rules designed to capture information about items that are frequently associated with each other; often used in business applications such as market-basket analysis to find relationships present among attributes in large datasets.

asynchronous Activities occurring at separate times, such as the capture and storage of healthcare data which is forwarded to healthcare providers for use at a later date.

B

Bayesian modeling Based on Bayes' theorem, it is used to estimate the conditional probability of a given data point belonging to a particular class using a probabilistic approach for data classification and is based on the assumption that attributes in the training examples are governed by probability distributions.

biometric identifiers Unique biological identification measures such as fingerprints and voice prints.

Boolean operators And, or, not; used to combine words or phrases in keyword searches.

breach A failure or disruption of a system.

business associate A person or organization that uses protected health information to perform activities on behalf of a covered entity but is not part of the covered entity's workforce.

business intelligence Using data to understand why buyers make purchasing decisions and developing well-defined techniques that increase a business's ability to understand what makes a business successful.

C

Census Data Mapper An application that allows users to create custom maps containing county-level demographic data.

Centers for Disease Control and Prevention (CDC) The national public health institute of the United States, whose main goal is to protect public health and safety through the control and prevention of disease, injury, and disability.

clinical decision rules Rules that inform clinical decision-support systems based on best practices.

clinical decision-support systems (CDSS) Computer systems designed to impact clinical decision making about individual patients at the moment those decisions are made.

clinical guidelines Evidence-based recommendations, which are usually generated from an authority group consisting of experts in the field and published regularly.

clinical informatics A broad term that encompasses all medical and health specialties, including nursing, and addresses the ways information systems are used in the day-to-day operations of patient care.

clinical microsystem A small group of people who work to provide care to a particular group of patients.

clinical vocabulary A common terminology that can be used globally in all computerized health information systems.

clustering rules A set of instructions used in descriptive algorithms to identify groupings in the data based on similarities in its attributes.

Cochrane Databases A library built by healthcare professionals who author Cochrane Reviews, which are the gold standard for preappraised research evidence.

commission An error caused by doing something wrong.

communication technologies Specialized equipment or technologies used to promote the transmission of information.

community Groups of people may be designated a community based on their own unique characteristics and dynamics. Those who reside in the community have similarities because they share a common greater environment and experience similar social interactions. Community residents may have shared histories, values, and concerns.

computerized provider order entry (CPOE) Refers to any system in which clinicians directly enter medication orders (and, increasingly, tests and procedures) into a computer system, which then transmits the order directly to the pharmacy.

conditional dependence The way in which two variables, or cases, can be related and dependent upon a third variable or case.

continuing education To stay current in practice, meet state-mandated continuing education units, and fulfill requirements for certification/recertification in specialty practice.

continuous quality improvement (CQI) The process of focusing upon every aspect of an organization for the purposes of improving care and/or services offered by the organization.

covered entity (1) Providers (ranging from an individual provider to a large organization), (2) health plans that provide or pay for health care, and (3) healthcare clearinghouses.

Cumulative Index to Nursing and Allied Health Literature (CINAHL) Database that indexes a comprehensive body of healthcare literature.

D

data (datum) Values or measurements, bits of information that can be collected and transformed, allowing one to answer a question or to create an end product, such as an image.

data analytics Data-based tools used to demonstrate or display visually the analysis of real or projected data such that it can be used in making decisions.

data display Data presented in an understandable manner, such as in flowcharts, Pareto charts, Gantt charts, run charts, control charts, scatterplots, force field analysis, and fishbone charts.

data mining An important component within the process of analytics, in which a particular mining algorithm is used to extract patterns from the dataset.

data quality and validity The state of completeness, validity, consistency, timeliness, and accuracy that makes data appropriate for a specific use; can be enhanced by using specific terminology and tools, such as drop-down menus.

data warehouse A collection of databases designed and optimized with specific applications in mind, consisting of several components including various external sources. Decision support systems are used in the warehouse to provide specific analyses, reports, mining, and other processing that users seek from the data. In a data warehouse, queries are optimized to provide efficient access to data for analysis, reporting, and mining. For example, a data warehouse of a healthcare system may keep aggregated data values of all its patient records.

database A collection of related data.

database management system (DBMS) Software that enables users to create and maintain a database.

decision tree Often used for patient protocols as an aid to decision making, and in analytical research; often represented as a tree-shaped diagram, with each branch used to represent a possible decision or occurrence. The structure of the branches can illustrate how one decision may lead to another.

decryption Translation or access to encrypted information.

defects Errors.

descriptive algorithm Generally used to explore data and identify patterns or relationships within them; examples of descriptive algorithms include clustering, summarization, and association rules.

dialogue Interaction between display of information and operation.

digital divide A technical divide based on the availability of infrastructure, and a social divide resulting from the skills required to manipulate and utilize health IT resources.

digital era Late 1980s; integrated computerized information that could transmit voice and video data at high speeds.

Directory of Open Access Journals (DOAJ) Database of journals that are open access.

E

effectiveness Accuracy and completeness with which users achieve specified goals.

efficiency Resources expended in relation to the accuracy and completeness with which users achieve goals.

electronic health record (EHR) A longitudinal electronic record of patient health information generated by one or more encounters in any care-delivery setting. Included in this information are patient demographics, progress notes, problems, medications, vital signs, past medical history, immunizations, laboratory data, and radiology reports. The EHR automates and streamlines the clinician's workflow.

electronic medical record (EMR) A longitudinal electronic record of a patient's medical record generated by one practice or healthcare facility.

embedded relational database Packaged as part of other software or hardware applications; for example, local databases used by a mobile application to store phone numbers can be considered an embedded relational database.

encryption Stored information frequently undergoes encryption, meaning that it cannot be interpreted by anyone unless it is translated by an authorized person who has a specialized key for decryption of the information.

end user The person who eventually uses the hardware or software product.

epidemiology A field of science that studies health and disease in defined populations or communities.

ergonomics The scientific discipline concerned with the understanding of the interactions among humans and other elements of a system, and the profession that applies theoretical principles, data, and methods to design in order to optimize human well-being and overall system performance.

errors Risks that pass through gaps in protective barriers that normally defend patients from harm.

ethics A branch of philosophy that is concerned with the values of human behavior; can be subjective; it incorporates moral values and requires examination of the issues involved.

evidence-based practice (EBP) A core skill necessary to improve nursing care and enhance the safety of patients; the components of EBP include a systematic and critical evaluation of the current literature, the nurse's clinical expertise and available resources, and patients' values and preferences. This information is used to make deliberate clinical decisions based on theory and relevant research to guide patient care.

F

fast healthcare interoperability resources (FHIR) A set of standards used to guide the electronic sharing of healthcare information.

flat database model Only one table is used, and the attributes are defined as separate columns of the table.

flowchart Graphical display tool used to show documents, tasks, decisions, and interactions associated with care delivery and/or to show work across time and roles; helpful for illustrating the relationship of tasks among providers.

forms The traditional interface to databases that offer a simple visual mechanism for users to insert new data into relational databases.

fragmentation Disconnected healthcare delivery; multiple healthcare providers may make decisions for a single patient resulting in fragmentation of care, which ultimately places patients at greater risk for poor outcomes, particularly if those patients have multiple or chronic conditions (e.g., patients with chronic diseases such as type 2 diabetes mellitus are at risk for multiple complications that often necessitate management by subspecialists, such as ophthalmologists, nephrologists, podiatrists, and cardiologists, making referrals and follow-ups for such patients an arduous task).

G

gap analysis The inefficiencies represent a gap between the current, inefficient workflow and the future, desired workflow with health IT; a formal report of this gap is the gap analysis.

Google Scholar A web-based search engine for scholarly literature across a broad range of disciplines, including literature from free and paid repositories, professional societies, academic publishers, and other sources across the web.

graphical user interface (GUI) A complex platform that allows users to interact with the computer through electronic devices or the computer mouse; interaction is facilitated by visual elements such as icons (symbols, pictograms).

H

hardware ergonomics Supplies the technical framework and sets the conditions for optimal human–computer interactions.

health information exchange (HIE) High-level systems that are designed to promote the rapid sharing of data across facilities.

health information technology (health IT) The comprehensive management of health information across computerized systems and its secure exchange between consumers, providers, government and quality entities, and insurers.

Health Information Technology for Economic and Clinical Health Act (HITECH) A section of the American Recovery and Reinvestment Act of 2009 that (1) modifies Health Insurance Portability and Accountability Act (HIPAA) regulations to make business associates directly liable for compliance with HIPAA regulations, to limit the use of protected health information (PHI) for marketing and fund-raising purposes, and to allow individuals to receive electronic copies of PHI; (2) establishes increased, tiered civil money penalties; (3) establishes an objective breach standard; and (4) prohibits health plans from using or disclosing genetic information for underwriting purposes.

Health Insurance Portability and Accountability Act (HIPAA) Federal law regarding ethical and regulatory guidelines for confidentiality; also includes sections promoting continuity of health insurance coverage for employed people, reducing Medicare fraud and abuse, simplifying health insurance administration, and protecting the privacy and security of health information.

health literacy The degree to which individuals can obtain, process, and understand the basic health information and services they need to make appropriate health decisions.

health maintenance A systematic program or procedure planned to prevent illness, maintain maximum function, and promote health; it is central to health care, especially nursing care.

healthcare providers (HCPs) Those who deliver health care, including doctors and nurses.

human–computer interaction (HCI) A natural way for users to interact with the system through information input, information processing, decision making, and information storage. The starting point is the perception of stimuli from the environment via visual, acoustic, and tactile stimuli.

I

index patient The first known case of a disease.

indexes Predefined record fields used in databases.

inefficiency The lack of ability to do something or produce something without wasting materials, time, or energy.

information Structured data that are understandable and meaningful.

information gain A measure of how well a given attribute separates a subset of the whole dataset (also known as training sample data) to achieve the target classification.

information management The process of collecting data, processing, and presenting and communicating the data as information or knowledge.

information processing Perceived information is subconsciously compared with an inner, dynamic perspective and used to initiate motor processes.

information systems The software and hardware systems that support data-intensive applications.

information technology Using computers or telecommunications systems for managing information.

instance-based learning classifiers As a new sample is presented to these classifiers, it is matched against a set of similar stored instances in order to assign a classification label.

integrity rules Rules that protect the validity of the data used in relational databases (e.g., if entity integrity is enforced, then every record will have its own specific identity and there will be no duplicate records).

interactivity A key component of computer applications depending on user input or given parameters.

interface Point at which separate systems meet and communicate.

interlibrary loan A service whereby a user of one library can borrow books or receive photocopies of documents that are owned by another library.

International Organization for Standardization (ISO) International standards are issued by the ISO and are based on firmly established scientific principles and are determined on an international level and adopted by majority decision.

Internet Worldwide broadcasting system, a mechanism for information dissemination, and a medium for collaboration and interaction between individuals and their computers without regard for geographic location.

Internet era 1990s–present; has enabled telehealth services such as videoconferencing, remote access to patient data and information, and rapid communication between patients and providers.

interoperability The ability of different information technology systems and software applications to communicate, exchange data, and use the information that has been exchanged.

interprofessional collaboration The process of building and sustaining relationships across healthcare disciplines for the purposes of improving patient care.

iterative Each step informs the next, resulting in health IT that is suited to the needs of healthcare providers.

K

K-means A partitional clustering algorithm where the desired number of clusters to partition the data is specified.

knowledge Information that has been synthesized so that relationships are identified and formalized.

knowledge base Essential elements to most clinical decision-support systems derived from research literature that are considered best evidence.

knowledge-based error Errors that occur when an individual does not possess the information needed to determine the appropriate action.

L

law An objective rule.

literature search A systematic approach to reviewing healthcare literature to improve practice.

logistics The organization of supplies and equipment to place them in the right locations at the right time for use.

M

Medical Subject Headings (MeSH) A controlled vocabulary thesaurus used in PubMed in place of keywords.

mobile health (mHealth) An emerging practice of medicine and public health and wellness enabled and supported by mobile communication devices such as smartphones and tablets.

mobile apps Software applications used on mobile devices such as smartphones.

mobile health monitoring Monitoring of particular health parameters from any location.

modeling A set of mathematical terms used to create a computer application capable of anticipating a response to a situation.

N

National Center for Biotechnology Information (NCBI) A branch of the National Library of Medicine, National Institutes of Health, designed to house multiple databases used in biotechnology and biomedicine; contains important resources for researchers who use them.

National Guideline Clearinghouse Evidence-based clinical practice guidelines and other related documents that are freely available to the public.

National Library of Medicine (NLM) As the world's largest medical library, it maintains both print and electronic collections of health resources on multiple topics, enabling billions of searches.

natural language processing (NLP) A method of taking free text from progress notes, nursing documentation, discharge summaries, or radiology reports, for example, and analyzing them for patterns and added meaning to create added rules and generate more individualized patient-specific alerts.

natural user interfaces User interfaces that avail themselves of the natural finger and hand movements of the user on a touch screen, allowing for intuitive use of interactive devices.

need to know Law requires that access to protected health information (PHI) be given only to those with a need to know, and that only the minimum amount of information needed to accomplish the purpose be released. (For example, a nurse would have a greater need for access to PHI than would a billing clerk; a nurse not involved in an individual's care would *not* have any need to know.)

Notice of Privacy Practices A document supplied to patients/consumers upon first contact with a covered entity, describing how the covered entity plans to use protected health information.

nursing informatics (NI) The science and practice that integrates nursing, its information, and knowledge with management of information and communication technologies to promote the health of people, families, and communities worldwide.

nursing intelligence data warehouse A collection of nursing-relevant data elements that can be mined to answer clinical questions, examine results of practice changes, and compare the effectiveness of different nursing interventions on patient outcomes.

O

omission Error caused by failing to do the right thing.

open access Freely available articles provided by publishers.

open source relational database Open source databases, such as MySQL (http://www.mySQL.com) and PostGIS (http://postgis.net), freely available for use.

out-of-range alarms Triggered when a patient's value is above or below a set parameter; these high and low limits can be set manually by the nursing staff or to a default determined by the institution.

P

patient empowerment The practice of maximizing the number of opportunities made available to patients to endow them with a better sense of control over their own health care, which can only lead to well-informed decisions and an improved collaborative dynamic with healthcare providers (HCPs).

patient engagement A set of reciprocal tasks performed by patients and healthcare providers (HCPs) in a collaborative effort to promote and support active patient involvement in their own health care.

patient safety Freedom from unacceptable risk of harm.

Patient Safety and Quality Improvement Act of 2005 (PSQIA) The PSQIA created a voluntary system for reporting medical errors without fear of liability. The patient safety information is considered a "patient safety work product" and can be shared by healthcare providers (HCPs) and organizations within a protected legal environment, with a common goal of improving patient safety and quality of care.

patient safety organization (PSO) A PSO can be public or private, for profit or not-for-profit organization. Insurance companies are not eligible to be designated as PSOs. It is designed to simulate an attack and identify weak areas in a system's security.

patient throughput The relationships between timeliness, efficiency, and coordination of patient care.

penetration testing A method that has been used in other areas of electronic information management to assess the security of systems.

personal health record (PHR) An electronic, universally available, lifelong resource of health information needed by individuals to make health decisions. Individuals own and manage the information in the PHR, which comes from healthcare providers and the individual. The PHR is maintained in a secure and private environment, with the individual determining rights of access. The PHR is separate from and does not replace the legal record of any provider.

Plan-Do-Study-Act (PDSA) A cyclical process that is made up of alternating phases of enacting changes and then assessing the effects of those changes.

point of care The time of care when healthcare providers deliver healthcare products and services to patients.

point-of-care data entry Allows the nurse to capture the activities of care as they occur, including the administration of medications, assessment of vital signs, physical exam, updating of medical histories, or other nursing duties.

population Those living in a specific geographic area or those in a particular group who experience a disproportionate burden of poor health outcomes.

predictive algorithm An algorithm that makes predictions about values of data using a set of known results.

privacy A patient's right to protection and confidentiality of health information.

procedures Tasks or sets of tasks commonly performed in healthcare settings.

process mapping Map of workflow.

productivity The rate at which work is completed.

proprietary relational database Licensed by vendors, proprietary relational databases provide a robust set of management tools that includes creation of a data warehouse.

protected health information (PHI) To be considered PHI three criteria must be met: (1) information that could reasonably identify the person such as name, address, date of birth, and social security number; (2) past, current, or future information about the patient's physical or mental conditions, information about the provision of care, and information about payment for care; and (3) it must be held or transmitted electronically by the covered entity or business associates.

protocols Sets of guidelines for care, based upon best-practice evidence, designed to improve uniformity of care, and updated regularly with the inclusion of new evidence.

public health informatics A specialized field of public health that uses informatics and communications technologies to address topics important to public health.

public health nursing A specialty held in nursing that combines populations, community, health, epidemiology, and informatics.

PubMed Database that indexes a comprehensive body of healthcare literature.

PubMed Advanced Search Builder An advanced search engine within PubMed with drop-down menus that can be set to Medical Subject Headings (MeSH) terms and uses Boolean operators.

PubMed Clinical Queries Displays citations filtered to a specific clinical study category and scope.

PubMed LinkOut A service that allows the user to link directly from PubMed and other National Center for Biotechnology Information (NCBI) databases to a wide range of information and services beyond the NCBI systems. LinkOut aims to facilitate access to relevant online resources in order to extend, clarify, and supplement information found in the NCBI database.

PubMed sidebar filters Filters that can be added to limit the search to a number that is more manageable, including categorizing by article type (clinical trials, systematic reviews, practice guidelines, etc.), text availability (abstract available, free full text available, or full text available), and publication date.

Q

qualitative method Use of interviews, focus groups, text, video, or audio to uncover why usability problems exist and sometimes how to fix them. Qualitative data can be converted to quantitative data by counting, for example, instances of users having difficulty finding information on a website.

quantitative method Produce numbers such as counts, frequencies, and ratios and might include assessments of tasks, surveys, usage logs, and error logs.

query An operation that is used to directly retrieve and update data from a database table.

R

read operation A question designed to extract specific information from a database.

real-time applications (live video synchronous) Take place when the capture and transfer of information occur simultaneously.

reasoning engine Essential elements to most clinical decision-support systems that function as a series of logic schemes for eventual output.

recovery capabilities Mechanisms to retrieve necessary data during downtime to carry on normal operating procedures and to prevent the loss of data when downtime occurs suddenly.

redundancy of data The repetition of a field in two or more places in a database.

reference maps Designed to show geographic locations and features such as rivers but do not contain demographic data.

relational database model A collection of tables linked together by relationship between attributes within the separate tables and/or operations within the tables.

remote access Users use their own computers to remotely access electronic health record (EHR) systems from their homes or offices.

remote patient monitoring (RPM) The transmission of an individual's personal health and medical data to the healthcare provider in a different location for diagnosis and treatment, such that patients can be monitored in nontraditional settings.

reports Documents generated by the rapid retrieval and display of selected data fields.

Rich Site Summary (RSS feeds) Simplified, aggregated summaries of the information provided on whole websites.

risk assessment Following a breach, a risk assessment must be conducted, which includes an assessment of the protected health information (PHI) involved, the person who used or to whom the PHI was disclosed, whether the PHI was actually viewed, and the extent of the risk.

rule-based error When a good rule is applied in the wrong situation.

S

satisfaction Freedom from discomfort; positive attitudes of the user of the product.

security Measures implemented to prevent unauthorized access.

security risk analysis Compares present security measures in the electronic health record (EHR) to those that are legally required to safeguard patient information, and the analysis can help in identifying high-priority threats and vulnerabilities; it is the initial step in creating an effective action plan for addressing threats and vulnerabilities of a system.

selective attention Ability to concentrate on relevant stimuli and ignore irrelevant information.

shared decision making A patient's increased involvement in decision making about his or her own health management, which may include lifestyle changes, diet modification, medication regimens, and regularly scheduled appointments with the healthcare provider (HCP).

simulation A model that uses mathematical terms to create a computer application capable of anticipating a response to a situation in order to imitate reality for purposes such as training or entertainment.

slip A type of error in which a person knows the correct actions, yet at the time care is delivered, an incorrect action is taken.

smartphones A mobile phone built on a mobile operating system, with more advanced computing capability and connectivity than a feature phone.

social media Web-based and mobile technologies that turn communication into interactive dialogues among many users.

software ergonomics Deals with the analysis, evaluation, and optimization of user interfaces by applying various strategies to meet the needs of the user and enhance the display of information and the interaction between information and subsequent operations. *See also* **human–computer interaction (HCI)**.

standardized/controlled data Accepted laboratory values, vital signs, and preaccepted items (typically made available via a drop-down menu).

store and forward applications Capture data and store it for review at a later date.

structured query language (SQL) A common database language that standardizes the ways to perform operations in various implementations of relational databases.

superusers Nurses who tend to display a positive attitude toward EHR use, are willing to take the time for extra training, and serve as a resource for others in the use of the system.

supply chain management A system of manufacturers or suppliers that is coordinated to move a product from production through distribution to consumers.

support vector machine modeling Informs the program to learn from the data; can be used in analyses of healthcare coverage in large populations of people.

synchronous Activity that is occurring between two remote operators at the same time, as in telehealth or telehealth nursing.

system development life cycle Employs user-centered design to meet the needs, desires, and limitations of users in order to create the optimal system design.

system downtime A system interruption that can occur for reasons as simple as short-term power outages, or can be prolonged if natural disasters, such as floods, affect healthcare facilities.

system fault alarms Triggered when there is an ineffective reading, potentially caused by displaced leads or other system malfunction(s).

systems thinking According to Trbovich (2014) the "dynamic interaction, synchronization, and integration of people, processes, and technology."

T

task analysis A qualitative and quantitative method for understanding the activities associated with a particular goal of patient care.

task design Requires user-centered tasks, versatility, completeness of job, significance, degree of autonomy, feedback, and opportunities for development.

telecommunications Communication over a distance by cable, telegraph, telephone, or other broadcasting mechanism; an essential component of telehealth.

telecommunications era 1970s–1980s; characterized by television and broadcast technologies.

teleconferencing Interactive electronic communication between multiple users at two or more sites that facilitates voice, video, and/or data transmission systems.

teleconsultation Remote consultation with a specialist by a healthcare provider.

telehealth The process of using technological communication systems in the assessment and management of patients.

telehealth nursing Nursing care that is delivered through various forms of communication technologies.

telemonitoring Patient data such as blood pressure, weight, and pulse are delivered to healthcare providers (HCPs) so that they can keep track of a patient's condition remotely.

telepresence Technologies that make individuals to feel as if they were present, to appear to be present, or to have an effect at a place other than their true location.

telerehabilitation The use of telecommunications and information technology to deliver rehabilitation services remotely.

teletrauma The remote treatment of trauma situations.

televisit An encounter involving a patient and a healthcare provider that is enabled by telecommunications technologies.

thematic maps Display of the socioeconomic, demographic, or business-related data about an area that may build on reference maps.

U

usability testing A technique used to evaluate a product or information system by testing it with representative users.

user experience (UX) A person's behaviors, attitudes, and emotions about using a particular product, system, or service.

user interface Input devices (e.g., keyboard or mouse) and output devices (e.g., screen, loudspeaker, or printer) that constitute the operational platform of a computer system in combination with software.

user-centered design (UCD) A method for assessing usability throughout the system development life cycle; UCD means that the needs, desires, and limitations of users are the driving factors for design, not the technology capabilities. UCD requires developers to understand human–computer interaction and to design a natural way for users to interact with the system that satisfies, rather than frustrates, them.

V

vendor Developers of electronic health record systems that in turn market them to healthcare settings, such as hospitals.

virtual private network (VPN) Enables the remote user to access the electronic health record (EHR) network remotely through a tightly configured firewall.

visual display terminal (VDT) The computer display; based on ergonomic guidelines, the dimensions of the workstation and the arrangement of the individual elements (e.g., table, chair, and computer) should reduce the demands on the musculoskeletal system and the eyes.

vital statistics Data points such as births, deaths, marriages, divorces, and fetal death.

voice user interfaces Human–machine interactions made possible through a voice or synthesized speech platform; input requires a speech recognition system, commonly called voice recognition (VR) software.

W

wearable sensors Sensors that transmit data by wireless technology to a patient's smartphone or other mobile communication device.

wisdom The proper use of knowledge to solve real-world problems and aid in continuous improvement.

work systems Humans and computers form a complex sociotechnical work system.

workarounds Nurses and other healthcare providers who experience workflow problems after implementation of health IT will often develop workarounds, which are unauthorized ways to use health IT.

workflow Clinical processes; the flow of people, equipment (including machines and tools), information, and physical and mental tasks, in different places, at different levels, at different timescales continuously and discontinuously, that are used or required to support the goals of the clinical work domain. Workflow also includes communication, coordination, searching for information, interacting with information, problem solving, and planning.

workflow analysis A method to avoid the consequences of poorly designed health IT and its impact on workflow.

workflow redesign The process of mapping out current workflows and analyzing how an organization gets work done (the current state) and planning for the future by mapping out how electronic health records (EHRs) will create new workflow patterns to improve the organization's efficiency and healthcare quality (the future state).

Z

Zotero A software program that can be added to a web browser and word-processing program to assist in citing while writing.

Index

Note: Page numbers followed by *b*, *f*, or *t* indicate material in boxes, figures, or tables, respectively.